Obstetrics: Maternal-Fetal Medicine

Obstetrics: Maternal-Fetal Medicine

Edited by Rosa Horton

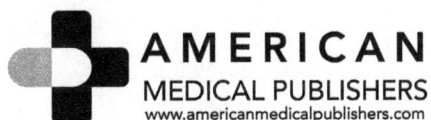

AMERICAN
MEDICAL PUBLISHERS
www.americanmedicalpublishers.com

American Medical Publishers,
41 Flatbush Avenue,
1st Floor, New York,
NY 11217, USA

Visit us on the World Wide Web at:
www.americanmedicalpublishers.com

ISBN: 978-1-63927-160-3

Cataloging-in-Publication Data

Obstetrics : maternal-fetal medicine / edited by Rosa Horton.
    p. cm.
Includes bibliographical references and index.
ISBN 978-1-63927-160-3
1. Obstetrics. 2. Obstetrical emergencies. 3. Maternity nursing. I. Horton, Rosa.
RG526 .O27 2022
618.2--dc23

Table of Contents

Preface

Obstetrics is the branch of medicine which specializes in the care of women during gestation and childbirth. The field encompasses both prenatal and postnatal care of the mother and the infant. Fetal screening helps to assess the viability of the fetus and investigate the presence of any congenital abnormalities. Other methods such as nonstress test, fetal karyotype, fetal haematocrit and oxytocin challenge test are used for fetal assessment. In case of fetal distress, placental malfunction, pre-eclampsis and intrauterine growth retardation, labor may be medically induced. Ectopic pregnancy, placental abruption, shoulder dystocia, obstetrical haemorrhage and puerperal sepsis are certain obstetrical emergencies which require immediate medical attention. Postnatal care is provided to the mother following parturition. The infant's health is also monitored and the mother is advised regarding babycare. This book aims to shed light on some of the unexplored aspects of obstetrics and the recent researches in this field. The various studies that are constantly contributing towards advancing investigative and interventional technologies and evolution of this field are examined in detail. For someone with an interest and eye for detail, this book covers the most significant topics in maternal-fetal medicine.

This book is the end result of constructive efforts and intensive research done by experts in this field. The aim of this book is to enlighten the readers with recent information in this area of research. The information provided in this profound book would serve as a valuable reference to students and researchers in this field.

At the end, I would like to thank all the authors for devoting their precious time and providing their valuable contribution to this book. I would also like to express my gratitude to my fellow colleagues who encouraged me throughout the process.

Editor

The impact of early outcome events on the effect of tranexamic acid in post-partum haemorrhage: an exploratory subgroup analysis of the WOMAN trial

Amy Brenner[1]*🆔, Haleema Shakur-Still[1], Rizwana Chaudhri[2], Bukola Fawole[3], Sabaratnam Arulkumaran[4], Ian Roberts[1] and on behalf of the WOMAN Trial Collaborators

Abstract

Background: In severe post-partum haemorrhage, death can occur within hours of bleeding onset so interventions to control the bleeding must be given immediately. In clinical trials of treatments for life-threatening bleeding, established treatments are given priority and the trial treatment is usually given last. However, enrolling patients in whom severe maternal morbidity or death is imminent or inevitable at the time of randomisation may dilute the effects of a trial treatment.

Methods: We conducted an exploratory analysis of data from the WOMAN trial, an international, randomised placebo-controlled trial of the effects of tranexamic acid on death and surgical intervention in 20,060 women with post-partum haemorrhage. We assessed the impact of early maternal death or hysterectomy due to exsanguination on the effect of tranexamic acid on each of these respective outcomes. We conducted repeated analyses excluding patients with these outcomes at increasing intervals from the time of randomisation. We quantified treatment effects using risk ratios (RR) and 99% confidence intervals (CI) and prepared cumulative failure plots.

Results: Among 14,923 women randomised within 3 h of delivery (7518 tranexamic acid and 7405 placebo), there were 216 bleeding deaths (1.5%) and 383 hysterectomies due to bleeding (2.8%). After excluding deaths from exsanguination at increasing time intervals following randomization, there was a significant reduction in the risk of death due to bleeding with tranexamic acid (RR = 0.41; 99% CI 0.19–0.89). However, after excluding hysterectomies at increasing time intervals post-randomization, there was no reduction in the risk of hysterectomy due to bleeding with tranexamic acid (RR = 0.79; 99% CI 0.33–1.86).

Conclusions: Findings from this analysis provide further evidence that tranexamic acid reduces the risk of death from exsanguination in women who experience postpartum haemorrhage. It is uncertain whether tranexamic acid reduces the risk of hysterectomy for bleeding after excluding early hysterectomies.

Keywords: Postpartum haemorrhage, Tranexamic acid, WOMAN trial, Hysterectomy, Death, Bleeding

* Correspondence: amy.brenner@lshtm.ac.uk
[1]Clinical Trials Unit, London School of Hygiene and Tropical Medicine, Keppel Street, London WC1E 7HT, UK
Full list of author information is available at the end of the article

Background

Tranexamic acid reduces bleeding by inhibiting the breakdown of fibrin blood clots. When given prior to incision, tranexamic acid reduces blood loss in elective surgery by about one third [1]. The CRASH-2 trial showed that early tranexamic acid administration reduces death due to bleeding in trauma patients with or at risk of significant haemorrhage [2]. The WOMAN trial assessed the effects of tranexamic acid on death, hysterectomy and other outcomes in 20,060 women with post-partum haemorrhage (PPH). There was a significant reduction in death due to bleeding with tranexamic acid (RR = 0·81, 95% CI 0·65–1·00; p = 0·045) [3]. As in traumatic haemorrhage, the reduction was greatest when treatment was given early (within 3 h of delivery), (RR 0·69, 95% CI 0·53–0·90; p = 0·007), with no apparent reduction after 3 h [3, 4]. There was also a decrease in laparotomy to control bleeding in women who received tranexamic acid (RR 0·64, 95% CI 0·49–0·85; p = 0·002). Based on these results, the World Health Organization has recommended the early use (within 3 h of birth) of tranexamic acid for the treatment of PPH [5].

In the WOMAN trial, tranexamic acid did not prevent hysterectomy due to bleeding (RR = 0.95 95%CI 0.78–1.16, p = 0.611). During the trial, we noticed that clinicians sometimes decided to perform a hysterectomy at or prior to the time of randomisation and so tranexamic acid could not influence the decision. We predicted that including such hysterectomies as 'outcome measures' in the trial would reduce or obscure the effect of tranexamic acid [6].

Inappropriate assumptions about the timing of an exposure's effect can cause bias towards the null [7]. Even when outcome events occur after randomisation, some will be imminent or inevitable at the time of randomisation and so cannot be prevented by the trial treatment. This is a particular problem in trials in life threatening emergencies when the trial treatment is usually given after the established treatments. Although a trial would ideally evaluate a treatment as it would be used in clinical practice, it is difficult to ensure that a treatment of uncertain effectiveness is given urgently, particularly when clinicians know that half of the patients will receive a placebo.

Given the extent of blood loss in PPH, many of the women enrolled in the WOMAN trial were probably critically ill at the time of randomisation: 59% of women had haemodynamic instability. As such, hysterectomy or death may have been imminent or inevitable in some women. Such outcomes would likely have occurred soon after randomisation. We hypothesised that the inclusion of imminent or inevitable outcome events in the analysis would dilute the treatment effect towards the null. To estimate an undiluted measure of effect, Rothman

proposed repeated analyses with varying assumptions about the timing of an exposure's effect [7]. We aimed to examine whether early outcome events diluted the effect of tranexamic acid on death due to bleeding and hysterectomy due to bleeding by conducting repeated analyses excluding outcomes at increasing intervals from randomisation.

Methods

The WOMAN trial was a randomised, placebo-controlled trial of the effect of tranexamic acid on death, hysterectomy and other morbidities in women with PPH. It included 20,060 women aged 16 years and older with a clinical diagnosis of PPH recruited from 193 hospitals in 21 countries between 2010 and 2016. We randomly allocated women to receive 1 g of tranexamic acid or placebo by slow intravenous injection. If bleeding continued after 30 min or restarted within 24 h of the first dose, we gave a second dose of 1 g of tranexamic acid or placebo. We obtained follow-up data for 99.8% of patients. We have published full details of the trial rationale, design, methods and results elsewhere [3, 6].

We conducted the trial in accordance with good clinical practice guidelines. The relevant ethics committees and regulatory agencies approved the consent procedures. We obtained informed consent from women if their physical and mental capacity allowed. If a woman could not give consent, we obtained proxy consent from a relative or representative. If no proxy was available, then if local regulation allowed, we deferred or waived the consent. In these cases, we told the woman about the trial as soon as possible and obtained consent for use of the data collected.

Analysis

We conducted exploratory analyses of the WOMAN trial dataset using the method proposed by Rothman [7]. Our primary outcome was death due to bleeding and our secondary outcome was hysterectomy due to bleeding. We prepared frequency bar charts of the time intervals between randomisation and death due to bleeding and between randomisation and hysterectomy due to bleeding in the treatment and placebo groups to show the time course of bleeding-related outcomes. We then examined the effect of tranexamic acid on these outcomes among women treated within 3 h of delivery since tranexamic acid only appears to be effective when given within this timeframe [3, 4]. We hypothesised that maternal deaths or hysterectomies due to bleeding that occurred soon after randomisation were imminent or inevitable at the time of randomisation. As such, we assessed the impact of early deaths or hysterectomies due to bleeding on the treatment effect by conducting repeated analyses excluding patients with these outcomes at increasing intervals from randomisation. We also excluded patients who died from any cause within the relevant exclusion period, as they could not contribute to the denominator. We increased the length of the exclusion period by one hour at a time, up to 10 h for deaths due to bleeding but 5 h for hysterectomy due to bleeding since there were few hysterectomies beyond 5 h. We excluded hysterectomies completed before randomisation. We conducted intention-to-treat and per-protocol analyses and quantified treatment effects using risk ratios and 99% confidence intervals. We used 99% rather than 95% confidence intervals due to the multiple number of between-group comparisons. We prepared plots of the cumulative percentage of death due to bleeding and hysterectomy due to bleeding in order to supplement the period-specific risk ratios, which can be susceptible to selection bias [8]. We assessed the proportional hazards assumption using the Grambsch-Therneau global test.

To assess the risk of selection bias from post-randomisation exclusions we examined the distribution of baseline characteristics by treatment group. We used stratified analyses to assess potential confounding factors including age, time to treatment, type and place of delivery, cause of haemorrhage, use of uterotonic prophylaxis, estimated blood loss, blood transfusion, and second dose of the trial treatment (or placebo). We adjusted for relevant factors using multivariable log binomial regression and selected a final model using likelihood ratio tests. We also conducted sensitivity analyses of women treated within an hour of delivery, women with uterine atony as the primary cause of haemorrhage, and women who underwent caesarean section.

Results

In the WOMAN trial, 20,060 women were randomly assigned to receive tranexamic acid ($n = 10,051$) or placebo ($n = 10,009$). After excluding 39 women who did not fulfil the eligibility criteria, withdrew consent or were lost to follow up, data on 20,021 women were available for analysis. Ten women (< 0.1%) had missing data on time of delivery or time of randomisation, so time to treatment was calculated in the remaining 20,011 women. Of these, 14,923 women were randomised within 3 h of delivery (7518 tranexamic acid and 7405 placebo), with a mean time from delivery to randomisation of 1 h (interquartile range = 0.4–1.5 h). Data on time of haemorrhage death were available for all women. Data on time of hysterectomy for bleeding or hysterectomy status were missing for 45 women (0.3%), leaving 14,878 patients for the hysterectomy analyses. Among women randomised within 3 h of delivery, there were 216 deaths due to bleeding (1.5%) and 383

hysterectomies due to bleeding (2.8%). Here we present the results of intention-to-treat analyses. In per-protocol analyses, we excluded 19 women who did not receive tranexamic acid ($n = 9$) or placebo ($n = 10$). The results of the per-protocol analysis were almost identical (see Additional file 1: Tables S1 and S2). The trial arms remained balanced by baseline characteristics (see Additional file 1: Tables S3 and S4), and there was no evidence of confounding (see Additional file 1: Tables S5 and S6).

Figure 1 shows a frequency bar chart of the interval between randomisation and death due to bleeding for the placebo group ($n = 173$) and tranexamic acid group ($n = 138$) over the 24 h after randomisation. The distribution was positively skewed, with 42% of all deaths from exsanguination occurring within 3 h of randomisation, 58% within 5 h, and 80% within 10 h. Thirty-five (10%) deaths from exsanguination occurred more than 24 h after randomisation.

Table 1 shows risk ratios for death due to bleeding in women treated within 3 h of delivery, excluding women who died at increasing intervals from randomisation. When all women were included, there was a 31% reduction in the risk of death due to bleeding with tranexamic acid (RR = 0.69, 99% CI 0.48–0.98). Excluding women who died soon after randomisation increased the treatment effect. The effect was largest after excluding women who died within 9 h of randomisation, with a 59% reduction in death due to bleeding (RR = 0.41, 99% CI 0.19–0.89). Although there was a decreasing trend in risk ratios, the 99% confidence intervals were wide and overlapping. In sensitivity analyses of women treated within an hour of delivery, women with uterine atony and women who underwent caesarean section, we observed the same decreasing trend in risk ratios (see Additional file 1: Tables S7-S9).

Figure 2 shows a plot of the cumulative percentage of deaths from bleeding by time from randomisation in the tranexamic acid and placebo groups. For the first few hours after randomisation the curves overlap but later they separate. The Grambsch-Therneau test for proportional hazards gave $p = 0.06$.

Figure 3 shows a frequency bar chart of the interval between randomisation and hysterectomy due to bleeding in the placebo group ($n = 263$) and tranexamic acid group ($n = 245$) for the 24 h after randomisation. Again, the distribution was positively skewed with 38% of hysterectomies for bleeding occurring within one hour of randomisation and 82% within 3 h. Less than 2% of hysterectomies for bleeding ($n = 9$) occurred more than 24 h after randomisation.

Table 2 shows risk ratios for hysterectomy due to bleeding for women treated within 3 h of delivery, excluding women who underwent hysterectomy at

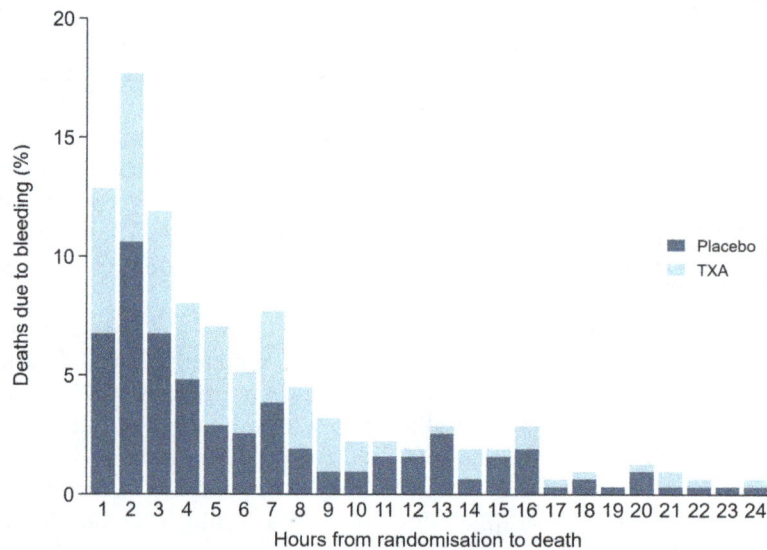

Fig. 1 Deaths due to bleeding within 24 h of randomisation by treatment group and hours since randomisation

increasing intervals from randomisation. When all women were included, there was no reduction in the risk of hysterectomy due to bleeding with tranexamic acid (RR = 0.95, 99% CI 0.73–1.23). Excluding women who had a hysterectomy for bleeding soon after randomisation resulted in a decrease in the risk ratio (RR = 0.79; 99% CI 0.33–1.86), however, the 99% confidence intervals overlapped the null at each exclusion interval.

Figure 4 shows a plot of the cumulative percentage of hysterectomy for bleeding by time from randomisation in the tranexamic acid and placebo groups. In the first hours after randomisation the curves were similar but with minimal separation later. The Grambsch-Therneau test for proportional hazards gave $p = 0.17$.

Discussion

In the original WOMAN trial, women who experienced PPH were randomized to receive tranexamic acid vs placebo. In the WOMAN trial, we observed a 19% reduction in the risk of death from exsanguination in women who received tranexamic acid compared to placebo, with a 31% reduction in women treated within 3 h of giving birth. In this secondary analysis of WOMAN trial data, after excluding deaths due to bleeding that occurred soon after randomisation, we observed a lower risk of death from exsanguination in women who received early tranexamic acid compared to placebo (RR = 0.41; 99% CI 0.19–0.89). Some women may have been so critically ill at the time of randomisation that death was imminent

Table 1 Impact of early deaths due to bleeding on the effect of tranexamic acid

Exclusion interval (hours from randomisation)	Exclusions[a]		N		Death due to bleeding		
	TXA (%)	Placebo (%)	TXA	Placebo	TXA (%)	Placebo (%)	Risk ratio (99% CI)
None	–	–	7518	7405	89 (1.2)	127 (1.7)	0.69 (0.48–0.98)
1	14 (0.2)	15 (0.2)	7504	7390	76 (1.0)	114 (1.5)	0.66 (0.45–0.96)
2	30 (0.4)	38 (0.5)	7488	7367	61 (0.8)	92 (1.3)	0.65 (0.43–1.00)
3	42 (0.6)	57 (0.8)	7476	7348	50 (0.7)	75 (1.0)	0.66 (0.41–1.05)
4	53 (0.7)	70 (1.0)	7465	7335	42 (0.6)	64 (0.9)	0.64 (0.39–1.07)
5	62 (0.8)	77 (1.0)	7456	7328	33 (0.4)	59 (0.8)	0.55 (0.31–0.96)
6	66 (0.9)	85 (1.2)	7452	7320	29 (0.4)	53 (0.7)	0.54 (0.30–0.97)
7	73 (1.0)	94 (1.3)	7445	7311	23 (0.3)	44 (0.6)	0.51 (0.26–0.99)
8	80 (1.1)	97 (1.3)	7438	7308	18 (0.2)	41 (0.6)	0.43 (0.21–0.89)
9	83 (1.1)	101 (1.4)	7435	7304	16 (0.2)	38 (0.5)	0.41 (0.19–0.89)
10	84 (1.1)	104 (1.4)	7434	7301	16 (0.2)	37 (0.5)	0.42 (0.20–0.91)

[a]% is the proportion of the original trial arm excluded (N = 7518 TXA, N = 7405 placebo). TXA = tranexamic acid. Includes women treated within 3 h of delivery only

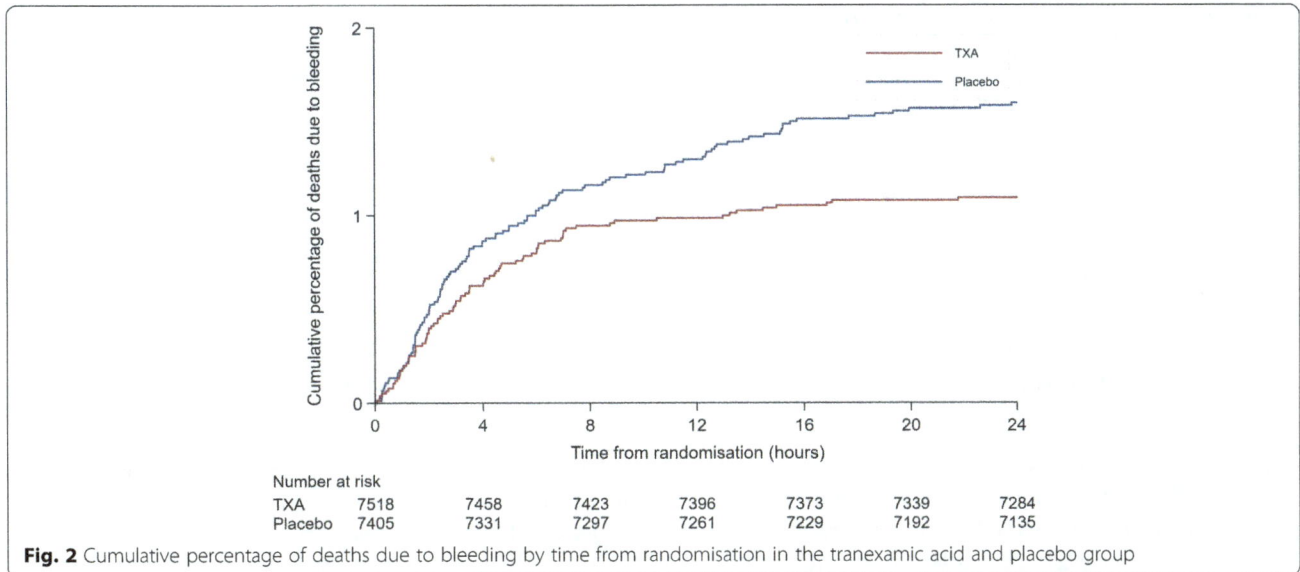

Fig. 2 Cumulative percentage of deaths due to bleeding by time from randomisation in the tranexamic acid and placebo group

and inevitable regardless of treatment. The findings of this secondary analysis extend those of the original WOMAN trial by further highlighting the importance of tranexamic acid as an early life-saving intervention for women who experience PPH.

The plasma concentration of tranexamic acid needed to inhibit fibrinolysis is around 5–15 mg/L and tranexamic acid has a half-life of 2–3 h [9–14]. After an intravenous injection of 1 g of tranexamic acid, the plasma concentration should exceed this range for several hours [13, 15]. Because it is eliminated by the kidneys, the concentration could remain elevated for much longer in women with severe bleeding and renal impairment [16]. Further research

on the pharmacokinetics and pharmacodynamics of tranexamic acid in obstetric bleeding will help to determine the optimal dosing regimen.

Our analysis has important limitations. Although the statistical analysis plan, which we prepared before seeing the trial results, anticipated that outcomes determined prior to randomisation would dilute the treatment effect, the exploratory analyses presented here were not pre-specified and comprise multiple between-group comparisons. The possibility of a type 1 error cannot be excluded and so our results require cautious interpretation. That said, in keeping with our hypothesis, we observed an increase in the treatment effect on death due to bleeding with an increasing exclusion interval. This

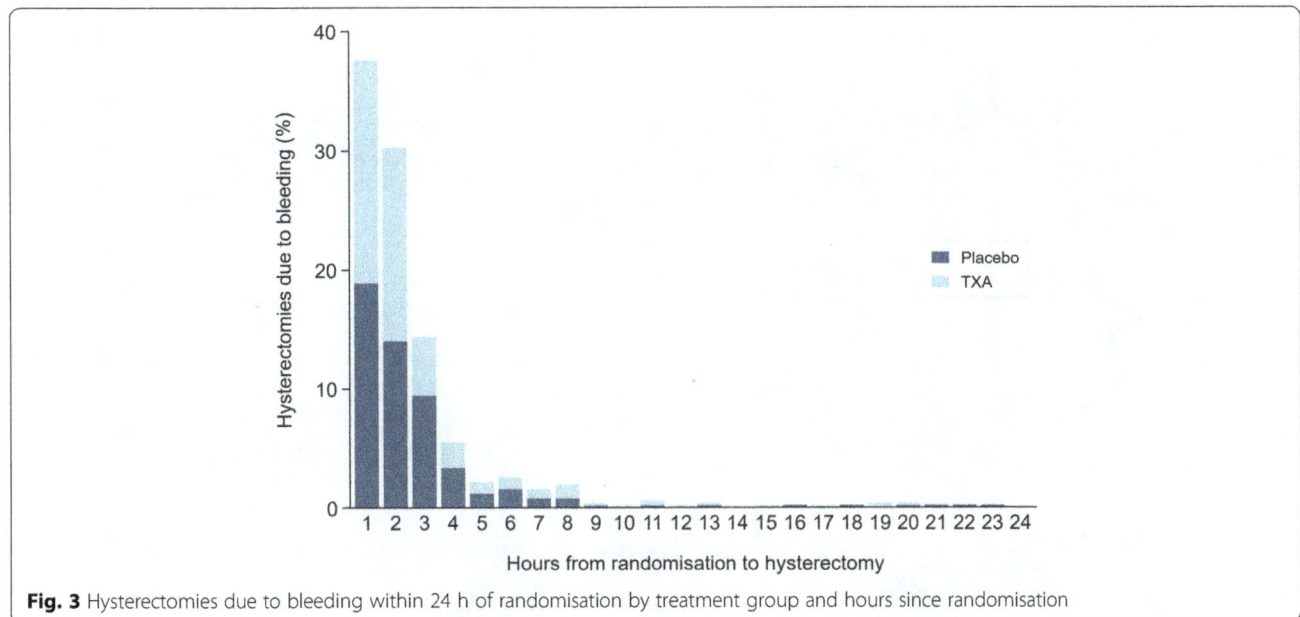

Fig. 3 Hysterectomies due to bleeding within 24 h of randomisation by treatment group and hours since randomisation

Table 2 Impact of early hysterectomies due to bleeding on the effect of tranexamic acid

Exclusion interval (hours from randomisation)	Exclusions[a]		N		Death due to bleeding		
	TXA (%)	Placebo (%)	TXA	Placebo	TXA (%)	Placebo (%)	Risk ratio (99% CI)
None	–	–	7494	7384	188 (2.5)	195 (2.6)	0.95 (0.73–1.23)
1	90 (1.2)	93 (1.3)	7404	7291	112 (1.5)	117 (1.6)	0.94 (0.67–1.32)
2	175 (2.3)	167 (2.3)	7319	7217	42 (0.6)	64 (0.9)	0.65 (0.39–1.08)
3	205 (2.7)	214 (2.9)	7289	7170	23 (0.3)	34 (0.5)	0.67 (0.33–1.33)
4	217 (2.9)	236 (3.2)	7277	7148	19 (0.3)	25 (0.4)	0.75 (0.34–1.63)
5	227 (3.0)	246 (3.3)	7267	7138	16 (0.2)	20 (0.3)	0.79 (0.33–1.86)

[a]% is the proportion of the original trial arm excluded ($N = 7494$ TXA, $N = 7384$ placebo). TXA = tranexamic acid. Includes women treated within 3 h of delivery only

finding was consistent in several sensitivity analyses. The temporal distribution of haemorrhage deaths allowed us to exclude women who died soon after randomisation. We did not observe a statistically significant decrease in the risk of hysterectomy for bleeding associated with tranexamic acid compared with placebo after excluding hysterectomies performed early after randomization. Although this finding suggests that tranexamic acid may not decrease the need for hysterectomy as a life-saving surgical intervention for PPH, it is possible that our sample size was inadequate to show a true treatment benefit when excluding early hysterectomies.

Period-specific risk ratios are susceptible to selection bias [8]. Because tranexamic acid reduces deaths due to bleeding, post-randomisation exclusions based on time-to-outcome are not independent of treatment. Indeed, we excluded 20 more deaths from the placebo group than from the treatment group. Although this might be expected to obscure rather than inflate the delayed effects of treatment, because we do not have data on patient characteristics at each time point selection bias remains a concern. Figure 2 provides some unbiased evidence of a lack of treatment benefit early on, in line with our hypothesis that early deaths due to bleeding may dilute the treatment effect, but this may be a spurious finding.

The validity of our results also depend on the accuracy of data on the time of randomisation (treatment) and the time of death but measurement error is inevitable. Although we urged investigators to give the trial treatment as soon as possible after randomisation, some outcomes would have occurred before the treatment was completed. Time of death could have been misclassified since there is often an interval between death and its formal confirmation.

Because maternal death can occur soon after major uncontrolled PPH, interventions to compensate for blood loss (e.g. blood transfusion) and control the bleeding (e.g. hysterectomy) may occur early after PPH diagnosis, often prior to administration of the trial

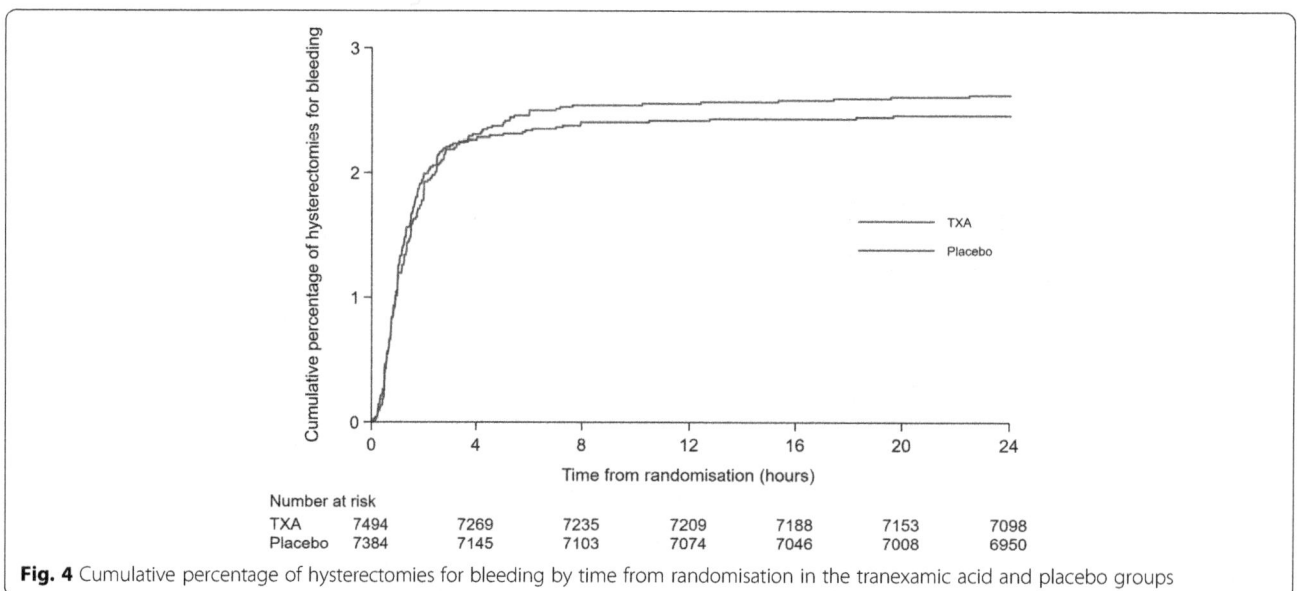

Fig. 4 Cumulative percentage of hysterectomies for bleeding by time from randomisation in the tranexamic acid and placebo groups

treatment. We conjecture that this may potentially explain the lack of any effect of tranexamic acid on blood transfusion and hysterectomy in the WOMAN trial. However, the results for hysterectomy were inconclusive and we did not have data on time of transfusion. Future studies are needed to examine the effect of tranexamic acid on haemorrhage-related morbidity, and should report the timing of relevant medical and surgical interventions, such as time to first transfusion, uterine balloon tamponade, interventional radiology, and surgical intervention (including hysterectomy and laparotomy).

Conclusions

In this secondary analysis of data from the WOMAN trial, we observed that tranexamic acid was associated with a reduced risk of maternal death from exsanguination after excluding early maternal deaths from the analysis. This finding is in line with the main findings from the WOMAN trial. Our results suggest that the inclusion of early deaths in the analysis may have diluted the treatment effect of tranexamic acid towards the null. Early outcome events could represent those that are imminent and inevitable. Therefore, the outcomes of some women with life-threatening PPH occurring soon after delivery may not be influenced by exposure to the study drug. These findings also raise the possibility that if we give women tranexamic acid as a first line treatment for PPH rather than a last resort, as now recommended by the World Health Organization [5], its effect on reducing the risk of death due to bleeding may exceed that observed in the WOMAN trial. However, these results should be viewed with caution due to the exploratory nature of this analysis. It remains uncertain whether tranexamic acid reduces the risk of hysterectomy for bleeding after excluding early hysterectomies post-randomisation. Further studies are needed to examine the effect of tranexamic acid on morbidity in PPH.

Additional file

Additional file 1: Supplementary data analyses. This file provides per protocol analyses (Tables S1 and S2); an assessment of potential selection bias (Tables S3 and S4); an assessment of potential confounding (Tables S5 and S6); a sensitivity analysis of women treated within an hour of delivery (Table S7); a sensitivity analysis of women with uterine atony as the primary cause of haemorrhage (Table S8); a sensitivity analysis of women who underwent caesarean section (Table S9).

Abbreviations

PPH: Post-partum haemorrhage; TXA: Tranexamic acid; WOMAN trial: World Maternal Antifibrinolytic trial

Acknowledgments
The authors want to thank all members of the WOMAN Trial Collaborative and all women who participated in the WOMAN trial.

Funding
Funding for the WOMAN trial was provided by London School of Hygiene & Tropical Medicine, Pfizer (provided the trial drug), the UK Department of Health (grant number HICF-T2–0510-007), the Wellcome Trust (grant number WT094947), and The Bill & Melinda Gates Foundation (grant number OPP1095618). The funders had no role in study design, data collection, analysis or interpretation, or the writing of the manuscript.

Authors' contributions
IR and HS conceived and designed the WOMAN trial. The WOMAN Trial Collaborators were responsible for conducting the study and for data collection. RC, BF, IR and HS contributed to the conception of this analysis. AB conducted the analysis. AB and IR drafted the manuscript. AB, HS, RC, BF, SA and IR participated in the interpretation of the data and the revising of the manuscript.

Ethics approval and consent to participate
Ethical approval was obtained from the London School of Hygiene and Tropical Medicine Ethics Committee and Berkshire Research Ethics Committee, in addition to the following local and national research ethics committees.
Albania: Komiteti Kombetar i Etikes.
Bangladesh: Ad-din Women's Medical College Ethics Committee; Ethical Review Committee Chittagong Medical College; Ethical Committee of Dhaka Medical College; Ethics Committee Ibn Sina Medical College Hospital; Rajshahi Medical College Hospital Ethical Committee.
Burkina Faso: Centre Hospitalier Regional de Dedougou; Centre Hospitalier Universitaire Yalgado Ouedraogo.
Cameroon: Comite d'Ethique de l'Hopital de District de Banyo; Comite d'ethique de l'hopital gyneco-obstetrique et pediatrique de Yaounde; Dschang District Hospital; Hopital Laquintinie de Douala; Kumba District Hospital; Limbe Regional Hospital; Le Comite d'ethique de l'Hopital de District de Sa'a; St Theresa's Catholic Hospital Local Ethics Committee; Yaounde Central Hospital; Comite d'ethique de l'hopital gyneco-obstetrique et pediatrique de Yaounde.
Colombia: Ethical and Biomedical Research Committee, Fundacion Valle del Lili.
Cote d'Ivoire: Direction Departementale d'Abobo-Est.
Democratic Republic of Congo: Le Comite d'Ethique du CSR Albert Barthel; Centre de Sante de Reference Kahembe; Centre Hospitalier Notre Dame d'Afrique; Le Comite d'Ethique Institutionnel, Centre Medical Abedeco; Le Comite d'Ethique du Centre Medical VUHE; Comite d'Ethique de CSR Carmel; Comite d'Ethique de GESOM; Comite d'Ethique de Hope Medical Center; Le Comite d'Ethique du Centre de l'Hopital Provincial du Nord Kivu/Goma; Le Comite d'Ethique du Centre de l'Hopital General de Reference Virunga.
Egypt: General Organisation for Teaching Hospitals and Institutes.
Ethiopia: Jimma University Ethics Committee; St. Paul's Hospital Millennium Medical College Ethics Committee.
Ghana: School of Medical Sciences Committee on Human Research Publications and Ethics.
Jamaica: UHWI/UWI/FMS Ethics Committee.
Kenya: AIC Kijabe Hospital Medical Education and Research; Bungoma District Hospital; Ministry of Medical Services Coast; Ministry of Health, Garissa; Kenyatta National Hospital/University of Nairobi Ethics and Research Committee; Moi Teaching and Referral Hospital Institutional Research and Ethics Committee; Ministry of Health & Sanitation, Mwingi District Hospital; Ministry of Health, Nakuru; Nairobi Hospital Bioethics and Research Committee.
Nepal: Biratnagar Aspataal & Research Center Ethics Committee; Institutional Ethical Review Board BPKIHS; Mid Western Regional Hospital Ethics Committee; Nepal Medical College Institutional Research/Review Committee.
Nigeria: Abubakar Tafawa Balewa University Teaching Hospital; Oyo State Research Ethical Review Committee; Aminu Kano Teaching Hospital; Ahmadu

Bello University Teaching Hospital Faculty of Medicine Ethical Committee; Braithwaite Memorial Specialist Hospital Ethics Committee; Delta State University Teaching Hospital Research Ethics Committee; University Teaching Hospital Ado-Ekiti Ethics and Research Committee; Federal Capital Territory Health Research Ethics Committee; Federal Medical Centre Abeokuta Research Ethics Committee; Federal Medical Centre Azare Health Research Ethics Committee; Federal Medical Centre Bida Ethical Committee; Federal Medical Centre Birnin-Kebbi Research Ethics Committee; Federal Medical Centre Gusau Ethic and Research Committee; Federal Medical Centre Ido-Ekiti Ethics and Research Committee; Federal Medical Centre Katsina Medical Research Ethics Committee; Federal Medical Centre Keffi Health Research Ethics Committee; Federal Medical Centre Lokoja Ethical Review Committee; Federal Medical Centre Makurdi Committee on Medical Ethics; Federal Medical Centre Owerri Ethical Committee; Federal Medical Centre Owo Ethical Review Committee; Federal Medical Centre, Umuahia; Federal Medical Centre, Yenagoa; Federal Teaching Hospital Abakaliki Research Ethics Committee; Irrua Specialist Teaching Hospital Research Ethics Committee; Jos University teaching Hospital Institutional Health Research Ethics Committee; Kogi State Specialist Hospital Research and Ethical Committee; Ladoke Akintola University of Technology Teaching Hospital Ethical Committee; Lagos Island Maternity Hospital Ethical Committee; Lagos State University Teaching Hospital Health Research and Ethics Committee; Lagos University Teaching Hospital Research & Ethics Committee; Mother & Child Hospital Akure Research Ethics Committee; National Hospital Abuja Ethics Committee; Nigeria National Health Research Ethics Committee; Nnamdi Azikiwe UTH Ethical Committee; Obafemi Awolowo University Teaching Hospital Ethics & Research Committee; Plateau State Specialist Hospital Health Research Ethics Committee; Seventh Day Adventist Hospital Internal Review Board and Ethics Committee; University of Ibadan/University College Hospital Ethics Committee; University of Abuja Teaching Hospital Health Research Ethics Committee; University of Calabar Teaching Hospital Ethical Committee; University of Ilorin Teaching Hospital Ethical Reveiw Committee; University of Maiduguri Teaching Hospital Ethics and research Committee; University of Nigeria Hospital Research Ethics Committee; University of Uyo teaching Hospital Institutional Review Committee; Usmanu Danfodiyo University Teaching Hospital Sokoto Ethical Research Committee; Obafemi Awolowo University Teaching Hospital Ethics & Research Committee.

Pakistan: Ayub Teaching Hospital Ethical Committee; Institutional Ethical Review Committee Bolan Medical College; Cantonment General Hospital Rawalpindi Ethics Committee; Institutional Ethics Committee, Combined Military Hospital Kharian; Combined Military Hospital Lahore Ethics Committee; Rawalpindi Medical College and Allied Hospitals Research and Ethics Committee; Fatima Bai Hospital Ethical Review Committee; Institutional Review Board Fatima Memorial Hospital; Ethical Committee Federal Government PolyClinic; Institutional Review Board Services Institute of Medical Sciences; Isra University Hospital Ethical Committee; AIMC/Jinnah Hospital Lahore Ethical Review Board; Ethical Review Committee Kahota Research Laboratory Hospital Islamabad; Institutional Review Board King Edward Medical University; Institutional Research & Ethics Board Lady Reading Hospital; Institutional Review Board King Edward Medical University; Liaquat Ethics Review Committee; Ethics Review Committee Liaquat University Hospital; Ethics Commitee MCH PIMS; Mian Muhammad Trust Hospital Ethics Committee; Research and Ethic Committee Islamabad Medical Complex Nescom; Institutional Ethical Review Committee Nishtar Medical College & Hospital Multan; Islamic International College Trust Pakistan Railway Hospital; Ethics Committee Patel Hospital; Ethical Review Committee People's University of Medical and Health Sciences; Rehman Medical Institute Peshawar Institutional Review Committee; Ethics Committee Shalamar Hospital; Ethical Committee Sharif Medical and Dental College; Institutional Review Board and Ethics Committee Shifa International Hospital; Sir Ganga Ram Hospital Lahore Ethics Committee; Zainab Panjwani Memorial Hospital Ethics Committee; Ziauddin Medical College.

Papua New Guinea: School of Medicine Research and Ethics Committee.

Sudan: National Medicines and Poisons Board.

Tanzania: Prime Ministers Office, Regional Administration and Local Government; Muheza Designated District Hospital; Muhimbili National Hospital; Mwananyamala Hospital; Temeke Municipal Council.

Uganda: Makerere University; Ugandan National Council of Science and Technology.

United Kingdom: Nottingham University Hospitals NHS Trust Research & Development Department; Liverpool Women's NHS Foundation Trust R&D Department; Central Manchester University Hospitals NHS Foundation Trust R&D; Guys and St Thomas NHS Foundation Trust Research and Development; City Hospitals Sunderland NHS Foundation Trust Research and Development; The Newcastle Upon Tyne NHS Foundation Trust Research and Development.

Zambia: Chipata General Hospital; Kabwe General Hospital Ethics Committee; University of Zambia Biomedical Ethics Committee; Livingstone General Hospital; St Paul's Mission Hospital, Kashikishi; St Francis Hospital Research Ethics Committee; University of Zambia Biomedical Ethics Committee.

The relevant ethics committees and regulatory agencies approved the consent procedures at each site. We obtained informed consent from women if their physical and mental capacity allowed. For fully competent women, an information sheet was provided, the study was discussed and written consent obtained. If the woman was unable to read or write then the information sheet was read to her and she then marked the consent form with either a cross or thumbprint. In this event, a witness not associated with the trial provided a full signature confirming the mark. If a woman could not give consent, we obtained proxy consent from a relative or representative in the same manner. If no proxy was available, then if local regulation allowed, we deferred or waived the consent. In these cases, we told the woman about the trial as soon as possible and obtained consent for use of the data collected. The consent procedures are described in detail in the trial protocol.

Competing interests
The authors declare that they have no competing interests.

Author details
[1]Clinical Trials Unit, London School of Hygiene and Tropical Medicine, Keppel Street, London WC1E 7HT, UK. [2]Holy Family Hospital, Gynaecology & Obstetrics Unit 1, F-762 Said Pur Road, Satellite Town, Rawalpindi, Pakistan. [3]Department of Obstetrics & Gynaecology, College of Medicine, University of Ibadan, Queen Elizabeth Road, Ibadan, Nigeria. [4]St George's University of London, Room 1.126, First Floor, Jenner Wing, Cranmer Terrace, London SW17 0RE, UK.

References
1. Ker K, Edwards P, Perel P, Shakur H, Roberts I. Effect of tranexamic acid on surgical bleeding: systematic review and cumulative meta-analysis. Br Med J. 2012;344:e3054.
2. CRASH-2 trial collaborators, Shakur H, Roberts I, Bautista R, Caballero J, Coats T, et al. Effects of tranexamic acid on death, vascular occlusive events, and blood transfusion in trauma patients with significant haemorrhage (CRASH-2): a randomised, placebo-controlled trial. Lancet. 2010;376:23–32.
3. WOMAN Trial Collaborators. Effect of early tranexamic acid administration on mortality, hysterectomy, and other morbidities in women with postpartum haemorrhage (WOMAN): an international, randomised, double-blind, placebo-controlled trial. Lancet. 2017;389:2105–16.
4. CRASH-2 collaborators, Roberts I, Shakur H, Afolabi A, Brohi K, Coats T, et al. The importance of early treatment with tranexamic acid in bleeding trauma patients: an exploratory analysis of the CRASH-2 randomised controlled trial. Lancet. 2011;377:1096–1101.e2.
5. World Health Organization. WHO recommendations for the prevention and treatment of postpartum haemorrhage. WHO 2017. Available from: http://www.who.int/reproductivehealth/publications/tranexamic-acid-pph-treatment/en/ Accessed 12 Jan 2018.
6. Shakur H, Roberts I, Edwards P, Elbourne D, Alfirevic Z, Ronsmans C. The effect of tranexamic acid on the risk of death and hysterectomy in women with post-partum haemorrhage: statistical analysis plan for the WOMAN trial. Trials BioMed Central. 2016;17:249.

7. Rothman KJ. Induction and latent periods. Am J Epidemiol. 1981;114:253–9.

8. Hernán MA. The hazards of hazard ratios. Epidemiology. 2010;21:13–5.

9. Andersson L, Nilsoon IM, Colleen S, Granstrand B, Melander B. Role of urokinase and tissue activator in sustaining bleeding and the management thereof with EACA and AMCA. Ann N Y Acad Sci. 1968;146:642–58.

10. Yee BE, Wissler RN, Zanghi CN, Feng C, Eaton MP. The effective concentration of tranexamic acid for inhibition of fibrinolysis in neonatal plasma in vitro. Anesth Analg. 2013;117:767–72.

11. Pilbrant A, Schannong M, Vessman J. Pharmacokinetics and bioavailability of tranexamic acid. Eur J Clin Pharmacol. 1981;20:65–72.

12. Fletcher DJ, Blackstock KJ, Epstein K, Brainard BM. Evaluation of tranexamic acid and   -aminocaproic acid concentrations required to inhibit fibrinolysis in plasma of dogs and humans. Am J Vet Res. 2014;75:731–8.

13. Fears R, Greenwood H, Hearn J, Howard B, Humphreys S, Morrow G, et al. Inhibition of the fibrinolytic and fibrinogenolytic activity of plasminogen activators in vitro by the antidotes   -aminocaproic acid, tranexamic acid and aprotinin. Fibrinolysis. 1992;6:79–86.

14. Godier A, Parmar K, Manandhar K, Hunt BJ. An in vitro study of the effects of t-PA and tranexamic acid on whole blood coagulation and fibrinolysis. J Clin Pathol. 2017;70:154–61.

15. Grassin-Delyle S, Theusinger OM, Albrecht R, Mueller S, Spahn DR, Urien S, et al. Optimisation of the dosage of tranexamic acid in trauma patients with population pharmacokinetic analysis. Anaesthesia. 2018; Available from: http://doi.wiley.com/10.1111/anae.14184. Accessed 10 Apr 2018.

16. Andersson L, Eriksson O, Hedlund PO, Kjellman H, Lindqvist B. Special considerations with regard to the dosage of tranexamic acid in patients with chronic renal diseases. Urol Res. 1978;6:83–8.

Barriers and facilitators to preventive interventions for the development of obstetric fistulas among women in sub-Saharan Africa

2

Eniya Lufumpa[1*], Lucy Doos[2] and Antje Lindenmeyer[1]

Abstract

Background: Obstetric fistula is a debilitating childbearing injury that results from poorly managed obstructed labour, leading to the development of holes between the vagina and bladder and/or rectum. Effects of this injury are long-lasting, as women become incontinent and are often marginalised from their communities. Despite continuous occurrence of this injury in lower-income countries, it is preventable, as evidenced in high-income countries. This systematic review aims to identify and understand barriers and facilitators to interventions aimed at the prevention of obstetric fistulas in sub-Saharan African women.

Methods: Electronic databases and grey literature were searched. We included studies written in English that discussed interventions to prevent obstetric fistulas implemented in sub-Saharan Africa, and their associated barriers and facilitators. Quality of the studies was assessed, and data including: country of implementation, preventive interventions, and barriers and facilitators to the interventions were extracted. They were then categorised based on the *Three Phase Delay Model*.

Results: Our search yielded 537 studies, of which 18 were included from sub-Saharan countries including Ethiopia, Nigeria, and Zambia. The most noted barrier to prevention addressed the first phase of delay: the decision to seek care, particularly lack of awareness of the dangers of unsupervised labours. The most noted facilitator addressed the decision to seek care and the quality of care received at a facility, through partnerships between health facilities and governments, and other organisations that provided both financial and resource support.

Conclusion: Despite being categorised by the three phases of the delay model, barriers and facilitators were found to play a role in multiple phases. The topic of obstetric fistula needs to be researched more extensively, particularly the effectiveness of preventive interventions.

Keywords: Obstetric fistula, Preventive interventions, Barriers, Facilitators, Basic and comprehensive emergency obstetric care

* Correspondence: ekl559@bham.ac.uk
[1]Institute of Applied Health Research, University of Birmingham, Edgbaston, Birmingham B15 2TT, UK
Full list of author information is available at the end of the article

Background

Obstetric fistula is a debilitating childbearing injury seen only in lower-income countries. It results predominantly from obstructed labour, but can also be iatrogenic and result from errors during surgeries such as caesarean sections. It represents a major public health issue for women and their communities, particularly in sub-Saharan Africa and Southeast Asia [1]. This injury results in holes between the vagina and bladder (vesicovaginal fistula), and/or vagina and rectum (rectovaginal fistula) [2]. These holes lead to incontinence of urine, and/ or faeces [3]. These have secondary effects such as the marginalisation and social exclusion of women from within their communities [4]. Social exclusion also decreases their likelihood of seeking treatment because they are less likely to be made aware of treatment options available to them [5]. Not seeking treatment results in difficulties in estimating the number of women currently suffering from this injury due to under-diagnosis. Current data reflect fistulas that have been accounted for mainly through clinical records, and there are still thousands of women who have yet to be accounted for [6, 7].

With an estimated number of more than two million women living with untreated fistulas worldwide, every year between 50,000 and 100,000 new cases of obstetric fistula occur [4]. Obstetric fistulas can be treated with reconstructive intravaginal surgery; however, the majority of affected women are unable to afford this treatment [8]. Conversely, fistulas are easily prevented through timely access to competent emergency obstetric care (EmOC) at the onset of labour complications such as prolonged labour [9]. As evidenced in high-income countries, this injury is completely preventable if proper measures are taken to educate women and healthcare providers about identifying and managing obstetric complications, while concurrently strengthening existing health systems within affected countries so as to ensure provision of adequate maternal care for all pregnant women [10]. This study focuses on prevention as the main means of ultimately eradicating this injury.

While preventive interventions in sub-Saharan Africa have already been identified in a previous systematic review by Banke-Thomas et al., included in this study, there is a need for a thorough assessment of the barriers to and facilitators of these interventions [11]. This is a critical component in making preventive interventions more accessible and effective. It is this knowledge gap which this systematic review aims to address.

Methods

Using the following databases: PubMed, EMBASE, MEDLINE, Cochrane Library, CINAHL, POPLINE, PsycINFO, and Web of Science for articles that identified barriers to and facilitators of interventions that aim to prevent the development of obstetric fistulas in sub-Saharan African women. Additional resources included official documents and grey literature—which included databases and websites of relevant organisations such as EngenderHealth, FistulaCare and the World Health Organization (WHO) (see Fig. 1). Search terms included both MESH terms and free text including: 'obstetric fistula', 'prevention', and 'sub-Saharan Africa'. A variation of these terms was used in the various databases listed above (Additional file 1).

We included articles written in English that met the following criteria: i) the setting of sub-Saharan Africa; ii) an intervention with the aim of preventing fistulas or its leading cause— obstructed labour— as well as its barriers and facilitators; and iii) fistulas that are a result of childbirth. The focus on sub-Saharan Africa is due to the highest prevalence in that continent; furthermore we also focused on obstetric fistulas as these are the most common types of fistulas within this region and allowed us to examine this topic with a context-specific approach [1]. We excluded studies that: i) were published in a language other than English; ii) discussed fistulas other than obstetric fistulas—vesicovaginal and rectovaginal—such as urethral fistulas, enterovaginal fistulas, and cervical fistulas; iii) discussed fistulas that are due to causes other than obstructed labour, for example, sexual trauma or radiation; and iv) focused on aspects other than prevention such as treatment, repair outcomes, experiences of living with this injury.

Articles were selected by two reviewers (EL, LD) using the process proposed by PRISMA, with a third reviewer resolving discrepancies (AL). We appraised included studies before the synthesis of the data, using either the relevant CASP checklist for qualitative studies or the AMSTAR checklist for systematic reviews. Descriptive studies were not appraised, as there was no applicable appraisal tool.

Reporting of the results was framed by the *Three Phase Delay Model*, proposed by Thaddeus and Maine [12]. The model identifies obstacles to the provision and timely utilisation of obstetric care—decision to seek care (first phase delay), accessibility of healthcare facilities (second phase delay), and receiving adequate care (third phase delay)— which are also applicable to preventive strategies.

Results

The search yielded a total of 537 studies, of which 70 studies were fully retrieved and read. A total of 16 studies met our inclusion criteria. These studies were then forward and backward referenced, which further identified two relevant studies, resulting in 18 studies identified as meeting the inclusion criteria (see Fig. 1).

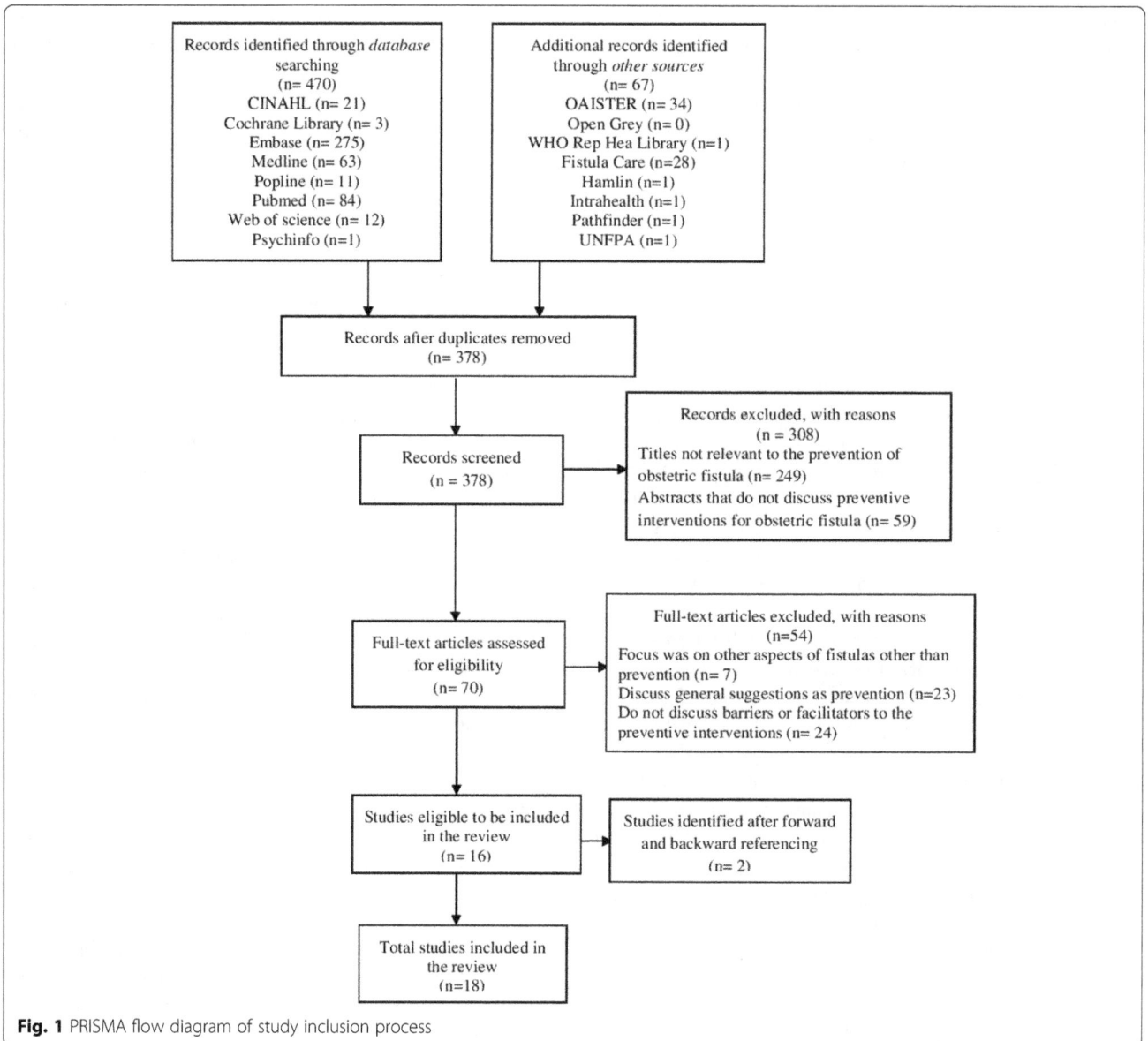

Fig. 1 PRISMA flow diagram of study inclusion process

Characteristics of included studies

All 18 included studies reflected: sub-Saharan Africa as a region (6), Nigeria (4), West Africa (1), Ethiopia (1), Eritrea (1), Guinea (1), Niger (1), Sierra Leone (1), Uganda (1) and Zambia (1), respectively. Nine studies were qualitative, eight descriptive, and one was a systematic review. Both barriers and facilitators were discussed to some extent in all 18 studies, with the exception of the study by Markos and Bogale which focused solely on barriers [13]. Barriers and facilitators were then characterised according to the Three Phase Delay Model. It is important to note that some of the included preventive interventions, mentioned in Table 1, do not have the primary aim of preventing fistulas but are instead basic and comprehensive maternity care that are not always readily available or accessible in lower-income countries, and as

such were included as preventive interventions by the authors [11].

Barriers

Phase one: Decision to seek care

Barriers were discussed in all studies (Table 2). The most frequently noted barrier was lack of awareness, as cited in four studies [14–17]. One study found that communities where fistulas are present were found to have limited knowledge of health issues, even more so with regard to the dangers of unsupervised births [16]. When a pregnant woman or members of her support system within her community were not aware of programmes that promote safe motherhood practices, they would not use the services that have been made available to them [16]. Two studies from Nigeria pointed out that this was

Table 1 Characteristics of included studies reporting on implemented fistula prevention interventions

Author(s)	Year	Country/ region of study	Preventive intervention implemented	Phase applicable to intervention
Bacon	2003	sub-Saharan Africa	Improving access to adequate medical care; Health education programs	All three phases
Banke-Thomas et al.	2014	sub-Saharan Africa	Community and Facility based interventions	All three phases
Fistula care[a]	2010	Guinea (Kissidougou)	Village safe motherhood committees; Financial partnerships; Maternal waiting homes; and Market Towns and Local Resource Mobilisation project	All three phases
Fistula care (a)[a]	2011	Sierra Leone	Aberdeen's Women's Centre: counselling, family planning, and a maternity care unit for pregnancy care, labour and delivery, and postpartum recovery (services to prevent fistulas)	All three phases
Fistula care (b)[a]	2011	sub-Saharan Africa	Partograph	Phase 3: Receiving adequate care
Fistula care[a]	2013	Uganda	Partograph	Phase 3: Receiving adequate care
Gerten et al.	2009	Nigeria	Patient educational brochure at a vesicovaginal hospital	Phase 1: Decision to seek care
Levin and Kabagema	2011	sub-Saharan Africa	Partograph	Phase 3: Receiving adequate care
Markos and Bogale	2015	Ethiopia (Bale zone)	Partograph	Phase 3: Receiving adequate care
Miller et al.	2005	sub-Saharan Africa	Fistula prevention centres; Community-based preventions; Maternal waiting homes; and Training course about screening for risk of fistula	All three phases
Nathan et al.	2009	West Africa	Femme pour Femme, community healthcare insurance plan	All three phases
Ngoma	2011	Zambia	EmOC and Safe Motherhood Actions Groups (SMAGs); and Income generating activities (IGA)	All three phases
Ojanuga	1991	Nigeria	Community health education programs; organizing transport for pregnant women in need; and training traditional birth attendants	All three phases
Ojanuga	1992	Nigeria	Health education programs	Phase 1: Decision to seek care
Seim et al.	2014	Niger	Community-mobilization program that arrange transport for women who experience complicated labours	All three phases
Tahzib	1989	Nigeria	Safe motherhood initiatives not specified but aimed at encouraging hospital deliveries, and the improvement of the perception of facilities by women seeking help	All three phases
Turan et al.	2007	Eritrea	Transport of women to healthcare facilities	Phase 2: Accessibility of care
UNFPA	2013	sub-Saharan Africa	Global midwifery program; All-terrain motorbikes (Women and Health Alliance International)	Phase 2: Accessibility of care; Phase 3: Receiving adequate care

[a]A six-year fistula repair and prevention program managed and implemented by Engender Health from 2007 to 2013

rooted in the fact that fistulas are most prevalent in remote areas where there are high levels of illiteracy which are exacerbated by low levels of education [14, 16]. As revealed through the use of an educational brochure in one study, Gerten et al. discuss the limited effectiveness of educational brochures published in English as some participants lived in remote areas and had very limited education resulting in their ability to only read and communicate in their native language, rendering brochures ineffective [14].

Lack of awareness was not limited to the knowledge of preventive interventions, but also applied to the perception of services provided at healthcare facilities [17]. Even when women were aware of preventive interventions some were still reluctant to seek care for obstetric complications due to their views regarding healthcare facilities which were shaped directly by the experiences of

other rural women who sought care at a facility [17]. The author further pointed out that this served as a barrier in cases when a woman had a negative experience at a healthcare facility.

Phase two: Accessibility of care

Accessibility of preventive interventions was identified as a barrier in seven studies [14, 15, 17–21]. In Ojanuga's study, longer distances between remote communities—where fistulas are prevalent—and preventive services—usually in urban settings—in Nigeria were identified as a phase two delay [16]. A further two studies based on Niger and Nigeria concluded that in areas where fistulas are most prevalent, dilapidated infrastructure made traveling to reach care nearly impossible [14, 20]. One study noted that conditions such as these were exacerbated during the rainy and harvest seasons, which further

Table 2 Barriers to interventions aimed at the prevention of obstetric fistulas categorised by the three phases of delay

Phase one: *Decision* to seek care	Phase two: *Reaching* a facility or preventive intervention	Phase three: *Receiving* adequate care through a preventive intervention

• Lack of awareness about health and preventive interventions
  ○ Ignorance among the villagers of the dangers associated with unsupervised delivery for women who are at risk
  ○ Negative experiences of other women at healthcare facilities
  ○ Illiteracy
• Lack of access to preventive interventions
• Lack of financial resources serve as a major disincentive to the use of modern health facilities
• Reluctance of women to be away from their homes for an undetermined period of time
• Language barrier, dependence on translation of a brochure into the reader's native language
	• Preventive strategies regarding birth plans are lagging
	• Lack of infrastructures such as paved roads, piped water, and electricity.
	  ○ Worsens accessibility during he rainy and harvest seasons
	• Lack of transport
	  ○ Large distances from the villages to healthcare facilities
	• Lack of financial resources to pay for transport
	• Lack of ambulance services and portable oxygen
	• Limited referral systems i.e. when emergency transport isn't available
		• Perception, healthcare practitioners view women with fistulas as a 'nuisance' and 'embarrassment'
		  ○ Affects their attitude towards them and in turn the experience of the patient
		• Limited services and manpower
		  ○ Doctors are preoccupied with high-tech practices, leaving their units overwhelmed with obstetric emergencies
		  ○ Overworked staff
		  ○ Staff shortages and high attrition rates
		• Lack of skilled healthcare providers
		  ○ High staff turnover at maternity units which results in the loss of valuable skills and training investments
		  ○ Absence of supervisory staff
		• Lack of financial resources, which leaves the facilities rarely self-sufficient
		• Lack of reimbursement for village practitioners
		• Improper/ limited use of the partograph
		  ○ Lack of essential supplies and equipment needed
		  ○ Lack of training

limited mobility and transport opportunities [18]. Moreover, Ojanuga's study highlighted that traveling such great distances and rough terrains were extremely costly and difficult to arrange, due to their limited financial resources [15].

As highlighted in five studies, financial limitations served as a barrier to women accessing preventive interventions [14–16, 22, 23]. Nathan et al. pointed out that within West Africa, limited financial resources was the most frequently noted barrier to intrapartum care, citing the example of Benin, where the yearly income per capita is about $1100 USD, which makes transport and medical care costs unaffordable [23].

Phase three: Receiving adequate care

Receiving care through preventive facilities and available services was the most frequently discussed issue as is evidenced in seven studies [11, 13, 17, 22, 24–26]. As discussed in five studies, limited manpower, and shortage of skilled healthcare workers was an important factor in third phase delay [11, 20, 24–26]. Two studies highlighted that this was further heightened by the lack of basic and essential supplies and equipment including access to running water and electricity, which had proven to be unreliable [17, 20, 24]. This was often the case as they had financial limitations. Two studies showed how this directly affected a facility as their financial resources were meant to maintain services through the provision of basic equipment and supplies, as well as the training and payment of the service providers [19, 22]. Fistula Care, and Seim et al. reported that this included transport systems that are meant to be provided through preventive interventions (Table 2) [19, 20].

Four studies highlighted the importance of a partograph—a pre-printed recording sheet on which progress of labour is documented and monitored by a healthcare provider— and its ability to greatly reduce maternal and foetal morbidity and mortality, when properly used [13, 19, 24, 25]. The most commonly cited barrier to the use of a partograph was the improper and poor use of it due to the difficulty of its use [13, 19, 24, 25]. One study highlighted that this was due to differences in the versions of partographs, as well as incompetent monitoring and recording of the necessary indicators [24]. Moreover, minimal training on how to use a partograph was referenced in the study [24]. This barrier was compounded with the lack of essential supplies such as the partograph forms, clocks, blood pressure monitors etc. further rendering this preventive intervention impossible to use effectively [24].

Facilitators
Phase one: Decision to seek care

Facilitators were discussed in 17 studies (Table 3). Increased awareness of maternal and child morbidities and how to prevent them, was noted as a facilitator in seven studies, particularly through health education programmes [14–16, 20–22, 27]. As Gerten et al. and Turan et al. reported, conducting programmes in the local languages addressed potential language barriers [14, 21]. The study conducted by Turan et al. also highlighted the use of figures and pictures as an aid which directly addressed the issue of illiteracy, which was often common in the areas where fistulas occur [21].

Another key element noted in eight studies based on Eritrea, Guinea, Niger, Nigeria, and sub-Saharan Africa as a region, was the involvement of key members within

Table 3 Facilitators to interventions aimed at the prevention of obstetric fistulas, categorised by the three phases of delay

Phase one: *Decision* to seek care	Phase two: *Reaching* a facility or preventive intervention	Phase three: *Receiving* adequate care through a preventive intervention

• Women with successful treatments acting as ambassadors and advocates for healthcare facilities
  ○ Women are provided with training on public speaking and interpersonal communication skills
• Increased awareness within communities through training
  ○ About maternal/ child morbidities, and the importance of seeking care
• Community involvement
  ○ Volunteer coordinator provides SMAGs with technical support, and schedule activities and training
  ○ Increased involvement of men, community leaders, and religious leaders, as they are decision-makers within these communities
• Financial support
  ○ Allowing women to participate in income-generating activities
  ○ Free healthcare services for pregnant women and children under 5 years old
	• Financial support
	  ○ Reimbursement for transport
	  ○ Insurance plan that provides transport costs
	  ○ Community generating money to assist with transport costs
	• Assistance with transport
	  ○ A politician procured an ambulance, which facilitated the evacuation of labouring women in need
	  ○ All-terrain motorbikes to facilitate transport to healthcare facilities
	• Volunteers initiate evacuation by phoning a midwife at a facility that has an ambulance available
	• Volunteers arrange transport to the closest facility
	• Relocation of midwives in rural areas where the most at-risk women and girls reside
	• Improved mobile coverage to arrange evacuation
		• Mobilisation of recognised experts
		• Training
		  ○ On the local needs as a means of improving the morale for the provision of preventive care
		  ○ On the improved use of the partograph
		  ○ Of patients so they educate women and their local communities when they return home
		• Financial support from international foundations and organisations
		  ○ Insurance plan that covers medical costs for pregnant women
		• Partnerships that provide funds for research, the purchase of essential equipment, and the development of basic infrastructure
		  ○ Donation of supplies and volunteers' time, which improves adequate staffing, space, equipment, and essential medication
		• Employment of more midwives
		• Mobile prenatal clinics serve remote villages

communities [11, 15–18, 20–22]. This included the involvement of men, and religious and community leaders, as they are the decision-makers and gatekeepers of their societies [16, 20, 22]. Miller et al. highlighted the Tostan program in which traditional and village leaders come together to publicly advocate the rights of girls and women, as well as the end of harmful cultural practices [22]. Also noted in five studies was the involvement of women who had previously used the service [11, 15, 17, 18, 21]. Women who had successful treatments would serve as advocates and community educators to encourage women to attend healthcare facilities when they experience complications during labour.

Phase two: Accessibility of care
Facilitating the accessibility of preventive interventions was addressed in seven studies [15, 18, 20, 22, 23, 26, 27]. Four studies discussed efforts by healthcare facilities and individuals to improve access to health services [15, 20, 22, 28]. UNFPA highlighted the use of motorbike ambulances within countries from West to East Africa, which are low cost and quickly transport women in labour to healthcare facilities [28]. In cases where emergency transport services were not available, three studies mentioned the use of mobile prenatal clinics and maternity waiting homes [15, 18, 22]. The use of mobile clinics addressed delays in receiving care, while maternity waiting homes provided pregnant women who have high-risk pregnancies with a place to stay that is within the vicinity of a facility that offers EmOC, if necessary [18, 22].

Financial support also served as a facilitator to the accessibility of care, as noted in five studies [15, 18, 20, 23, 27]. The studies discussed community-led programs—in the West African region, Guinea, Nigeria, and Zambia,

respectively—that acted as insurance plans and provided financial support for women in need. Seim et al. identified a program in Niger that subsidised the cost of fuel that ambulances used to transport pregnant women to hopsitals [20]. Two studies carried out by Fistula Care and Ngoma highlighted the importance of Safe Motherhood Committees [18, 27]. These committees participate in income-generating activities which provide financial support for women needing emergency care. Fistula Care pointed out the importance of income-generating activities in the Guinean community of Kissidougou through which a minimum of 5% of generated income is allocated to their local fistula programs [18].

Phase three: Receiving adequate care
Receiving adequate care was facilitated through financial support from partnerships with the government, and international organisations and foundations, as mentioned in three studies [17, 19, 25]. Financial support was provided to hospitals and other preventive interventions, particularly with essential equipment needed to provide care for women with labour complications.

Miller et al. and Seim et al. note the employment of more midwives, and their relocation to rural communities where fistulas are most prevalent as a facilitator [20, 22]. Moreover, two studies discussed the use of mentoring and training programs as a means of improving the competence of care providers as well as their morale [17, 25]. Mentoring and training was also provided on the use of the partograph—a pre-printed recording sheet on which the progression of labour is documented and monitored by a healthcare provider. This training would enable healthcare providers to take timely and appropriate decisions in response to the progression of labour [25].

Discussion

Numerous barriers and facilitators were identified, and categorised by the *Three Phase Delay Model*– the decision to seek preventive care, accessing preventive care, and receiving adequate preventive care. Our analyses demonstrate that despite being categorised by the three phases of the delay model, barriers and facilitators were found not to be limited to one phase. More specifically, barriers— limited finances, limited education and awareness, and location of services— were also found to be interlinked. Fistulas are most prevalent in remote communities far from educational and health facilities. Characteristic of these areas are low levels of education and financial instability, as these communities rely on subsistence farming [16]. We also found that facilitators discussed in the literature, unlike barriers, were not found to be as clearly interlinked as they were more diverse. The main facilitators to interventions aimed at the prevention of fistulas— increased awareness of maternal and child morbidities, involvement of key members of the community, and financial support—were also not limited to one phase, but instead affected all three phases of delay. Accordingly, they were examined across phases.

Barriers

Despite numerous countries adopting recommendations of United Nations agencies and the African Union to subsidize the cost of maternal care, women are still required to pay for some costs [29]. Our review highlighted limited finances as the most cited barrier, which was echoed in relevant studies as affecting all three phases of delay [29]. Our findings mirror the study of Melberg et al. in rural Burkina Faso, and found that expectant women were reluctant to leave their homes for an unknown duration due to their inability to attend to their responsibilities at home and participate in income-generating activities [30]. Additionally, limited finances led to a lack of basic necessities such as scissors, blood pressure monitors, and ambulances which greatly impaired the services that health facilities could provide. They further point out that these are exacerbated by a lack of basic amenities such as beds, adequate lighting, or running water which makes the provision of quality care difficult as issues such as sterility arise [30].

Our systematic review confirms that limited education was found not only with regard to people living in remote communities where fistulas are found, but also applied to the skills of health care providers. Our findings concur with Wall's study of fistula patients in Jos, Nigeria, which reported that they were unaware of obstetric care available to them at the time [31]. Our study is also in line with Melberg et al. who attributed lack of skilled health care workers to high turnover rates within maternity units, which leads to the loss of skills and training investments [30]. Their study also reinforced barriers as being interlinked, as they pointed out that childbearing injuries are most common in women who are living far away from health centres and consequently may be unable to understand advantages of care at health facilities [30]. Another barrier linked to distance was the inability to afford transport from the areas they reside to health care facilities. Lori et al. point out that it is often worsened by the location of health facilities, being situated in more populated and urban areas [32]. Due to these longer distances, transport costs are unaffordable and this is compounded by unreliable transport.

Most barriers to receiving care were noted with regard to the partograph, specifically its improper use. Improper use was noted as a result of different versions of the partograph used in various facilities as well as inadequate monitoring of indicators required to use a partograph. Health care providers were unable to constantly monitor progress of labour [30]. This also resulted from lack of essential supplies required to monitor the necessary indicators, such as partograph forms, blood pressure machines, watches etc. Improper use leads to an increase in number of interventions that labouring women will go through, resulting in a more negative experience for them. Additionally, lack of adequate training on how to use the partograph also is a barrier to its use.

Facilitators

Similarly, facilitators were found to contribute to all phases of delay particularly the first and second phases. Our finding that involvement of key community members—traditional leaders, religious leaders, and husbands— facilitate the use of preventive services concurs with a study which examined delays in accessing EmOC in Bangladesh; husbands were found to make half of the decisions on seeking care, as opposed to women deciding to seek care themselves in only one-eighth of the cases [33]. Furthermore, a study carried out in Zambia highlighted the importance of men being aware of and having a positive attitude towards the use of maternity waiting homes, as this results in them encouraging the use of such preventive services [34, 35]. Our findings also mirrored De Allegri's study which identified the influence that village leaders carry in Burkina Faso. Through village leaders advocating for user fees reduction, a reduction occurred in the costs of facility deliveries [29]. Their involvement is a key facilitator as communities in which fistulas occur, are male centric societies in which they hold decision power.

Our findings showed that financial support through government partnerships, communities, and international donors served as a major factor in all three phases of the delay model through making resources available to labouring women, their communities, and health facilities they visit. Our study was in line with De Allegri et al. who highlighted that as a result of UN recommendations to subsidise obstetric care, there has been an increase in facility deliveries and a decrease in births at home [29].

Strengths and limitations

To our knowledge, this review is the first to examine and synthesise barriers and facilitators associated with preventive interventions in sub-Saharan Africa, within the region with the highest prevalence of this injury. Moreover, it is the first to do so with the theoretical underpinning of the *Three Phases Delay Model*. Publication bias was reduced through a thorough search for unpublished literature using grey literature databases and websites of relevant organisations. A limitation of this review is its restriction to interventions in sub-Saharan Africa only. However, as Africa has the highest regional concentration of obstetric fistulas worldwide, the majority of interventions targets that population. Inclusion of descriptive studies also served as a limitation, as we were not able to carry out a full quality assessment due to the lack of an appropriate tool. We used our personal discretion when deciding whether to include a descriptive study, and were informed by the inclusion and exclusion criteria.

Implications for practice and policy

- Future policies and initiatives should focus on increasing awareness of preventive interventions through training programs, and should not only be addressed to women but even more so to men and the leaders of communities.
- Simultaneously, the capability of health facilities to provide EmOC should be strengthened through appropriate and regular training on management of complicated labours, as well as through the provision of basic and essential tools and amenities.
- Lastly, financial support is required both in relation to the provision and payment of services, but also to improve transport and infrastructure, allowing labouring women to arrive sooner at facilities offering preventive care.

Conclusion

This systematic review found that although barriers and facilitators were identified according to the phase of delay, they were found to play a role in all three phases of the delay model. Main barriers were found to be clustered and interlinked, while facilitators were less related. As the literature currently reflects a focus on preventive interventions aimed at either the decision to seek care or receiving adequate care, our review indicates that there is a need for more research on preventive interventions that target issues with regard to the second phase of delay, reaching a facility. Furthermore, there is a need to assess these preventive interventions as it will generate evidence reflecting their efficacy.

Abbreviations

AMSTAR: A measurement tool to assess systematic reviews; CASP: Critical Appraisal Skills Programme; EmOC: Emergency obstetric care; IGA: Income generating activities; SMAGs: Safe Motherhood Action Groups; WHO: World Health Organization

Author's contributions

The systematic review was written by EL, with substantial contributions made by LD and AL. The article selection process was carried out by EL and LD, with AL resolving differences. Both LD and AL contributed significantly to the drafting of the manuscript. All authors read and approve the final manuscript.

Competing interests

The authors declare that they have no competing interest.

Author details

[1]Institute of Applied Health Research, University of Birmingham, Edgbaston, Birmingham B15 2TT, UK. [2]Institute for Research into Superdiversity, University of Birmingham, Edgbaston, Birmingham B15 2TT, UK.

References

1. Adler A, Ronsmans C, Calvery C, Filippi V. Estimating the prevalence of obstetric fistula: a systematic review and meta-analysis. BMC Pregnancy Childbirth. 2013;13:246–59.
2. Bangser M. Obstetric fistula and stigma. Lancet. 2006;367(9509):535–6.
3. Banke-Thomas A, Kouraogo S, Siribie A, Taddese H, Mueller J. Knowledge of obstetric fistula prevention amongst young women in urban and rural Burkina Faso: a cross-sectional study. PLoS One. 2013;8(12):1–8.
4. WHO. 10 facts on obstetric fistula. Geneva: World Health Organization; 2014. http://www.who.int/features/factfiles/obstetric_fistula/en/. Accessed 13 Apr 2016.
5. Wegner M, Ruminjo J, Sinclair E, Pesso L, Mehta M. Improving community knowledge of obstetric fistula prevention and treatment. Int J Gynaecol Obstet. 2007;99(Suppl 1):108–11.
6. Capes T, Ascher-Walsh C, Abdoulaye I, Brodman M. Obstetric fistula in low and middle income countries. Mt Sinai J Med. 2011;78(3):352–61.
7. Ramphal S, Moodley J. Vesicovaginal fistula: obstetric causes. Curr Opin Obstet Gynecol. 2006;18(2):147–51.
8. UNFPA. http://www.unfpa.org (2016). Accessed 19 Apr 2016.
9. Fistula Foundation. http://fistulafoundation.org (2014). Accessed 19 Apr 2016.
10. Cron J. Lessons from the developing world: obstructed labor and the vesicovaginal fistula. MedGenMed. 2003;5(3):24–30.
11. Banke-Thomas A, Wilton-Waddell O, Kouraogo S, Mueller J. Current evidence supporting obstetric fistula prevention strategies in sub Saharan Africa: a systematic review of the literature. Afr J Reprod Health. 2014;18(3): 118–27.
12. Thaddeus S, Maine D. Too far to walk: maternal mortality in context. Soc Sci Med. 1994;38(8):1091–110.
13. Markos D, Bogale D. Documentation status of the modified World Health Organization partograph in public health institutions of bale zone, Ethiopia. Reprod Health. 2015;12:81–6.

14. Gerten K, Venkatesh S, Norman A, Shu'Aibu J, Richter H. Pilot study utilizing a patient educational brochure at a vesicovaginal fistula hospital in Nigeria, Africa. Int Urogynecol J Pelvic Floor Dysfunct. 2009;20(1):33–7.

15. Ojanuga D. Preventing birth injury among women in Africa: case studies in northern Nigeria. Am J Orthop. 1991;61(4):533–9.

16. Ojanuga D. Education: the key to preventing vesicovaginal fistula in Nigeria. World Health Forum. 1992;13(1):54–6.

17. Tahzib F. An initiative on vesicovaginal fistula. Lancet. 1989;1(8650):1316–7.

18. Fistula C. Beyond repair: involving communities in fistula prevention and social reintegration—experience from Kissidougou, Guinea. New York: Fistula Care/EngenderHealth; 2010. https://fistulacare.org/archive/files/1/1.1/guinea_brief_beyond_repair.pdf. Accessed 20 Apr 2016.

19. Fistula C. Integrating fistula treatment and prevention: the launch of a maternity unit in Sierra Leone. New York: Fistula Care/EngenderHealth; 2011. https://www.engenderhealth.org/files/pubs/fistula-care-digital-archive/2/2.2/Integrating-Fistula-Treatment-sierra_Leone_tech_brief.pdf. Accessed 20 Apr 2016

20. Seim A, Alassoum Z, Bronzan R, Mainassara A, Jacobsen J, Gali Y. Pilot community-mobilization program reduces maternal and perinatal mortality and prevents obstetric fistula in Niger. Int J Gynaecol Obstet. 2014;127(3):269–74.

21. Turan J, Johnson K, Polan M. Experiences of women seeking medical care for obstetric fistula in Eritrea: implications for prevention, treatment, and social reintegration. Glob Public Health. 2007;2(1):64–77.

22. Miller S, Lester F, Webster M, Cowan B. Obstetric fistula: a preventable tragedy. J Midwifery Womens Health. 2005;50(4):286–94.

23. Nathan L, Rochat C, Grigorescu B, Banks E. Obstetric fistulae in West Africa: patient perspectives. Am J Obstet Gynecol. 2009;200(5):40–2.

24. Fistula C. Force MHT. Revitalizing the Partograph: does the evidence support a global call to action. New York: EngenderHealth/Fistula Care; 2012. https://fistulacare.org/wp-fcp/wp-content/uploads/pdf/program-reports/EngenderHealth-Fistula-Care-Partograph-Meeting-Report-9-April-12.pdf. Accessed 20 Apr 2016

25. Fistula C. Improving partograph use in Uganda through coaching and mentoring. New York: Fistula Care/EngenderHealth; 2013. https://fistulacare.org/archive/files/2/2.3/Uganda_Partograph_technical_brief.pdf. Accessed 20 Apr 2016

26. Levin K, Kabagema J. Use of the Partograph: effectiveness, training, modifications, and barriers- a litearature review. New York: EngenderHealth/Fistula Care; 2011. https://fistulacare.org/archive/files/2/2.2/partograph_literature_review.pdf. Accessed 20 Apr 2016.

27. Ngoma J. Prevention of Vesicovaginal fistula: a literature review and experience from Zambia. 2011. http://www.theseus.fi/handle/10024/26462; https://www.theseus.fi/bitstream/handle/10024/26462/Josephine%20ngoma%20thesis.pdf?sequence=1&isAllowed=y. Accessed 2 May 2016.

28. UNFPA. Obstetric fistula needs assessment report: findings from nine African countries. New York: United Nations Population Fund; 2015. https://www.unfpa.org/sites/default/files/pub-pdf/fistula-needs-assessment.pdf. Accessed 19 Apr 2016.

29. De Allegri M, Tiendrebeogo J, Muller O, Ye M, Jahn A, Ridde V. Understanding home delivery in a context of user fee reduction: a cross-sectional mixed methods study in rural Burkina. BMC Pregnancy Childbirth. 2015;15:330–42.

30. Melberg A, Diallo A, Tylleskar T, Moland K. 'We saw she was in danger, but we couldn't do anything': missed opportunities and health worker disempowerment during birth care in rural Burkina Faso. BMC Pregnancy Childbirth. 2016;16(1):292–302.

31. Wall L, Karshima J, Kirschner C, Arrowsmith S. The obstetric vesicovaginal fistula: characteristics of 899 patients from Jos, Nigeria. Am J Obstet Gynecol. 2004;190(4):1011–9.

32. Lori J, Munro-Kramer M, Mdluli E, Musonda G, Boyd C. Developing a community driven sustainable model of maternity waiting homes for rural Zambia. Midwifery. 2016;41:89–95.

33. Nahar S, Banu M, Nasreen H. Women-focused development intervention reduces delays in accessing emergency obstetric care in urban slums in Bangladesh: a cross-sectional study. BMC Pregnancy Childbirth. 2011;11:11.

34. Sialubanje C, Massar K, Kirch E, van der Pijl M, Hamer D, Ruiter R. Husbands' experiences and perceptions regarding the use of maternity waiting homes in rural Zambia. Int J Gynaecol Obstet. 2016;133(1):108–11.

35. van Lonkhuijzen L, Stekelenburg J, van Roosmalen J. Maternity waiting facilities for improving maternal and neonatal outcome in low-resource countries. Cochrane Database Syst Rev. 2012;10:CD006759.

3

Maternal death and delays in accessing emergency obstetric care in Mozambique

Leonardo Antonio Chavane[1*], Patricia Bailey[2], Osvaldo Loquiha[3], Martinho Dgedge[4], Marc Aerts[5] and Marleen Temmerman[6,7]

Abstract

Background: Despite declining trends maternal mortality remains an important public health issue in Mozambique. The delays to reach an appropriate health facility and receive care faced by woman with pregnancy related complications play an important role in the occurrence of these deaths. This study aims to examine the contribution of the delays in relation to the causes of maternal death in facilities in Mozambique.

Methods: Secondary analysis was performed on data from a national assessment on maternal and neonatal health that included in-depth maternal death reviews, using patient files and facility records with the most comprehensive information available. Statistical models were used to assess the association between delay to reach the health facility that provides emergency obstetric care (delay type II) and delay in receiving appropriate care once reaching the health facility providing emergency obstetric care (delay type III) and the cause of maternal death within the health facility.

Results: Data were available for 712 of 2,198 maternal deaths. Delay type II was observed in 40.4% of maternal deaths and delay type III in 14.2%.and 13.9% had both delays. Women who died of a direct obstetric complication were more likely to have experienced a delay type III than women who died due to indirect causes. Women who experienced delay type II were less likely to have also delay type III and vice versa.

Conclusions: The delays in reaching and receiving appropriate facility-based care for women facing pregnancy related complications in Mozambique contribute significantly to maternal mortality. Securing referral linkages and health facility readiness for rapid and correct patient management are needed to reduce the impact of these delays within the health system.

Keywords: Maternal deaths, Delays type II & III, Mozambique

Background

Maternal death and delays in accessing emergency obstetric care in Mozambique

Delays in access to quality care have been identified as one of the important determinants of preventable maternal death [1, 2]. Thaddeus and Maine's three delays model that describes the multiple factors that drive maternal mortality has proven to be an effective tool to evaluate the circumstances surrounding access to and appropriateness of emergency obstetric and newborn care (EmONC) [3]. The model has been helpful identifying barriers and potential points of intervention along the continuum from home to hospital for more than 20 years [4–6].

According to this framework 3 delays in access to quality emergency care are defined. The first delay occurs at the household and community level and reflects the delay in deciding to seek care for pregnancy complications. The second delay (delay II) refers to the delay to reach the facility that provides emergency obstetric care (EmONC) and, the third delay (delay III) refers to the delay that occurs in receiving care after arrival at the health facility [3].

In Mozambique, estimates based on the 2007 population census indicate that around 46% of maternal deaths occur within health institutions [7], a substantial proportion considering that these women reached a health facility.

Maternal mortality ratio in Mozambique has declined from more than 1600 estimated deaths per 100.000 live births in 1990 [8] to 403 in 2003 [9] and DHS 2011 [10].

* Correspondence: leochavane@gmail.com
[1]Jhpiego Mozambique, Rua A.W. Bayly, 61 Maputo, Mozambique
Full list of author information is available at the end of the article

Despite considerable reduction over time, the latest estimations available show that the ratio still is very high, even when compared with the neighboring countries [2].

Several factors have been identified at the health care facility level that interfere with the readiness to deal adequately with obstetric emergencies. Knight described six groups of factors, namely drugs and equipment, policy and guidelines, human resources, facility infrastructure, patient-related and referral-related aspects [11].

A near miss study, an approach to evaluate maternal quality of care and learning from women that survived severe maternal complications [12, 13] covered 564 survival women and 71 maternal deaths, conducted in Mozambique's Maputo Province, found delay II in 21.3% and delay III in 69.7% (women could experience multiple delays [14]. In some cases these delays followed the woman's path throughout the referral system from admission to a peripheral health facility and then on to the referral facility [14].

With this paper we aim to examine the relationship between the cause of maternal death and delays II and III.

Methods
Study setting
Mozambique is a low income country located in the Sub-Saharan Africa region with an estimated population of 26.4 million in 2016, based on projections of the 2007 population census. The public sector is the main provider of health care services [15]. Childbirth services are provided throughout 4 levels of care. At peripheral level services are available in the smallest type 2 health centers, with 1 MCH nurse as provider and 3 maternity beds. The different layers of care are connected by a network referral system based on ambulances managed at the referral health facilities. Usually a health facility covering an average population of 300.000 inhabitants has 1 to 2 ambulances to serve a network of 10 to 15 health facilities. In the district capitals maternity services are available in large type 1 health centers, with more than 10 maternity beds; at this level the staff include at least 3 MCH nurses and in some facilities, a general practitioner physician. The District, Provincial, General and Central hospitals are more complex facilities with different specialties, wards and operating rooms. Health centers type 1 and 2 should have capacity to offer Basic Emergency Obstetric Care (BEmOC). According to the Annual Joint Assessment Report in 2012, in average 2.3 health facilities were available with BEmOC services per 500 thousand inhabitants. When needed, the health centers refer patients to hospitals with capacity to offer Comprehensive Emergency Obstetric Care (CEmOC).

This paper draws on secondary data analyses of a large health facility needs assessment on maternal and neonatal health care services, which included 427 health facilities nationwide. The sample was designed to be representative of the mix of the health facilities at national and provincial levels. Data collection was done between November 2007 and January 2008 by health providers previously trained to undertake this task. Service statistics were collected from registers and logbooks and covered a period of 12 months, from November 2006 to October 2007.

The national survey identified a total of 2,198 maternal deaths in the 427 health facilities out of 312,537 deliveries, corresponding to an estimated facility based maternal mortality ratio of 703 deaths per 100.000 deliveries. At each facility, a detailed maternal death review was conducted if the patient's records were available. A maternal death review was completed for 712 maternal deaths for which there was sufficient information in the files. Prior to data entry, these were reviewed by a committee of experts composed of 6 ObGyn Medical doctors. The committee reviewed the circumstances of death to determine: 1) the final cause of death, 2) if evidence existed to suggest that the woman experienced a delay in arriving at the health facility providing emergency obstetric care services (delay II). Women that faced delay in the referral process reaching the second health facility was considered as delay II. and 3) if evidence suggested a delay in receiving adequate health care services after reaching the health facility with emergency obstetric care services (delay III).

For each maternal death, the time of arrival at the initial health facility was collected as well as the time of treatment initiation, time of arrival at the referral (second) facility and time of death. The delay was defined based on assessment of each woman's individual story since her arrival at the initial health facility. This included the combination of the clinical status on admission in the health facility, and the time taken for action at peripheral and referral facilities. Women presenting life threatening condition at admission of ether initial facility or at the referral facility were considered facing delay type II. In all these steps the quality of care was assessed relating the decision (diagnosis and or to refer to next level of care) and the treatment prescribed and or initiated. The 712 maternal deaths were found in 93 of the 427 facilities included in the survey, including health centers and hospitals, located in rural and urban areas of the 11 provinces of Mozambique. Approval from the Mozambican national bioethical committee was received before starting the survey implementation.

Statistical analysis
Data were analyzed using the SAS-STAT software, version 9.4. A bivariate binary mixed effects model was applied to examine if and how the probability for delay type II and delay type III depends on the main cause of maternal death and other risk factors and covariates, while accounting for the correlation between both types of delay. Specifically, as in Wilson and Lorenz (2015)

[16],we used one logistic regression model for each outcome variable (delay type II and III), both models consisting of fixed effects related to observed covariates and a random intercept related to unobserved effects affecting both delay types specific to each woman.

The advantage of such model specification is that it allows the logistic regressions to be modelled simultaneously, for which, conditional on the latent variable, delay type II and III were assumed as independent outcomes. This allows the estimation of the correlation between the outcomes while also controlling for the main cause of death and other observed covariates such as age, parity, referrals, type of health facility and availability of human resources. The potential covariates were selected for the final model using logistic regression for each outcome separately in a backwards selection procedure with removal rob of 0.2. The initial model didn't include any interaction between the risk factors.

Inference was based on 95% confidence intervals and p-values for odds ratio estimates, and these were only valid if the missing data mechanism was known to be missing completely at random, (MCAR) [17, 18]. About 13% of cases with missing data for either outcome were excluded from the analysis (see Table 1 for more details), and considered to be MCAR, since being missing was not related to any covariate investigated in this study. The latter was based on a logistic regression model on the missing indicator for both delay types (results not shown), for which no significant association was found between the missing indicator and the covariates [17].

Results

Table 1 below presents the women's demographic characteristics, previous obstetric history, facility characteristics, timing and cause of death (direct or indirect). Also this table presents the distribution of proportion of delays within the selected characteristics.

Most women (62.1%) were between 20 and 34 years old at the time of their death. The median age was 25 years and only 18.4% were nulliparous. Most women arrived at the health facility with an obstetric complication (78.4%), and 53.1% were referred from another health facility. Delay II (reaching the health facility where she died) was observed in 40.4% of deaths and delay III (receiving treatment after arrival at the health facility) was registered in 14.2% of cases, 13.9 faced the both type of delays and in 18.5% of cases no evidence of delay was identified. Direct obstetric complications were registered as the main cause of death for most cases (73.7%).

Around 10% of women developed complications after admission in the health facilities. Out of this group, 53% of deaths occurred at the tertiary hospitals while 35% at the health Centers and 12% at the Central Hospitals. The main causes of death in this group were post-partum hemorrhage which accounted for 28% followed by uterine rupture responsible of 14% of deaths. Uterine rupture was the first cause at the health centers level.

Table 2 summarizes the causes of death in relation to the type of delay. Amongst the direct causes of death, hemorrhage was observed in 60.6% of cases, followed by sepsis in 20.8%, while HIV/AIDS was frequent amongst the indirect causes, observed in 40.6% of the cases.

Around 40.4% of women suffered delay type II but not delay type III, 13.9% experienced both delay type II and type III and 18.5% did not experienced any type of delay at the referral facility.

The modelling results in Table 3 show a significant association between the main cause of death and delay type III after controlling for other risk factors. Pregnant women who died of a direct pregnancy complication were twice more likely to have experienced a delay type III than pregnant women who died due to indirect causes. However, no significant association between delay type II and cause of death was observed.

Experience of delay type II was strongly and positively associated with having been referred due to complications, and with care-seeking at central hospitals compared to seeking care at a health center. The odds of delay type II among women who were referred were roughly two times that of women not referred.

A negative correlation was estimated between the probability of experiencing both delays type II and III. Delay type III is less likely to occur in a woman who experienced delay type II and vice-versa. A test on the overall effect of risk factors based on contrasts between model parameters showed that the significant effects on Table 3 were different between Delay II and Delay III.

Discussion

This study evaluated the associations between two types of delays for a women experiencing pregnancy complications and the cause of death: delays type II, reaching a facility with capacity to manage pregnancy related complications and delays type III, delay in receiving appropriate treatment. This study focused on type II and III delays and therefore only provided the analysis of the deaths that occurred within health facilities.

The second delay was shown to be more frequent in this setting when compared with the third delay regardless of cause of death (direct or indirect). It was observed in more than 60% of women who died. The delay type II has been described in other studies [18–20]. Patient referral from a peripheral facility was strongly associated with the delay type II. This finding suggests that part of the delay in reaching the appropriate facility to treat the complication may occur at the peripheral health facility. At these facilities we often find junior and less qualified staff with critical limitations with regard to decision-making (diagnosis

Table 1 Summary of selected characteristics of maternal deaths

		Neither delay II nor delay III		Delay III only		Delay II only		Both delay II and delay III		Missing		Total	
		Count	Row N %	Count	Row N %	Count	Row N %	Count	Row N %	Count	Row N %	Count	Column N %
Age recoded	< 20	25	18.7%	22	16.4%	46	34.3%	21	15.7%	20	14.9%	134	18.8%
	20 – 34	90	20.4%	54	12.2%	190	43.0%	56	12.7%	52	11.8%	442	62.1%
	> 35	14	15.9%	17	19.3%	37	42.0%	13	14.8%	7	8.0%	88	12.4%
	Missing	3	6.3%	8	16.7%	15	31.3%	9	18.8%	13	27.1%	48	6.7%
Parity	Nullipara	29	22.1%	20	15.3%	37	28.2%	18	13.7%	27	20.6%	131	18.4%
	> 1	96	19.1%	76	15.1%	205	40.8%	68	13.5%	57	11.4%	502	70.5%
	Missing	7	8.9%	5	6.3%	46	58.2%	13	16.5%	8	10.1%	79	11.1%
Previous cesarean	No	101	19.3%	77	14.8%	207	39.7%	69	13.2%	68	13.0%	522	73.3%
	Yes	11	22.0%	8	16.0%	21	42.0%	5	10.0%	5	10.0%	50	7.0%
	Missing	20	14.3%	16	11.4%	60	42.9%	25	17.9%	19	13.6%	140	19.7%
Complication after admission	No	88	15.8%	67	12.0%	262	47.0%	88	15.8%	53	9.5%	558	78.4%
	Yes	29	39.2%	21	28.4%	6	8.1%	2	2.7%	16	21.6%	74	10.4%
	Missing	15	18.8%	13	16.3%	20	25.0%	9	11.3%	23	28.8%	80	11.2%
Referred from another facility	No	62	19.7%	61	19.4%	113	35.9%	30	9.5%	49	15.6%	315	44.2%
	Yes	67	17.7%	39	10.3%	171	45.2%	67	17.7%	34	9.0%	378	53.1%
	Missing	3	15.8%	1	5.3%	4	21.1%	2	10.5%	9	47.4%	19	2.7%
Type of Health facility	Central Hospital	40	19.7%	13	6.4%	96	47.3%	39	19.2%	15	7.4%	203	28.5%
	Hospital (Prov, Gen, & Dist.)	64	16.6%	64	16.6%	153	39.6%	48	12.4%	57	14.8%	386	54.2%
	Health Centers	28	22.8%	24	19.5%	39	31.7%	12	9.8%	20	16.3%	123	17.3%
Moment of death	While pregnant	31	14.2%	28	12.8%	101	46.1%	32	14.6%	27	12.3%	219	30.8%
	During delivery	10	10.3%	21	21.6%	26	26.8%	18	18.6%	22	22.7%	97	13.6%
	Postpartum	88	23.5%	50	13.3%	154	41.1%	48	12.8%	35	9.3%	375	52.7%
	Missing	3	14.3%	2	9.5%	7	33.3%	1	4.8%	8	38.1%	21	2.9%
*Cause of death	Direct	98	18.7%	85	16.2%	200	38.1%	86	16.4%	56	10.7%	525	73.7%
	Indirect	34	18.2%	16	8.6%	88	47.1%	13	7.0%	36	19.3%	187	26.3%
	Total	132	18.5%	101	14.2%	288	40.4%	99	13.9%	92	12.9%	712	100.0%

*Cause of death: Direct = Maternal death from direct pregnancy related complications; Indirect = Maternal deaths due to non-obstetric causes aggravated by the pregnancy
Prov Province, Gen general, Dist district

Table 2 Delays type II and type III by cause of death

	Neither delay II nor III		Delay III only		Delay II only		Both delay II and III		Missing		Total	
	n	%	n	%	n	%	n	%	n	%	n	%
Direct causes	98	18.7	85	16.2	200	38.1	86	16.4	56	10.7	525	73.7
Hypertension	21	23.3	12	13.3	40	44.4	10	11.1	7	7.8	90	17.1
Hemorrhage	59	18.6	53	16.7	116	36.5	50	15.7	40	12.6	318	60.6
Sepsis/Infections	14	12.8	18	16.5	44	40.4	25	22.9	8	7.3	109	20.8
Other direct causes	4	50	2	25	0	0	1	12.5	1	12.5	8	1.5
Indirect causes	34	18.2	16	8.6	88	47.1	13	7	36	19.3	187	26.3
Malaria	8	15.4	7	13.5	22	42.3	7	13.5	8	15.4	52	27.8
HIV/AIDS	14	18.4	2	2.6	50	65.8	0	0	10	13.2	76	40.6
Malaria/HIV-AIDS	2	16.7	0	0	7	58.3	1	8.3	2	16.7	12	6.4
Severe anemia	1	7.7	2	15.4	4	30.8	3	23.1	3	23.1	13	6.9
Other indirect causes	6	26.1	3	13	5	21.7	1	4.4	8	34.8	23	12.3
Unknown/Undetermined	3	27.3	2	18.2	0	0	1	9.1	5	45.5	11	5.9
Total	132	18.5	101	14.2	288	40.4	99	13.9	92	12.9	712	100%

Table 3 Parameter estimates for the bivariate logistic regression model (with random intercepts)

	Delay II		Delay III		Overall effect
Effect	O.R. (95% C.I)	p-value	O.R. (95% C.I)	p-value	p-value
Age					
< 20	Ref.		Ref.		
20 – 34	1.32 (0.82 – 2.12)	0.2565	**0.59** (0.37 – 0.96)	**0.0324**	**0.0345**
> 35	1.21 (0.62 – 2.37)	0.5729	0.73 (0.38 – 1.42)	0.3545	0.3586
Parity					
Nullipara	Ref.		Ref.		
> 1	0.80 (0.51 – 1.26)	0.3343	1.17 (0.74 – 1.84)	0.5109	0.297
Referred					
No	Ref.		Ref.		
Yes	**1.76** (1.18 – 2.62)	**0.0055**	0.67 (0.45 – 1.00)	0.0506	**0.0019**
Type of Health Facility					
Health Centers (I;II)	Ref.		Ref.		
Central Hospital	**2.37** (1.30 – 4.33)	**0.0049**	0.89 (0.49 – 1.62)	0.6957	**0.0279**
Prov, Gen & Dist Hosp.	1.52 (0.90 – 2.58)	0.1207	1.16 (0.68 – 1.99)	0.5839	0.4603
Cause of death					
Indirect	Ref.		Ref.		
Direct	0.66 (0.42 – 1.05)	0.0771	**2.11** (1.29 – 3.46)	**0.0031**	**0.0018**
Lack of staff for surgical care					
No	Ref.		Ref.		
Yes	1.35 (0.66 – 2.76)	0.4118	1.25 (0.65 – 2.41)	0.5103	0.8833
Within-subject correlation between delay type II and III	**−0.745**		**p-value < .0001**		

and treatment) in the face of an obstetric emergency. Another source of delays is related to the referral process management which is characterized by frequent fuel stock out and lack of ambulance maintenance or even inexistence of one functioning in the District. This slows down the decision-making to transfer patients and results in an inefficient functioning referral system. Referral has been noted elsewhere in Mozambique to be a risk factor for stillbirth outcomes [21]. A combination of factors such as the perception of poor quality of care and the lack of availability of skilled personnel have been identified in other studies to influence the choice of where to deliver and ultimately contributes to the delay for women to reach the health facility [22–25]. Elsewhere lack of transportation, prolonged travel time and seeking care at more than one facility were also identified as contributing factors to the delay type II [20].

Delay type II was identified and potentially contributed to one third of facility based maternal deaths. Women who died of acute direct obstetric complications were more likely to have faced delay type III. This might be interpreted as a lack of adequate emergency response from health services. Appropriate and timely complication management requires specific midwifery and specialist skills from the health providers as well as adequate availability of EmOC services [26–28]. Thus, availability of qualified services providers in right quantity must be combined with the availability of supplies for emergency care (e.g. drugs, blood), and the structural functioning of the health facilities such as the referral system and the functionality of the operating room [6, 27, 29–31].

We identified a negative relationship between delay II and delay III. A woman experiencing a delay in reaching the health facility may trigger a quick response from the health system when she arrives at the health facility and is less likely to experience a third delay. This correlation has been noted elsewhere [11]. This emphasizes the importance of ensuring the availability of services to identify and effectively manage the emergency resulting from pregnancy complications. Measures to improve delay type II tend to contribute to a reduction in delay III as well [32].

In a study in Brazil of maternal near miss cases the occurrence of any delay increased the severity of maternal outcome, particularly leading to maternal death [5]. Other authors have found an association between delays and severe pregnancy outcomes and maternal death [33].

In our study, direct obstetric causes were the most important causes of maternal deaths and hemorrhage the most frequent among this group followed by sepsis. HIV/AIDS was the most common cause of death among indirect causes. This finding aligns with the pattern of causes of maternal deaths in the developing world described elsewhere [5, 34].

In this national study 44% of the reviewed cases went directly from home to a health facility where they died. Another study conducted in a more urbanized setting in Mozambique found that 29% of near miss cases went directly from home to the health facility evaluated [14]. It is important to note that around 10% of the women who died were admitted to health facilities without any complication. Data from this group of women showed hemorrhage and obstructed labor as responsible of 42% of deaths. This results may indicate inadequate labor and delivery management including the issue of referral system discussed previously. Women still face important risk of dying even arriving in the maternities in healthier status [11]. The health facilities in this setting suffer from the same challenges described for the developing world in relation to human resources and the overall health services provision. A comprehensive effort to improve health system responsiveness is desirable for better maternal health outcomes.

Study limitations

The absence of information on survival limited the analysis that might have further clarified factors that were determinants of maternal deaths. Also the fact that only part of the facility based data was available, limits the generalization of the conclusions to all country but rather to the covered facilities.

The quality of hospital and health center registers and medical charts was poor, as were storage and retrieval systems, which reduced our access to the files of all maternal deaths and to more complete information on the circumstance surrounding maternal deaths and the actions taken. The analysis done by the expert group helped reduce the inconsistency in the data from the files that were accessible.

This survey found that only 55% of the maternal deaths registered in the health facilities were reported in the national health information system. This study covered the analysis of around 32% of total institutional maternal deaths during the evaluation period.

Conclusions

Investment is needed to strengthen referral linkages and secure hospital and health center readiness to rapidly diagnose and manage pregnancy related complications, and thus, lessen the impact of delays II and III, and ultimately reduce institutional maternal mortality. Further studies that include women who survive will be important to understand the broader impact of the delays on maternal health outcomes in this setting.

Abbreviations
AIDS: Acquired immunodeficiency syndrome; BEmOC: Basic emergency obstetric care; CEmOC: Comprehensive emergency obstetric care; EmONC: Emergency obstetric neonatal care; HIV: Human immunodeficiency virus; MCH: Maternal and child health; ObGyn: Obstetric and gynecologist; SAS-STAT: Statistical analysis system

Acknowledgements
Not applicable.

Consent to participate
Not applicable as this study review secondary aggregated data.

Funding
No funding was received for this study.

Authors' contributions
LC conceived and designed the study protocol and developed the first manuscript draft, OL and MA did the statistical analysis, MD, PB and MT provided feedback on the protocol design and inputs on the manuscript development. All the authors have read and approved the manuscript.

Competing interests
The authors declare that they have no competing interests.

Author details
[1]Jhpiego Mozambique, Rua A.W. Bayly, 61 Maputo, Mozambique. [2]RMNCH Unit, Global Health Programs, FHI, Durham, NC 360, USA. [3]Department of Mathematics and Informatics, Eduardo Mondlane University, Maputo, Mozambique. [4]Faculty of Medicine, Eduardo Mondlane University, Maputo, Mozambique. [5]Interuniversity Institute for Biostatistics and Statistical Bioinformatics (I–BioStat), Hasselt University, Hasselt, Belgium. [6]Centre of Excellence in Women and Child Health- East Africa, Aga Khan University, Karachi, Pakistan. [7]Ghent University Belgium, Ghent, Belgium.

References
1. Kerber KJ, de Graft-Johnson JE, Bhutta ZA, Okong P, Starrs A, Lawn JE. Continuum of care for maternal, newborn, and child health: from slogan to service delivery. Lancet. 2007;370:1358–69.
2. Kassebaum NJ, Barber RM, Bhutta ZA, Dandona L, Gething PW, Hay SI, et al. Global, regional, and national levels of maternal mortality, 1990–2015: a systematic analysis for the global burden of disease study 2015. Lancet. 2016;388:1775–812. Available from: http://www.thelancet.com/journals/lancet/article/PIIS0140-6736(16)31470-2/fulltext.
3. Thaddeus S, Maine D. Too far to walk : maternal mortality in context. Soc Sci Med. 1994;38:1091–110.
4. Combs Thorsen V, Sundby J, Malata A. Piecing together the maternal death puzzle through narratives: the three delays model revisited. PLoS One. 2012;7
5. Pacagnella RC, Cecatti JG, Parpinelli MA, Sousa MH, Haddad SM, Costa ML, et al. Delays in receiving obstetric care and poor maternal outcomes: results from a national multicentre cross-sectional study. BMC Pregnancy Childbirth. 2014;14:159. Available from: https://bmcpregnancychildbirth.biomedcentral.com/articles/10.1186/1471-2393-14-159 http://www.pubmedcentral.nih.gov/articlerender.fcgi?artid=4016777&tool=pmcentrez&rendertype=abstract
6. Pacagnella RC, Cecatti JG, Osis MJ, Souza JP. The role of delays in severe maternal morbidity and mortality: expanding the conceptual framework. Reprod. Health matters. Reprod. Health Matters. 2012;20:155–63.
7. Saúde IN de E, da M. MORTALIDADE EM MOÇAMBIQUE Inquérito Nacional sobre Causas de Mortalidade, 2007/8. Maputo: Instituto Nacional de Saúde; 2009.
8. Instituto Nacional de Estatistica. Inquérito Demográfico e de Saúde 1997. Maputo: Macro International Inc.; 1998.
9. INE & MISAU. Moçambique, Inquerito Demográfico e de Saúde 2003. Maputo: Macro International Inc.; 2003.
10. Instituto Nacional de Estatística & Ministério da Saúde. Inquêrito Demográfico e de Saúde 2011. Maputo: ICF International/MEASURE DHS program; 2011.
11. Knight HE, Self A, Kennedy SH. Why are women dying when they reach hospital on time? A systematic review of the "third delay". PLoS One. 2013;8:51.
12. Pattinson R, Say L, Souza JP, Van Den Broek N, Rooney C. Evaluating the quality of care for severe pregnancy complications: the WHO near-miss approach for maternal health. Bull World Health Organ. 2011;87:1–29.
13. Say L, Souza JP, Pattinson RC. Maternal near miss - towards a standard tool for monitoring quality of maternal health care. Best Pract Res Clin Obstet Gynaecol. 2009;23:287–96.
14. David E, Machungo F, Zanconato G, Cavaliere E, Fiosse S, Sululu C, et al. Maternal near miss and maternal deaths in Mozambique: a cross-sectional, region-wide study of 635 consecutive cases assisted in health facilities of Maputo province. BMC Pregnancy Childbirth. 2014;14:401.
15. Long Q, Kempas T, Madede T, Klemetti R, Hemminki E. Caesarean section rates in Mozambique. BMC Pregnancy Childbirth. 2015;15:253. Available from: https://bmcpregnancychildbirth.biomedcentral.com/articles/10.1186/s12884-015-0686-x
16. Wilson JR, Lorenz KA. Modeling binary correlated responses using SAS, SPSS and R. Heidelberg C, editor. Switzerland: Springer International Publishing; 2015.
17. Molenberghs G, Verbeke G. Models for discrete longitudinal data. New York: Springer; 2005.
18. Montfort K Van, Oud J, Satorra A. Longitudinal research with latent variables. London and New York: Springer; 2010.
19. Jammeh A, Sundby J, Vangen S. Barriers to emergency obstetric care services in perinatal deaths in rural Gambia: a qualitative in-depth interview study. ISRN Obstet Gynecol. 2011;2011:1–10. Available from: http://www.hindawi.com/journals/isrn/2011/981096/
20. Cham M, Sundby J, Vangen S. Maternal mortality in the rural Gambia, a qualitative study on access to emergency obstetric care. Reprod Health. 2005;2:3.
21. Seljeskog L, Sundby J, Chimango J. Factors influencing Women's choice of place of delivery in rural Malawi-an explorative study. African J Reprod Heal. 2006;10:66–75.
22. Geelhoed D, Stokx J, Mariano X, Lázaro CM, Roelens K. Risk factors for stillbirths in Tete, Mozambique. Int J Gynecol Obstet. 2015:148–52.
23. Machira K, Palamuleni M. Factors influencing women's utilization of public health care services during childbirth in Malawi public health facility utilization. Afr Health Sci. 2017;17:400–8.
24. Asseffa NA, Bukola F, Ayodele A. Determinants of use of health facility for childbirth in rural Hadiya zone, southern Ethiopia. BMC pregnancy childbirth [internet]. BMC Pregnancy Childbirth. 2016;16:355. Available from: http://bmcpregnancychildbirth.biomedcentral.com/articles/10.1186/s12884-016-1151-1
25. Fisseha G, Berhane Y, Worku A, Terefe W. Distance from health facility and mothers ' perception of quality related to skilled delivery service utilization in northern Ethiopia. Int J Women's Heal. 2017:749–56.
26. Cavallaro FL, Marchant TJ. Responsiveness of emergency obstetric care systems in low- and middle-income countries: a critical review of the "third delay". Acta Obstet Gynecol Scand. 2013;92:496–507.
27. Paxton A, Maine D, Freedman L, Fry D, Lobis S. The evidence for emergency obstetric care. Int J Gynecol Obstet. 2005;88:181–93.
28. Cabero-Roura L, Rushwan H. An update on maternal mortality in low-resource countries. Int J Gynaecol Obstet. 125:175–80. International Federation of Gynecology and Obstetrics; 2014 [cited 2015 Jan 13]; Available from: http://www.ncbi.nlm.nih.gov/pubmed/24642275
29. Essendi H, Mills S, Fotso JC. Barriers to formal emergency obstetric care services' utilization. J Urban Heal. 2011;88(Suppl 2):S356–69. Available from: http://www.ncbi.nlm.nih.gov/pmc/articles/PMC3132235/pdf/11524_2010_Article_9481.pdf
30. Kongnyuy EJ, Mlava G, van den Broek N. Facility-based maternal death review in three districts in the central region of Malawi. An analysis of causes and characteristics of maternal deaths. Women's Heal. 2009;19:14–20. Issues [Internet]. Jacobs Institute of Women's Health; Available from: https://doi.org/10.1016/j.whi.2008.09.008.
31. Kruk ME, Leslie HH, Verguet S, Mbaruku GM, Adanu RMK, Langer A. Quality of basic maternal care functions in health facilities of five African countries:

an analysis of national health system surveys. Lancet Glob Heal. 2016;4:845–55. Available from: http://www.thelancet.com/journals/langlo/article/PIIS2214-109X(16)30180-2/fulltext.

32. Holmer H, Oyerinde K, Meara JG, Gillies R, Liljestrand J, Hagander L. The global met need for emergency obstetric care: a systematic review. BJOG An Int J Obstet Gynaecol. 2015;122:183–9.

33. Filippi V, Richard F, Lange I, Ouattara F. Identifying barriers from home to the appropriate hospital through near-miss audits in developing countries. Best Pract. Res. Clin. Obstet. Gynaecol. 2009;23:389–400.

34. Say L, Chou D, Gemmill A, Tunçalp Ö, Moller AB, Daniels J, et al. Global causes of maternal death: a WHO systematic analysis. Lancet Glob Heal. 2014;2:323–33.

4

Resolution of maternal Mirror syndrome after successful fetal intrauterine therapy

Angel Chimenea[1], Lutgardo García-Díaz[1], Ana María Calderón[1], María Moreno-De Las Heras[1]
and Guillermo Antiñolo[1,2]*

Abstract

Background: Mirror syndrome (MS) is a rare obstetric condition usually defined as the development of maternal edema in association with fetal hydrops. The pathogenesis of MS remains unclear and may be misdiagnosed as pre-eclampsia.

Case presentation: We report a case series of MS in which fetal therapy (intrauterine blood transfusion and pleuroamniotic shunt) resulted in fetal as well as maternal favourable course with complete resolution of the condition in both mother and fetus.

Conclusions: Our case series add new evidence to support that early diagnosis of MS followed by fetal therapy and clinical maternal support are critical for a good outcome.

Keywords: Mirror syndrome, Ballantyne syndrome, Parvovirus B19, Hydrops fetalis, Fetal therapy

Background

Mirror syndrome (MS) is a rare complication of fetal hydrops appearing as a triple edema (fetal, placental as well as maternal) [1], in which the mother "mirrors" the hydropic fetus. This syndrome was first described in 1892 by the Scottish obstetrician John William Ballantyne [2].

There have been multiple feto-placental diseases related to MS, that can be classified into diverse groups based on different etiologies [3]: cardiac failure associated with fetal anemia (e.g. Parvovirus B19 [4], erytroblastosis [5], fetal alloimmune thrombocytopenia [6], hemoglobin Bart's disease [7]); high-output cardiac failure associated with shunting (e.g. chorioangioma [8], twin to twin transfusion syndrome [9–13]); and fetal anomalies (e.g. fetal arrhythmias [14], CHAOS syndrome [15]).

MS maternal clinical picture includes peripheral edema, uterine distension and rapid weight gain [3]. Those non-specific clinical features may lead to a misdiagnosis of pre-eclampsia, delaying diagnosis and therapy of MS and worsening fetal and maternal condition. MS does not usually present with hypertension, but blood pressure can be elevated and proteinuria can appear, resembling the clinical features of pre-eclampsia [3, 16]. Like in pre-eclampsia, laboratory findings may include proteinuria, low platelet count and elevation of creatinine, hepatic enzymes and uric acid levels [3].

The treatment of choice for MS is the resolution of the fetal hydrops. If correction of the fetal condition is not possible, delivery usually results in a favourable maternal outcome [17]. Vaginal delivery may be preferred, but complications as maternal pulmonary edema or deterioration of the fetal condition can lead to an emergent caesarean section [18–20].

Case presentation
Case 1

A 31-year-old G1P0 caucasian woman was referred to our centre at 27 + 2 gestational weeks for evaluation of fetal hydrops. Her medical and obstetric record as well as the previous fetal ultrasound at 20 weeks were unremarkable.

* Correspondence: gantinolo@us.es
[1]Department of Genetics, Reproduction, and Fetal Medicine, Institute of Biomedicine of Seville (IBIS), Hospital Universitario Virgen del Rocio/CSIC/ University of Seville, Seville, Spain
[2]Centre for Biomedical Network Research on Rare Diseases (CIBERER), Seville, Spain

On admission the patient was normotensive, with stable vital signs. Physical examination showed a significant edema in both lower extremities and sacrum. Blood analysis results revealed a hemoglobin of 105 g/L, and a hematocrit of 28.8% with normal platelet count. Liver function test was abnormal: ALT 68 mU/ml ($N < 40$ mU/ml), AST 44 mU/ml ($N < 37$ mU/ml). LDH was elevated (240 UI/L; $N < 225$ UI/L) as well as uric acid levels (8.4 mg/dL; $N < 7$ mg/dL). Renal function was normal with a creatinine of 0.87 mg/dL ($N < 1.1$ mg/dL) and a urea of 39 mg/dL ($N < 40$ mg/dL). Her 24-h urinary protein excretion was 2925 mg.

Ultrasound revealed a single fetus with hydrops including severe ascites, pericardial effusion, subcutaneous tissue edema, a slightly thickened placenta (Figure 1), and normal amniotic fluid index (AFI). No fetal anomalies were detected. Middle cerebral artery peak systolic velocity (MCA-PSV) value was 77.5 cm/s (2.19 MoM [21, 22]) with an estimated hemoglobin of 38.6 g/L (0.31 MoM [22]). The EFW was 1.073 g. Initial evaluation of fetal anemia included indirect Coomb's test, serology for Parvovirus B19 and TORCH. Fetus was diagnosed as having a hydrops related to severe anemia and a MS was diagnosed.

Forty-eight hours following patient admission, intrauterine blood transfusion (IBT) was performed as described elsewhere [8]. Before the procedure, a single course of corticosteroid therapy was administered to accelerate fetal pulmonary maturity, and tocolysis with atosiban was started. During the intervention, fetal blood samples for genetic, anemia and infection studies were obtained, and a Kleihauer-Betke test was requested. Following IBT, fetal hemoglobin increased from 43 g/L to 109 g/L, and fetal hematocrit from 14% to 34%. Anti-D Ig 300 μg IM was administered after transfusion to prevent Rh(D) alloimmunization. The next day MCA-PSV value decreased to 36.9 cm/s (1.02 MoM) [21, 22]. In both maternal and fetal blood Indirect Immunofluorescence Test (IIFT) a positive IgM for Parvovirus B19 were found, confirming the etiology of the fetal anemia.

Fetal and maternal follow up revealed a progressive reduction of fetal hydrops (Figure 2) together with a progressive resolution of maternal clinical picture including normalization of laboratory tests.

At 29 + 4 gestational weeks, a preterm premature rupture of membranes occurred. At 34 gestational weeks a healthy male infant was born by vaginal delivery, with Apgar score of 8/9/10 at 1, 5 and 10 min. Both mother and child were discharged without complications and are currently doing well 2 years after delivery.

Case 2

A 37-year-old G1P0 caucasian woman was admitted to our centre at 31 gestational weeks due to nausea, vomiting and severe abdominal pain refractory to the medical treatment. Premature labor with progressive cervical shortening was diagnosed and tocolysis with atosiban was started. Physical examination showed a significant skin edema in both lower extremities. Her vital signs and laboratory results were within normal range except for anemia (hemoglobin 89 g/L). Further laboratory test showed a marked increase in C-reactive protein to 82.3 mg/L ($N < 5$ mg/dL).

Fetal ultrasound revealed a bilateral hydrothorax with a structural and functionally normal heart and vessels. A large hyperechoic placenta and placental edema were observed as well. No fetal anomalies were detected, and AFI was in normal range. MCA-PSV was 51.9 cm/s (1.21 MoM), consistent with an estimated fetal hemoglobin of 111.1 g/L (0.85 MoM [22]).

MS was diagnosed and a pleuroamniotic shunt (rocket catheter) was placed in right hemithorax to resolve fetal hydrops. Shunting was followed by bilateral lung parenchyma expansion (Figure 3).

On post-operative day#1, a deterioration of maternal clinical status with respiratory distress associated with increasing edema and diuresis volume reduction were observed. In addition, maternal echocardiography showed evidence of moderate pericardial effusion and tricuspid insufficiency. Treatment was started with furosemide, spironolactone, seroalbumine and potassium. In the next 72 h following maternal treatment and fetal hydrops resolution, an improvement of maternal clinical condition ocurred, with progressive disappearance of maternal peripheral edema, respiratory distress and anemia.

At 35 + 2 gestational weeks preterm premature rupture of membranes occurred, followed by delivery of a healthy

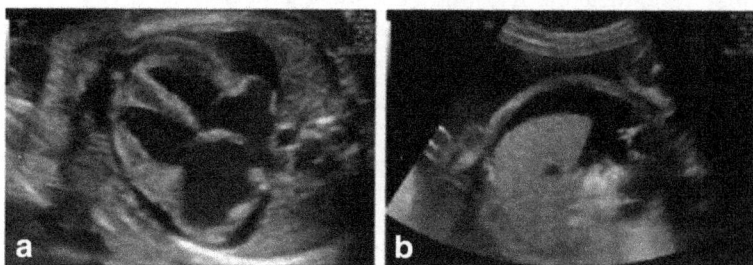

Fig. 1 Case 1. GA: 27 + 3 weeks. Pleural effusion (**a**), ascites (**b**)

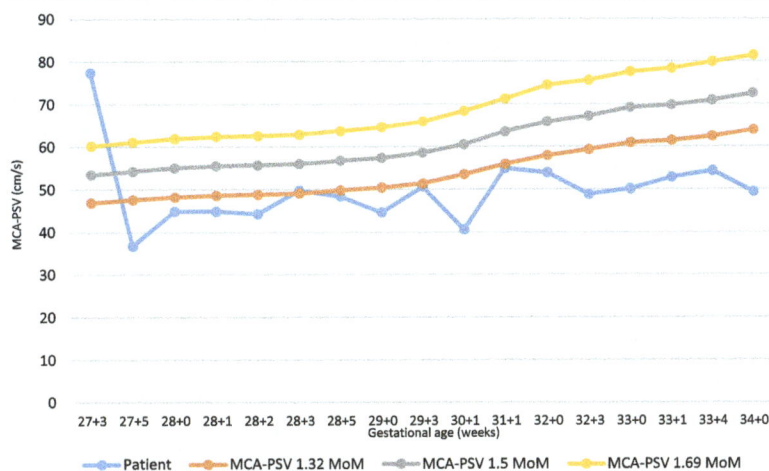

Fig. 2 Case 1. MCA-PSV evolution. IBT was performed at 27 + 4 weeks. Blue line represents patient values. Red line represents 1.32 MoM of normal fetal MCA-PSV. Grey line represents 1.5 MoM of normal fetal MCA-PSV. Yellow line represents 1.69 MoM of normal fetal MCA-PSV

male newborn with Apgar score 10/10/10 at 1, 5 and 10 min. At birth no lesions in newborn costal grid related to intrauterine shunt placement were observed. Both mother and newborn were discharged without complications and are currently doing well one year after delivery.

Discussion and conclusions

MS is a condition wherein the mother "mirrors" the edema present in the fetus. This entity was first described in association with rhesus-immunization, although MS is most commonly associated with non-immune fetal hydrops (NIHF) of an unknown etiology [19]. Anemia related to Parvovirus B19 is the most frequent reported infectious cause of NIHF. Therefore, complete serology including Parvovirus B19 is mandatory in the differential diagnosis of the fetal hydrops etiology related to anemia.

MS has many similarities to pre-eclampsia [23], sharing clinical features that may be caused in both cases by an imbalance between angiogenic and anti-angiogenic

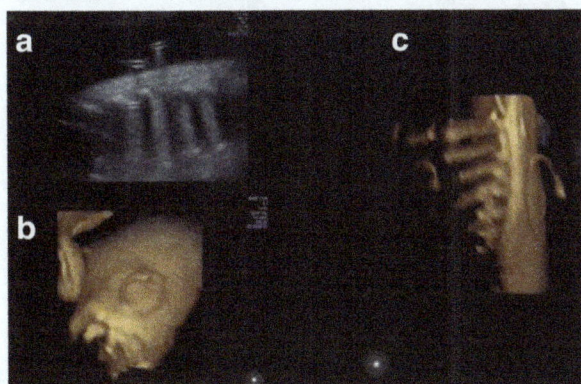

Fig. 3 Case 2. 2-D (**a**) and 4-D (**b**, **c**) ultrasound images of the catheter pigtail correctly inserted inside and outside of the fetal hemithorax

factors [24]. In pre-eclampsia there exists evidence of placental underperfusion caused by failure of trophoblastic invasion into the spiral arteries, with a subsequent increasing of circulating sFLT-1 levels and decreasing of PlGF levels [25, 26], being the second one a mechanism proposed as well as responsible for the maternal clinical findings in MS [27–31].

The association of edema, oliguria, and hemodilution might be characteristic of MS [32]. In addition, it has been suggested that the presence of hemodilution might be criteria for diagnosis of MS, as opposed to pre-eclampsia with low haematocrit [33]. MS does not usually present with oligohydramnios or hypertension [34], and unlike pre-eclampsia may be reversed if fetal hydrops is resolved. Fetal prognosis in MS is usually worse than in pre-eclampsia, resulting in many cases in intrauterine fetal demise [3], and being 56% the currently reported rate of intrauterine fetal death in MS [33].

In MS fetal hydrops successful therapy has been claimed as a key step to maternal clinical picture resolution [3, 5, 9, 10, 12, 31, 35]. According to a recent systematic review, interventions to correct the fetal hydrops related to anemia were significantly associated with improved fetal survival [35]. However, sometimes delivery is required when it is not possible to perform fetal therapy or when it is not successful [3, 12, 17, 20, 33, 36–38]. Different strategies have been described for the resolution of fetal hydrops, [3, 5, 9, 13, 14, 31, 39]. In our case series, fetal therapy (IBT and pleuroamniotic shunt) led to a slow but consistent reversal of maternal clinical picture following fetal hydrops resolution, resulting in a good fetal and maternal outcome.

Current data and experience from clinical practice support that fetal hydrops therapy, regardless etiology, improves fetal survival as well as maternal evolution in

MS. The cases we described show the need for an early diagnosis of MS, followed by an adequate treatment of the fetal condition, which improves maternal condition as well as perinatal morbidity and mortality. When the underlying fetal insult is corrected, we can expect a slow but sustained recovery of maternal condition, that may require an adequate intensive support.

Abbreviations
AFI: Amniotic Fluid Index; EFW: Estimated Fetal Weight; IBT: Intrauterine Blood Transfusion; IIFT: Indirect Immunofluorescence Test; MCA-PSV: Middle Cerebral Artery Peak Systolic Velocity; MS: Mirror Syndrome; NIHF: Non-Immune Fetal Hydrops; NST: Nonstress Test

Acknowledgements
All persons that contributed to this study are listed authors and meet the criteria for authorship.

Funding
There was no funding for this study.

Authors' contributions
AC, LG-D and GA drafted the manuscript, and AMC and MMD collaborated with valuable contributions to the manuscript. All authors have read and approved the final manuscript.

Competing interests
The authors declare that they have no competing interests.

References
1. Ballantyne KIH. triple edema. Am J Obstet Gynecol. 1971;110:115–20.
2. Ballantyne JW. The disease and deformities of the fetus. Edinburgh: Oliver & Boyd; 1892.
3. Braun T, Brauer M, Fuchs I, Czernik C, Dudenhausen JW, Henrich W, Sarioglu N. Mirror syndrome: a systematic review of fetal associated conditions, maternal presentation and perinatal outcome. Fetal Diagn Ther. 2010;27(4):191–203.
4. Desvignes F, Bourdel N, Laurichesse-Delmas H, Savary D, Gallot D. Ballantyne syndrome caused by materno-fetal parvovirus B19 infection: about two cases. J Gynecol Obstet Biol Reprod (Paris). 2011;40(3):262–6.
5. Valsky D, Daum H, Yagel S. Reversal of mirror syndrome after prenatal treatment of diamond-Blackfan anemia. Prenat Diagn. 2007;27(12):1161–4.
6. Jain V, Clarke G, Russell L, McBrien A, Hornberger L, Young C, Chandra SA. Case of alloimmune thrombocytopenia, hemorrhagic anemia-induced fetal hydrops, maternal mirror syndrome, and human chorionic gonadotropin-induced thyrotoxicosis. AJP Rep. 2013;3(1):41–4.
7. Zhang Z, Xi M, Peng B, You Y. Mirror syndrome associated with fetal hemoglobin Bart's disease: a case report. Arch Gynecol Obstet. 2013;288(5):1183–5.
8. García-Díaz L, Carreto P, Costa-Pereira S, Antiñolo G. Prenatal management and perinatal outcome in giant placental chorioangioma complicated with hydrops fetalis, fetal anemia and maternal mirror syndrome. BMC Pregnancy and Childbirth. 2012;12:72.
9. Masakuzu M, Masahiko N, Murata S, Sumie M, Sugino N. Resolution of mirror syndrome after successful fetoscopic laser photocoagulation of communicating placental vessels in severe twin–twin transfusion syndrome. Prenat Diagn. 2008; 28(12):1167–8.
10. Chang YL, Chao AS, Chang SD, Wang CN. Mirror syndrome after fetoscopic laser therapy for twin-twin transfusion syndrome due to transient donor hydrops that resolved before delivery. A case report. J Reprod Med. 2014;59(1- 2):90–2.
11. Chai H, Fang Q, Huang X, Zhou Y, Luo Y. Prenatal management and outcomes in mirror syndrome associated with twin-twin transfusion syndrome. Prenat Diagn. 2014;34(12):1213–8.
12. Brandão AM, Domingues AP, Fonseca EM, Miranda TM, Moura JP. Mirror syndrome after Fetoscopic laser treatment - a case report. Rev Bras Ginecol Obstet. 2016;38(11):576–9.
13. Nassr AA, Shamshirsaz AA, Belfort MA, Espinoza J. Spontaneous resolution of mirror syndrome following fetal interventions for fetal anemia as a consequence of twin to twin transfusion syndrome. Eur J Obstet Gynecol Reprod Biol. 2017;208:110–1.
14. Sherer DM, Sadovksy E, Menashe M, Mordel N, Rein AJ. Fetal ventricular tachycardia associated with nonimmunologic hydrops fetalis. A case report. J Reprod Med. 1990;35:292–4.
15. Ren S, Bhavsar T, Wurzel JCHAOS. In the mirror: Ballantyne (mirror) syndrome related to congenital high upper airway obstruction syndrome. Fetal Pediatr Pathol. 2012;31(6):360–4.
16. Paternoster DM, Manganelli F, Minucci D, Nanhornguè KN, Memmo A, Bertoldini M, Nicolini U. Ballantyne syndrome: a case report. Fetal Diagn Ther. 2006;21(1):92–5.
17. Heyborne KD, Chism DM. Reversal of Ballantyne síndrome by selective second-trimester fetal termination. A case report. J Reprod Med. 2000;45(4):360–2.
18. Tayler E, DeSimone C. Anesthetic management of maternal mirror syndrome. Int J Obstet Anesth. 2014;23(4):386–9.
19. Society for Maternal-Fetal Medicine. (SMFM), Norton ME, Chauhan SP, Dashe JS. Society for Maternal-Fetal Medicine (SMFM) clinical guideline #7: nonimmune hydrops fetalis. Am J Obstet Gynecol. 2015;212(2):127–39.
20. Li H, Gu WR. Mirror syndrome associated with heart failure in a pregnant woman: a case report. Int J Clin Exp Med. 2015;8(9):16132–6.
21. Detti L, Oz U, Guney I, Ferguson JE, Badaho-Singh RO, Mari G. Collaborative Group for Doppler Assessment of the blood velocity in anemic fetuses. Doppler ultrasound velocimetry for timing the second intrauterine transfusion in fetuses with anemia from red cell alloimmunization. Am J Obstet Gynecol. 2001;185(5):1048–51.
22. Mari G, Deter RL, Carpenter RL, Rahman F, Zimmerman R, Moise KJ Jr, Dorman KF, Ludomirsky A, González R, Gómez R, Oz U, Detti L, Copel JA, Badaho-Singh R, Berry S, Martínez-Poyer J, Blackwell SC. Noninvasive diagnosis by Doppler ultrasonography of fetal anemia due to maternal red-cell alloimmunization. Collaborative Group for Doppler Assessment of the blood velocity in anemic fetuses. N Engl J Med. 2000;342(1):9–14.
23. Wu LL, Wang CH, Li ZQ. Clinical study of 12 cases with obstetric mirror syndrome. Zhonghua Fu Chan Ke Za Zhi. 2012;47(3):175–8.
24. Bixel K, Silasi M, Zelop CM, Lim KH, Zsengeller Z, Stillman IE, Rana S. Placental origins of angiogenic dysfunction in mirror syndrome. Hypertens Pregnancy. 2012;31(2):211–7.
25. Maynard SE, Min JY, Merchan J, Lim KH, Li J, Mondal S, Libermann TA, Morgan JP, Sellke FW, Stillman IE, Epstein FH, Sukhatme VP, Karumanchi SA. Excess placental soluble fms-like tyrosine kinase 1 (sFlt1) may contribute to endothelial dysfunction, hypertension, and proteinuria in preeclampsia. J Clin Invest. 2003;111(5):649–58.
26. Levine RJ, Maynard SE, Qian C, Lim KH, England LJ, Yu KF, Schisterman EF, Thadhani R, Sachs BP, Epstein FH, Sibai BM, Sukhatme VP, Karumanchi SA. Circulating angiogenic factors and the risk of preeclampsia. N Engl J Med. 2004;350(7):672–83.
27. Prefumo F, Pagani G, Fratelli N, Benigni A, Frusca T. Increased concentrations of antiangiogenic factors in mirror syndrome complicating twin-to-twin transfusion syndrome. Prenat Diagn. 2010;30(4):378–9.
28. De Oliveira L, Sass N, Boute T, Moron AF. sFlt-1 and PlGF levels in a patient with mirror syndrome related to cytomegalovirus infection. Eur J Obstet Gynecol Reprod Biol. 2011;158(2):366–7.
29. Stepan H, Faber R. Elevated sFlt1 level and preeclampsia with parvovirus-induced hydrops. N Engl J Med. 2006;354(17):1857–8.
30. Lee JY, Hwang JY. Mirror syndrome associated with fetal leukemia. J Obstet Gynaecol Res. 2015;41(6):971–4.

31. Llurba E, Marsal G, Sánchez O, Domínguez C, Alijotas-Reig J, Carreras E, Cabero L. Angiogenic and antiangiogenic factors before and after resolution of maternal mirror syndrome. Ultrasound Obstet Gynecol. 2012;40(3):367–9.
32. Carbillon L, Oury JF, Guerin JM, Azancot A, Blot P. Clinical biological features of Ballantyne syndrome and the role of placental hydrops. Obstet Gynecol Surv. 1997;52(5):310–4.
33. Espinoza J, Romero R, Nien JK, Kusanovic JP, Richani K, Gomez R, Kim CJ, Mittal P, Gotsh F, Erez O, Chaiworapongsa T, Hassan S. A role of the anti-angiogenic factor sVEGFR-1 in the 'mirror syndrome' (Ballantyne's syndrome). J Matern Fetal Neonatal Med. 2006;19(10):607–13.
34. Giacobbe A, Grasso R, Interdonato ML, Laganà AS, Valentina G, Triolo O, Mancuso A. An unusual form of mirror syndrome: a case report. J Matern Fetal Neonatal Med. 2013;26(3):313–5.
35. Allarakia S, Khayat HA, Karami MM, Aldakhil AM, Kashi AM, Algain AH, Khan MA, Alghifees LS, Alsulami RE. Characteristics and management of mirror syndrome: a systematic review (1956-2016). J Perinat Med. 2017;45(9):1013–21.
36. Eiland S, Cvetanovska E, Bjerre AH, Nyholm H, Sundberg K, Nørgaard LN. Mirror syndrome is a rare complication in pregnancy, characterized by oedema and hydrops fetalis. Ugeskr Laeger. 2017;10:179(15).
37. Iciek R, Brazert M, Klejewski A, Pietryga M, Ballantyne Syndrome BJ. (Mirror syndrome) associated with severe non-immune fetal hydrops. A case report. Ginekol Pol. 2015;86(9):706–11.
38. Xu Z, Huan Y, Zhang Y, Liu Z. Anesthetic management of a parturient with mirror syndrome: a case report. Int J Clin Exp Med. 2015;8(8):14161–5.
39. Okby R, Mazor M, Erez O, Beer-Weizel R, Hershkovitz R. Reversal of mirror syndrome after selective feticide of a hydropic fetus in a dichorionic diamniotic twin pregnancy. J Ultrasound Med. 2015;34(2):351–3.

5

A systematic review of non-antibiotic measures for the prevention of urinary tract infections in pregnancy

Flavia Ghouri, Amelia Hollywood[*] ⓘ and Kath Ryan

Abstract

Background: Urinary tract infections (UTIs) are common in pregnancy and account for the highest proportion of primary care antibiotic prescriptions issued to pregnant women in the UK. It is well known that antibiotic use is associated with increased antimicrobial resistance and therefore measures to minimise antibiotic use for UTI prevention have been studied. The efficacy and safety of these measures in pregnancy have not been addressed and therefore the aim of this study was to systematically review the literature to identify and evaluate potential measures to prevent UTIs in pregnant women.

Methods: Ten databases (EMBASE, AMED, BNI, CINAHL, Medline, PubMed, PsycINFO, Cochrane Trials, Scopus and Science Direct) were systematically searched in July 2017 for studies reporting non-antibiotic measures to prevent UTIs in pregnancy. The terms ("urinary tract infection" or UTI or bacteriuria or cystitis) AND (prevention) AND (pregnan*) were used. The quality of the publications was appraised using the Critical Appraisal Skills Programme (CASP) checklists for cohort study, case-control study and randomised controlled trial. The results were synthesised using a textual narrative approach.

Results: Search results yielded 3276 publications and after reviewing titles and removing duplicates, 57 full text articles were assessed for eligibility and eight were included in the review. Five different approaches (hygiene measures, cranberry juice, immunisation, ascorbic acid and Canephron® N) have been identified, all of which are reported to be safe in pregnancy.

Conclusion: The quality of the evidence varied considerably and only hygiene measures were supported by evidence to be recommended in practice. Future work needs to concentrate on strengthening the evidence base through improved design and reporting of studies with a focus on immunisation, ascorbic acid and Canephron® N.

Keywords: Systematic review, Non-antibiotic measures, Prevention, Urinary tract infection, Antimicrobial resistance, Pregnancy, Behaviour change

Background

Urinary tract infections (UTIs) account for the highest proportion of primary care antibiotic prescriptions issued to pregnant women in the UK [1]. Pregnant women have an increased susceptibility to UTIs because of physiological changes. The growing uterus can result in urinary retention which predisposes the woman to infection. In addition, hormonal fluctuations relax the ureteral muscle and cause accumulation of urine in the bladder which also increases the chance of developing a UTI [2].

Treatment of UTIs is recommended in pregnancy if bacteria are detected in the urine even if there are no accompanying symptoms i.e. in asymptomatic bacteriuria (ASB) [3]. Both ASB and symptomatic UTIs in pregnancy are risk factors for the development of pyelonephritis which can result in severe maternal morbidity [4]. It is estimated that 20–30% of women with bacteriuria in the first trimester go on to develop pyelonephritis in later trimesters [5]. Therefore, although ASB on its own is not treated in the general population, guidelines

---
* Correspondence: a.hollywood@reading.ac.uk
School of Pharmacy, University of Reading, PO Box 226, Whiteknights, Reading RG6 6AP, UK

published by the European Urological Association (EAU) [3] and Scottish Intercollegiate Guidelines Network (SIGN) [6] recommend screening and treating bacteriuria with or without symptoms. The current management strategy according to these guidelines is to use a short course of antibiotics.

Whilst antibiotics are vital in eradication of UTIs, antimicrobial resistance due to their use is a global health threat [7, 8]. Antimicrobial resistance means that bacteria can survive antibiotic treatment and cause serious or life threatening infections. Use of antibiotics is strongly associated with increasing emergence of resistant bacteria and subsequent redundancy of antibiotics i. e. previously effective antibiotics are losing their efficacy [8, 9]. Unlike the general population, the choice of safe antibiotics in pregnancy is limited because of teratogenic potential e.g. quinolones should be avoided in pregnancy because of a risk of joint malformations in the foetus. Therefore antibiotics becoming ineffective due to antimicrobial resistance is a particular concern in pregnancy as it further limits the range of drugs available to treat infections safely [10]. An example of this in practice is the replacement of trimethoprim with nitrofurantoin as the first line antibiotic to treat UTIs [11] because of an increase in resistance due to its widespread use in the UK [12]. Use of antibiotics can also result in carriage of resistant bacteria by individuals for a period of several months to a year after completing a course of antibiotics [13]. The resistant bacteria can transfer to close physical contacts and may colonise and infect subsequent hosts. This is especially of concern in pregnancy as women can pass on resistant bacteria to the neonate during birth, which is when they are most vulnerable to infection. An example of resistance specific to obstetric practice is the increase in ampicillin resistant neonatal infections due to maternal use of ampicillin [14, 15].

As well as contributing to antimicrobial resistance, antibiotic use in pregnancy also carries the risk of being harmful to the foetus. Recently, a study has found a link between antibiotic use and increased risk of spontaneous miscarriages [16]. Another study assessing the effects of nitrofurantoin, trimethoprim-sulfamethoxazole and cephalosporins which are used to treat UTIS, found an increased risk of birth defects such as oral clefts, oesophageal and anorectal abnormalities in the offspring [17]. In addition, research has also found an association with antibiotic use in pregnancy and functional impairment in children later on in life [18].

In light of the risks, it is essential that the use of antibiotics in pregnancy is carefully considered with a balance struck between the risks and benefits of these drugs. The UK's 5 year antimicrobial resistance strategy [19] developed by the Department of Health (DH) and Department for Environment Food and Rural Affairs (Defra) identifies seven key areas where action is needed to tackle antimicrobial resistance. One of these key areas is 'improving infection prevention and control practices' which will lead to a reduction in the use of antibiotics as infection rates will be minimised. Improving infection prevention is also one of the main recommendations of 'The Review on Antimicrobial Resistance' (2016), chaired by economist Jim O'Neill [8]. Non-antibiotic measures to minimise antibiotic use for UTI prevention have been studied but the efficacy and safety of these measures in pregnancy have not been addressed [20]. Therefore, the aim of this systematic review is to identify alternate measures reported in scientific literature which may be used to prevent UTIs in pregnancy. The benefits of non-antibiotic measures to prevent UTIs in pregnancy are two-fold. Firstly, the reduced use of antibiotics will mean that they remain effective for longer, and secondly, medication which is potentially harmful in pregnancy can be avoided.

Methods

Ten databases (EMBASE, AMED, BNI, CINAHL, Medline, PubMed, PycINFO, Cochrane Trials, Scopus and Science Direct) were searched and the final search string was conducted in July 2017. The inclusion criteria according to PICOS (see Table 1) consisted of studies reporting non-antibiotic measures for the prevention of UTIs in pregnant women.

Studies conducted exclusively in non-pregnant groups or in conditions such as diabetes or spinal cord injury were excluded. Search terms were; **P**: (pregnan*), **I**: (prevention or control or management), **O**: ("urinary tract infection" or UTI or bacteriuria or cystitis) as shown in Table 2.

The search terms 'control' or 'management' were initially used but these terms did not yield relevant results therefore this paper focuses on prevention only. The final search strategy is available in Additional file 1.

A manual search of references from included studies was also conducted. The quality of the publications was appraised using the Critical Appraisal Skills Programme (CASP) checklists for cohort study, case-control study and randomised controlled trial [21–23]. The results

Table 1 Inclusion criteria (PICOS)

Population	Pregnant Women
Intervention	Non-antibiotic prevention measures
Comparator	Any e.g. a placebo
Outcome	Incidence of bacteriuria or UTI
Study Design	Any e.g. randomised control trial (RCT) or observational study

Table 2 Search strategy

Database	Search terms	Results
EMBASE	("urinary tract infection" or UTI or bacteriuria or cystitis) AND (prevention or control or management) AND pregnan*	744
AMED	("urinary tract infection" or UTI or bacteriuria or cystitis) AND (prevention or control or management) AND pregnan*	0
BNI	("urinary tract infection" or UTI or bacteriuria or cystitis) AND (prevention or control or management) AND pregnan*	10
CINAHL	("urinary tract infection" or UTI or bacteriuria or cystitis) AND (prevention or control or management) AND pregnan*	66
Medline	("urinary tract infection" or UTI or bacteriuria or cystitis) AND (prevention or control or management) AND pregnan*	397
PubMed	("urinary tract infection" or UTI or bacteriuria or cystitis) AND (prevention or control or management) AND pregnan*	942
PsycINFO	("urinary tract infection" or UTI or bacteriuria or cystitis) AND (prevention or control or management) AND pregnan*	4
Cochrane Trials	("urinary tract infection" or UTI or bacteriuria or cystitis) AND (prevention or control or management) AND pregnan*	102
SCOPUS	(TITLE-ABS-KEY ("urinary tract infection" OR UTI OR bacteriuria OR cystitis) AND TITLE-ABS-KEY (prevention or control or management) AND TITLE-ABS-KEY (pregnan*) AND NOT TITLE-ABS-KEY (catheter OR catheter AND associated) AND NOT TITLE-ABS-KEY (antibacterial* OR antibiotic* OR antimicrobial*) Note: additional terms searched using 'NOT' due to too many results	1008
ScienceDirect	("urinary tract infection" or UTI or bacteriuria or cystitis) AND (prevention or control or management) AND pregnan*	3
Manual search		0
Total		3276

were analysed and discussed using a narrative synthesis approach.

Results

Search results yielded 3276 publications and after reviewing titles and removing duplicates, 56 full text articles and one conference abstract were assessed for eligibility by FG and eight were included in the review as shown in Fig. 1. The results identified five different measures (hygiene behaviour, cranberry juice, immunisation, ascorbic acid and Canephron® N) which can be used for the prevention of UTIs in pregnancy. Quality appraisal of the included publications using the CASP checklists is shown in Tables 3, Table 4 and Table 5.

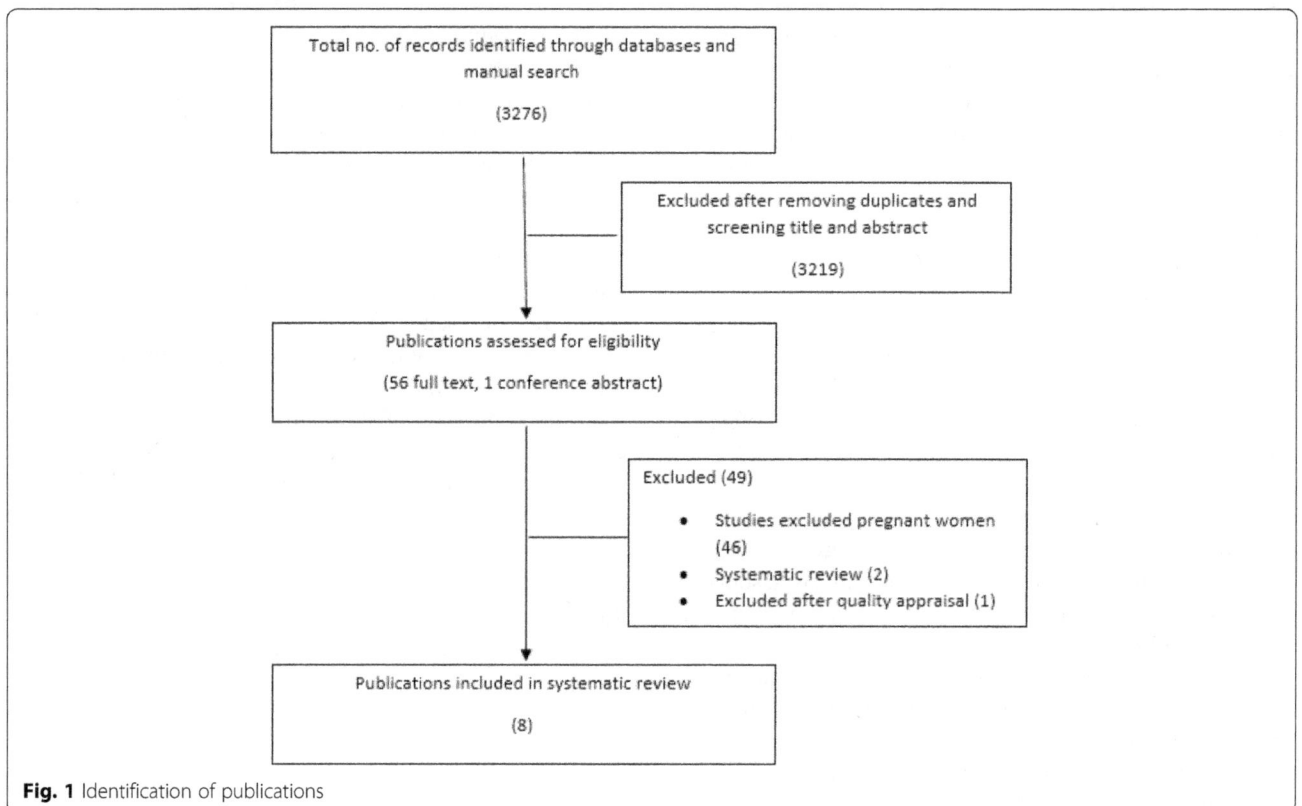

Fig. 1 Identification of publications

Table 3 Quality appraisal using CASP checklist for cohort studies

CASP cohort study checklist			
	Elzayat et al. 2017 [26]	Baertschi et al. 2003 [29]	Ordzhonikidze et al. 2009 [32]
Did the study address a clearly focused issue?	Yes	Yes	Yes
Was the cohort recruited in an acceptable way?	Yes	Yes	Can't tell
Was the exposure accurately measured to minimise bias?	Yes	Yes	Can't tell
Was the outcome accurately measured to minimise bias?	Yes	Yes	Can't tell
(a) Have the authors identified all important confounding factors?	Yes	Yes	Yes
(b) Have they taken account of the confounding factors in the design and/or analysis?	Yes	Yes	Yes
(a) Was the follow up of subjects complete enough?	Not applicable	Yes	Yes
(b) Was the follow up of subjects long enough?	Not applicable	Yes	Yes
How precise are the results?	Can't tell (no CI given)	Can't tell (no CI given)	Can't tell (no CI given)
Do you believe the results?	Yes	Yes	Yes
Can the results be applied to the local population?	Yes	Yes	No (study population not clearly defined)
Do the results of this study fit with other available evidence?	Yes	Yes	Yes
Does the study have implications for practice?	Yes	Yes	Yes

CI Confidence interval. Significance: $p \leq 0.05$

The characteristics of the publications are included in Table 6.

Hygiene behaviour

Three observational studies were identified which investigated the association between sexual and genital hygiene behaviours of pregnant women and the incidence

Table 4 Quality appraisal using CASP checklist for case-control studies

CASP case-control study checklist	
	Amiri et al. 2009 [25]
Did the study address a clearly focused issue?	Yes
Did the authors use an appropriate method to answer their question?	Yes
Were the cases recruited in an acceptable way?	Yes
Were the controls selected in an acceptable way?	Yes
Was the exposure accurately measured to minimise bias?	Yes (but questionnaire completed by midwives)
Have the authors taken account of the potential confounding factors in the design and/or in their analysis?	Yes
Were the results and risk estimate precise?	Yes
Do you believe the results?	Yes
Can the results be applied to the local population?	Yes
Do the results of this study fit with other available evidence?	Yes

of asymptomatic bacteriuria (defined as $> 10^5$ colony forming units/ml of urine) or symptomatic UTIs. One study by Badran et al. [24] was not included in the review due to repetition of results from a previously conducted study.

The study by Amiri et al. [25] was a case-control study which included 100 cases matched to 150 controls i.e. total of 250 pregnant women. The two groups were compared in terms of differences in genital hygiene or sexual activity. The study by Elzayat et al. [26] was an observational cohort study that included 170 pregnant women between the ages of 18–41. Participants in this study were administered a questionnaire about their hygiene behaviours and a urine sample was tested to determine the prevalence of bacteriuria. Both studies show that hygiene behaviours are associated with the incidence of UTIs.

Cranberry juice

There were two studies that assessed the effectiveness of cranberry juice in preventing UTIs during pregnancy. Wing et al. [27] conducted a randomised controlled trial with 188 pregnant women under 16 weeks of pregnancy and compared the efficacy of cranberry juice with a placebo. There was a 57% reduction in bacteriuria and 41% reduction in all UTIs reported in this trial. Essadi et al. [28] conducted a randomised controlled trial that compared cranberry juice with water in 760 pregnant women. They also reported positive results for the effectiveness of cranberry juice and 70.5% of the participants who drank cranberry juice showed a significant

Table 5 Quality appraisal using CASP checklist for randomised controlled trials

CASP randomised control study checklist

	Ochoa-Brust et al. 2007 [31]	Grischke et al. 1987 [30]	Wing et al. 2008 [27]	Essadi et al. 2010 [28]
Did the trial address a clearly focused issue?	Yes	Yes	Yes	Yes
Was the assignment of patients to treatments randomised?	Yes	N (although described as randomised)	Yes	Can't tell
Were all of the patients who entered the trial properly accounted for at its conclusion?	No	No	Yes	Yes
Were patients, health workers and study personnel 'blind' to treatment?	No	No (only patients were blinded)	Yes	No (able to differentiate between juice and water)
Were the groups similar at the start of the trial?	Yes	No (different pregnancy status)	Yes	Yes
Aside from the experimental intervention, were the groups treated equally?	Yes	Yes	Yes	Can't tell
How large was the treatment effect?	Significant ($p = 0.03$)	Significant ($p \leq 0.001$)	Not significant ($p = 0.71$)	Significant ($p < 0.05$)
How precise was the estimate of the treatment effect?	Precise (95% CI used)	Can't tell (no CI limits)	Precise (95% CI used)	Can't tell (no CI limits)
Can the results be applied in your context? (Or to the local population)	Yes	Probable	Yes	Yes
Were all clinically important outcomes considered?	Yes	Yes	Yes	Yes
Are the benefits worth the harms and costs?	Yes	Yes	N (due to stomach disturbances)	No (due to stomach disturbances)

CI Confidence interval. Significance: $p \leq 0.05$

reduction in UTIs compared to 32.16% of women who drank water.

Immunisation

Immunisation as a means of preventing UTIs in pregnancy was assessed by two studies. Baertschi et al. [29] conducted a before-after study using a bacterial extract in 62 women who were 16–28 weeks pregnant. Use of the extract significantly reduced the incidence of UTIs and recurrence rates fell from 52.5% prior to using the extract to 19.4% after women started using the extract. Grischke and Ruttgers [30] investigated the effectiveness of an intramuscular vaccine in an open randomised trial. A total of 400 women were included in the trial and a significant difference was seen in the incidence of UTIs in the trial (28 infections) and control groups (84 infections) suggesting a beneficial effect of the vaccine.

Ascorbic acid

Ochoa-Brust et al. [31] conducted a RCT to evaluate whether daily intake of ascorbic acid (100 mg) prevented UTIs in pregnancy. There was a total of 110 pregnant women, 55 in the trial group and 55 in the control group. The infection percentage was 12.7% in women who were given daily ascorbic acid compared with 29.1% in women who received the comparator.

Canephron® N

Ordzhonikidze et al. [32] conducted a cohort study in 300 pregnant women using Canephron® N which is a

herbal product. Women were divided into two groups, those who had a current UTI and those who suffered with chronic urinary tract problems but did not have a current exacerbation. The results show that the frequency of pyelonephritis was 1.5 times less in the first group and 1.3 times less in the second group due to use of this product.

Discussion

The five different measures (hygiene behaviour, cranberry juice, immunisation, ascorbic acid and Canephron® N) highlighted in the review vary in the evidence supporting their use for the prevention of UTIs in pregnancy.

Hygiene behaviour

The EAU guideline for urological infections states that studies investigating hygiene behaviours have not found any association with the incidence of UTIs [3]. The two observational studies included in this review, however, provide evidence that hygiene behaviours are associated with the incidence of UTIs. Results show that increased sexual activity of greater than two or three times a week was linked to a high frequency of UTIs. However, washing the genital area and voiding the bladder after intercourse had a protective effect. The direction of wiping the genital area after voiding the bladder was also found to be important and women who wiped from back to front had a higher incidence of UTIs according to both studies. Lastly, Amiri et al. [25] also found that drinking

Table 6 Characteristics of included publications

Author, Year, Country	Wing et al., 2008, USA [28]
Design	Pilot randomised control trial comparing cranberry juice with placebo. Participants were divided into three groups and asked to drink 240 ml of either cranberry or placebo juice. A. cranberry juice three times daily B. cranberry juice once and placebo twice daily C. placebo three times daily Note: High withdrawal led to modification of dose frequency to twice daily in the middle of the trial. Randomisation was stratified by site.
Aim	To determine effectiveness of cranberry juice at reducing the frequency of ASB.
Participants	188 pregnant women < 16 weeks gestation
Key findings	Results report a 57% reduction in bacteriuria and 41% reduction in all UTIs. Authors concluded that cranberries provide protection against ASB as well as symptomatic infections.
Limitations	Small sample size as it was a pilot. About 39% participants dropped out due to gastrointestinal issues.
Author, Year, Country	Essadi et al., 2010, Libya [29]
Design	Randomised control trial comparing cranberry juice to placebo (water). Participants were divided into two groups and asked to drink 250 ml of cranberry juice or water. A: cranberry juice four times daily B: water four times daily Note: This publication is from a conference poster and full details were not available.
Aim	To determine the effectiveness of cranberry juice at reducing the frequency of UTIs.
Participants	760 pregnant women
Key findings	Results report that 70.5% of patients who drank cranberry juice showed a significant reduction ($p < 0.05$) in frequency of UTI compared to 32.16% who drank water. Of women who developed symptomatic UTI, 4.12% delivered prematurely. Authors concluded that cranberry juice has a protective effect in UTI prevention.
Limitations	There was no blinding as cranberry juice is distinguishable from water. High withdrawal rate of participants (28%) attributed to gastrointestinal upset. It is not clear whether authors used intention to treat analysis which may distort results in favour of cranberry juice.
Author, Year, Country	Elzayat et al., 2017, Egypt [26]
Design	An observational study to determine prevalence of ASB and the risk factors associated with it in pregnancy. Urine specimens were collected and analysed to determine ASB. A survey was conducted using a pre-tested questionnaire to gather data for the associated risk factors.
Aim	To determine the prevalence of ASB and identify risk factors associated with it in terms of socioeconomic status or personal hygiene.
Participants	170 pregnant women between the ages of 18–41.

Table 6 Characteristics of included publications *(Continued)*

Key findings	The prevalence of ASB was 10% (CI 95% 5.93% to 15.53%) in this sample of pregnant women. There was an association between sexual activity and incidence of ASB and 14% of women with ASB reported sexual activity > twice per week ($p = 0.01$). There was also an association between direction of wiping and 15% of women with ASB reported wiping their genitals from back to front ($p = 0.03$). No other significant association was found. Authors recommended educating women on the significance of personal hygiene to prevent UTI during pregnancy.
Limitations	This is an observational study and data was collected by questionnaire which is subject to accurate participant recall. Confidence intervals were not reported for all the categories.
Author, Year, Country	Amiri et al., 2009, Iran [25]
Design	An observational case-control study. Cases (women with UTI) and controls (no UTI) were matched and compared in terms of difference in genital hygiene or sexual activity. The women were administered a questionnaire by a midwife following which a urine sample was taken for analysis.
Aim	To determine association of genital hygiene and sexual activity with the frequency of UTIs in pregnant women.
Participants	250 pregnant women (100 cases and 150 controls)
Key findings	The authors investigated multiple factors. Of note is the significant association seen with: Sexual activity > thrice a week (OR = 5.62 95% CI: 3.10–10.10) Not voiding the bladder after intercourse (OR = 8.62 95% CI: 6.66–16.66) Washing genital area from back to front (OR - 2.96 95% CI: 1.66–5.28)
Limitations	This was an observational study and data was collected using a questionnaire which is subject to accurate participant recall. Matching of cases and controls is not reported in detail.
Author, Year, Country	Baertschi et al., 2003, Switzerland [33]
Design	A before and after study testing a bacterial extract's (OM-8930) efficacy and safety in preventing the incidence of UTIs during pregnancy.
Aim	To determine the effect of immunisation on the number of UTI recurrences, the number and duration of antibiotic treatment used and establish the safety of the vaccine (in women or new born).
Participants	62 women 16–28 weeks pregnant
Key findings	The extract significantly reduced the recurrence of UTIs from 52.5% to 19.4% ($p = 0.002$). Number of people needing antibiotic treatment reduced from 55.7% to 12.9% ($p = 0.0002$) Duration of antibiotic treatment reduced from a mean of 3.2 to 2 days ($p = 0.0016$) The authors concluded that OM-8930 reduced the number of UTI recurrences but a larger trial was needed to confirm this result.
Limitations	

Table 6 Characteristics of included publications *(Continued)*

	The study compares data from the trial to the 6 month period prior to the study instead of comparison with a control group. There is a risk of bias due to this because women's pregnancy status would likely be different at the two times. Also, The study was a pilot and had a small sample size.
Author, Year, Country	Grischke & Ruttgers, 1987, Germany [35]
Design	An open comparative randomised trial comparing effectiveness of a vaccine preparation, Solco-Urovac®, to standard antibiotic therapy for prevention of UTIs. The participants were divided into two groups
Group 1: 200 participants given Solco-Urovac® (68 were pregnant)
Group 2: 198 participants given nitrofurantoin or another appropriate antibiotic
Aim	To establish the effectiveness of Solco-Urovac® in reducing the frequency of UTIs.
Participants	400 pregnant and non-pregnant women
Key findings	There were 28 infections in the trial group and 84 infections in the control group – this was a significant difference ($p \leq 0.001$).
Average duration of the infection was significantly longer than in the control group.
No adverse effects were observed in the offspring.
Limitations	The study was not conducted exclusively in pregnant women and their proportion in each group is not specified.
Randomisation was not done appropriately as the treating physician may have allocated patients with acute symptoms to the antibiotic group.
Author, Year, Country	Ochoa-Brust et al., 2007, Mexico [36]
Design	A randomised trial to assess the prophylactic role of ascorbic acid in preventing UTIs during pregnancy. Participants were divided into two groups.
Group A: treatment with ferrous sulphate 200 mg, folic acid 5 mg and ascorbic acid 100 mg daily for 3 months
Group B: treatment with ferrous sulphate 200 mg and folic acid 5 mg daily for 3 months.
Aim	To determine the role of ascorbic acid in reducing the frequency of UTIs.
Participants	110 pregnant women, 55 in each group.
Key findings	The infection percentage was 12.7% in Group A and 29.1% in Group B ($p = 0.03$, OR 0.35, CI 95% 0.13–0.91).
The relative risk reduction was 56.5% and absolute risk reduction was 16.3%,
The number needed to treat was 6.
The authors concluded that pregnant women in areas with high rates of antimicrobial resistance should take ascorbic acid during gestation to prevent UTIs.
Limitations	Patients were excluded from study if they were not compliant, had serious side effects or if they had a UTI recurrence which may have distorted the results in favour of ascorbic acid.
Author, Year, Country	Ordzhonikidze et al., 2009, Russia [38]
Design	

Table 6 Characteristics of included publications *(Continued)*

	Two groups of pregnant women were treated with Canephron® N.
Group 1: 160 women with an exacerbation of pyelonephritis were given Canephron® N in combination with standard therapy (antibiotics).
Group 2: 140 women with chronic history of urinary tract disease who were given Canphron® N alone for prevention.
The dose of Canephron® N was two tablets three times a day.
Aim	To assess the role of Canephron® N in the management of urinary tract diseases in pregnant women.
Participants	300 pregnant women
Key findings	Group 2 seemed to show more favourable results compared to Group 1. The percentage frequency of exacerbation of pyelonephritis was 10–6.25 in Group 1 and 3–2.1 in Group 2.
The authors state in the results section that there was a 1.5-fold decrease in the frequency of infectious complications in the first group and a 1.3-fold decrease in the second group when comparing results to previous years.
Limitations	The methods, results and analysis have not been reported clearly.
Canephron® N was not compared to a placebo or to antibiotics.

inadequate amounts of fluid and delaying voiding of the bladder also increased the likelihood of UTIs.

The overall evidence from these studies supports the adoption of protective hygiene behaviours, which may seem intuitive, as good hygiene is well known to protect against all types of infections. Women should be provided with specific recommendations because they may get upset if they get advised to 'just keep clean' as evidenced by a qualitative study conducted by Flower et al. [33].

Cranberry juice
Both RCTs [27, 28] assessing the efficacy of cranberry juice to prevent UTIs in pregnancy concluded that it has the potential to be effective. However, both studies had limitations which shed doubt on the effectiveness of this intervention. The study by Wing et al. [27] was underpowered with a small sample size (188 women). Essadi et al. [28] had a larger cohort (760 women) but compared cranberry juice to water which led to inadequate blinding giving rise to a risk of performance bias i.e. systemic differences between the groups. In addition, it is not clear if they used intention-to-treat analysis which may have distorted the results in favour of cranberry juice. A point to note with regards to Essadi et al. [28] is that it was published as a conference poster and full details were not available but it was included because the abstract reported data in sufficient detail to determine the significance of the results.

A limitation of cranberry juice seen in both studies was the high volume of juice that needed to be ingested (240 ml [27] and 250 ml [28]). Both trials had a high withdrawal rate mostly due to gastrointestinal disturbances which can limit its use on grounds of acceptability to women. These results point to a need to investigate a standardised content of cranberries in alternative formulations such as tablets and capsules which may help with improving adherence and tolerability of this intervention.

Both these trials view cranberry juice as potentially effective at preventing UTIs in pregnancy but a Cochrane review by Jepson et al. [34] included both these studies in a meta-analysis and found cranberries to be ineffective in preventing UTIs in pregnancy. Thus, although there has been interest in using cranberries for UTI prevention, the evidence does not support its efficacy. It can still be used as a self-care option, if preferred by women, because of its known safety in pregnancy [35, 36].

Immunisation

Both studies investigating the role of immunisation to safely reduce the recurrence of UTIs in pregnancy found favourable results, however both had significant limitations. Baertschi et al. [29] used a bacterial extract consisting of different strains of *Escherichia coli (E.coli),* which is the most common uropathogen [37], however this vaccine would not be effective against any other type of bacteria. Furthermore it was an open pilot study and did not have a control group to compare the effectiveness of the vaccine. Therefore, the results need to be confirmed by a RCT, as noted by the authors themselves. Grischke and Ruttgers [30] conducted their study in a sample where 68 pregnant women were given the intramuscular vaccine but the number of pregnant women in the control group was not specified. Blinding was not clearly described either and so there is an unclear risk of bias. Therefore, immunisation as an approach to prevent UTIs in pregnancy needs further exploration to assess its feasibility in practice.

Ascorbic acid

Ochoa-Brust et al. [31] concluded that daily ascorbic acid was beneficial especially in areas with a high incidence of UTIs and antimicrobial resistance. This is a promising result but requires additional trials to strengthen the evidence before it can be recommended. It is not clear whether the authors used intention-to-treat analysis because they did not specify the withdrawal rate and there was a selection bias as they excluded women who were non-adherent or had 'serious side effects' from the medication. Excluding these results from analysis may distort the results in favour of ascorbic acid. It is worth noting, however, that no harmful effects were observed in the offspring of women who ingested ascorbic acid daily.

Canephron® N

Canephron® N is a phytotherapeutic medicine with antibacterial properties and contains three herbs namely rosemary, lovage and centaury [38]. It is manufactured by a German company, Bionorica®, which focuses on researching and developing plant-based medicines. Ordzhonikidze et al. [32] conducted a study with pregnant women using this product, to optimise management of urinary tract diseases including ASB and pyelonephritis, which concluded that it could be recommended for prevention of urinary tract complications in pregnancy. The reporting of results was not comprehensive so it was not possible to determine how the study was conducted in sufficient detail (see Table 3). A review by Naber et al. [38] assessing the efficacy of Canephron® N suggests that there might be some benefit from its use in pregnant women because it included evidence from additional studies which have not been discussed here as they were conducted in pregnant women with co-morbidities and so did not meet the inclusion criteria of this review. It is worth noting that the safety of Canephron® N in pregnancy has been established [39, 40] but in order to make an evidence based recommendation, its efficacy needs to be confirmed by a randomised controlled trial.

Strengths and limitations

A total of ten databases were searched and search terms were mutually agreed by the authors and an independent colleague to ensure a comprehensive process. The studies included in the review were assessed independently by the authors using CASP checklists. Any disagreement was resolved by meeting and discussing the relevant studies. A limitation of this review is that only English language publications were included therefore there might be options which have not been identified. The results of this review have been discussed using a narrative synthesis approach due to the heterogeneous design of the included studies and the differing nature of the interventions identified.

Conclusion

All the approaches identified in this review are reported to be safe and effective. However apart from hygiene behaviours, the evidence behind these approaches is not robust enough to be recommended in practice. Future work needs to focus on strengthening the evidence base through improved design and reporting of clinical trials, in particular for the use of immunisation, ascorbic acid and Canephron® N. It is important that evidence based non-antibiotic measures to prevent UTIs in pregnancy are discovered to combat the danger that antimicrobial resistance poses to the health of this vulnerable patient group as well as the wider population.

Abbreviations
ASB: Asymptomatic bacteriuria; Defra: Department for Environment Food and Rural Affairs; DH: Department of Health; EAU: European Association of Urology; RCT: Randomised control trial; SIGN: Scottish Intercollegiate Guidelines Network; UTI: Urinary tract infection

Acknowledgements
We would like to thank all the authors of the original studies, and Tim Chapman, the pharmacy division's liaison librarian at the University of Reading, for his support with conducting the literature search.

Funding
This work was supported by the University of Reading as a PhD studentship for F.G.

Authors' contributions
FG conducted the literature search and screened the papers for eligibility for this review. All authors (FG, AH and KR) screened the publications for quality assessment. The final manuscript was prepared by FG, then edited and approved by AH and KR.

Competing interests
The authors declare that they have no competing interests.

References
1. Petersen I, Gilbert R, Evans S, Ridolfi A, Nazareth I. Oral antibiotic prescribing during pregnancy in primary care: UK population-based study. J Antimicrob Chemother. 2010;65:2238–46. https://doi.org/10.1093/jac/dkq307.
2. Johnson EK, Wolf JS, Edward K, editors. Urinary tract infections in pregnancy: Medscape; 2016. https://emedicine.medscape.com/article/452604-overview. Accessed 20 Nov 2017
3. Bonkat G, Pickard R, Bartoletti R, Bruyère F, Geerlings S, Wagenlehner F, Wult B. Guideline: urological infections. Eur Assoc Urol. 2017; http://uroweb.org/guideline/urological-infections. Accessed 20 Nov 2017
4. Cunningham FG, Morris GB, Mickal A. Acute pyelonephritis of pregnancy: a clinical review. Obstet Gynecol. 1973;42(1):112–7.
5. Nicolle LE. Asymptomatic bacteriuria when to screen and when to treat. Infect Dis Clin N Am. 2003;17:367–94. https://doi.org/10.1016/S0891-5520(03)00008-4.
6. Scottish Intercollegiate Guidelines Network (SIGN). Management of suspected bacterial urinary tract infection in adults. 2012. (SIGN publication no. 88). http://www.sign.ac.uk/assets/sign88.pdf. Accessed 20 Nov 2017.
7. Fair RJ, Tor Y. Antibiotics and bacterial resistance in the 21st century. Perspect Med Chem. 2014;6:25–64. https://doi.org/10.4137/PMC.S14459.
8. O'Neill J. Tackling drug-resistant infections globally: final report and recommendations. Rev Antimicrob Resist. 2016; https://amr-review.org. Accessed 20 Nov 2017
9. Hillier S, Roberts Z, Dunstan F, Butler C, Howard A, Palmer S. Prior antibiotics and risk of antibiotic-resistant community-acquired urinary tract infection: a case–control study. J Antimicrob Chemother. 2007;60(1):92–9. https://doi.org/10.1093/jac/dkm141.
10. Rizvi M, Khan F, Shukla I, Malik A, Shaheen. Rising prevalence of antimicrobial resistance in urinary tract infections during pregnancy: necessity for exploring newer treatment options. J Lab Physicians. 2011;3(2):98–103. https://doi.org/10.4103/0974-2727.86842.
11. Public Health England. Managing common infections: guidance for primary care. 2017. https://www.gov.uk/government/publications/managing-common-infections-guidance-for-primary-care. Accessed 10 Apr 2018.
12. Winstanley TG, Limb DI, Eggington R, Hancock F. A 10 year survey of the antimicrobial susceptibility of urinary tract isolates in the UK: the Microbe Base project. J Antimicrob Chemother. 1997;40:591–4. https://doi.org/10.1093/jac/dkg028.
13. Costelloe C, Metcalfe C, Lovering A, Mant D, Hay AD. Effect of antibiotic prescribing in primary care on antimicrobial resistance in individual patients: systematic review and meta-analysis. BMJ. 2010;340:c2096. https://doi.org/10.1136/bmj.c2096.
14. Towers CV, Carr MH, Padilla G, Asrat T, Beach L. Potential consequences of widespread antepartal use of ampicillin. Am J Obstet Gynecol. 1998;179(4):879–83. https://doi.org/10.1203/00006450-199804001-00946.
15. Mercer BM, Carr TL, Beazley DD, Crouse DT, Sibai BM. Antibiotic use in pregnancy and drug-resistant infant sepsis. Am J Obstet Gynecol. 1999;181(4):816–21. https://doi.org/10.1016/S0002-9378(99)70307-8.
16. Muanda FT, Sheehy O, Bérard A. Use of antibiotics during pregnancy and risk of spontaneous abortion. Can Med Assoc J. 2017;189(17):E625–33. https://doi.org/10.1503/cmaj.161020.
17. Ailes EC, Gilboa SM, Gill SK, Broussard CS, Crider KS, Berry RJ, et al. Association between antibiotic use among pregnant women with urinary tract infections in the first trimester and birth defects, National Birth Defects Prevention Study 1997 to 2011. Birth Defects Res A Clin Mol Teratol. 2016;106(11):940–9. https://doi.org/10.1002/bdra.23570.
18. Kenyon S, Pike K, Jones D, Brocklehurst P, Marlow N, Salt A, et al. Childhood outcomes after prescription of antibiotics to pregnant women with spontaneous preterm labour: 7-year follow-up of the ORACLE II trial. Lancet. 2008;372(9646):1319–27. https://doi.org/10.1016/S0140-.
19. Department of Health, Department for Environment Food and Rural Affairs. UK five year antimicrobial resistance strategy 2013 to 2018. 2013. https://www.gov.uk/government/uploads/system/uploads/attachment_data/file/244058/20130902_UK_5_year_AMR_strategy.pdf. Accessed 18 Dec 2017.
20. Beerepoot MAJ, Geerlings SE, Van Haarst EP, Mensing Van Charante N, Ter Riet G. Nonantibiotic prophylaxis for recurrent urinary tract infections: a systematic review and meta-analysis of randomized controlled trials. J Urol. 2013;190:1981–9.
21. Critical Appraisal Skills Programme. CASP Cohort Study Checklist. 2017. http://www.casp-uk.net/casp-tools-checklists. Accessed 15 Dec 2017.
22. Critical Appraisal Skills Programme. CASP Case Control Study Checklist. http://www.casp-uk.net/casp-tools-checklists. Accessed 15 Dec 2017.
23. Critical Appraisal Skills Programme. CASP Randomised Controlled Trial Checklist. 2017. http://www.casp-uk.net/casp-tools-checklists. Accessed 15 Dec 2017.
24. Badran YA, El-Kashef TA, Abdelaziz AS, Ali MM. Impact of genital hygiene and sexual activity on urinary tract infection during pregnancy. Urol Ann. 2015;7(4):478–81. https://doi.org/10.4103/0974-7796.157971.
25. Amiri FN, Rooshan MH, Ahmady MH, Soliamani MJ. Hygiene practices and sexual activity associated with urinary tract infection in pregnant women. East Mediterr Health J. 2009;15(1):104–10.
26. Elzayat MA, Barnett-vanes A, Farag M, Dabour E, Cheng F. Prevalence of undiagnosed asymptomatic bacteriuria and associated risk factors during pregnancy : a cross-sectional study at two tertiary centres in Cairo, Egypt. BMJ Open. 2017:1–7. https://doi.org/10.1136/bmjopen-2016-013198.
27. Wing DA, Rumney PJ, Preslicka CW, Chung JH. Daily cranberry juice for the prevention of asymptomatic bacteriuria in pregnancy: a randomized, controlled pilot study. J Urol. 2008;180(4):1367–72. https://doi.org/10.1016/j.juro.2008.06.016.
28. Essadi F, Elmehashi MO. Efficacy of cranberry juice for the prevention of urinary tract infections in pregnancy [abstract]. Poster Session. J Matern Fetal Neonatal Med. 2010;23(sup1):378. https://doi.org/10.3109/14767051003802503.
29. Baertschi R, Balmer JA, Eduah SB, Liechti A, Lurie D, Schams H. Bacterial extract for the prevention of recurrent urinary tract infections in pregnant women: a pilot study. Int J. Immunotherapy. 2003;19(1):25–31.
30. Grischke EM, Rüttgers H. Treatment of bacterial infections of the female urinary tract by immunization of the patients. Urol Int. 1987;42:338–41. https://doi.org/10.1159/000281988.
31. Ochoa-Brust GJ, Fernández AR, Villanueva-Ruiz GJ, Velasco R, Trujillo-Hernández B, Vásquez C. Daily intake of 100 mg ascorbic acid as urinary tract infection prophylactic agent during pregnancy. Acta Obstet Gynecol Scand Suppl. 2007;86(7):783–7. https://doi.org/10.1080/00016340701273189.
32. Ordzhonikidze N, Yemelyanova A, Petrova S. Prevention and treatment of complications in pregnant women and peurperas with urinary tract diseases. Akush Ginekol (Mosk). 2009;6:41–5.

33. Flower A, Bishop FL, Lewith G. How women manage recurrent urinary tract infections: an analysis of postings on a popular web forum. BMC Fam Pract. 2014;15:162. https://doi.org/10.1186/1471-2296-15-162.

34. Jepson RG, Williams G, Craig JC. Cranberries for preventing urinary tract infections. Cochrane Database Syst Rev. 2012;10 https://doi.org/10.1002/14651858.CD001321.pub5.

35. Dugoua J-J, Seely D, Perri D, Mills E, Koren G. Safety and efficacy of cranberry (vaccinium macrocarpon) during pregnancy and lactation. Can J Clin Pharmacol. 2008;15(1):e80–6.

36. Heitmann K, Nordeng H, Holst L. Pregnancy outcome after use of cranberry in pregnancy – the Norwegian mother and child cohort study. BMC Complement Altern Med. 2013;13:345. https://doi.org/10.1186/1472-6882-13-345.

37. Bartoletti R, Cai T, Wagenlehner FM, Naber K, Bjerklund Johansen TE. Treatment of urinary tract infections and antibiotic stewardship. Eur Urol. 2016;15(4):81–7. https://doi.org/10.1016/j.eursup.2016.04.003.

38. Naber KG. Efficacy and safety of the phytotherapeutic drug Canephron® N in prevention and treatment of urogenital and gestational disease: review of clinical experience in Eastern Europe and Central Asia. Res Rep Urol. 2013;5:39–46. https://doi.org/10.2147/RRU.S39288.

39. Medved VI, Islamova EV. To the question on safety of the preparation Canephron N in the obstetric practice. Med Asp Women's Health. 2009;4:32–5.

40. Medved V. Safety of Canephron® N for the treatment of urinary tract infections in the first trimester of pregnancy. Clin Phytoscience. 2015;1:11. https://doi.org/10.1186/s40816-015-0012-1.

6

Adverse obstetric and neonatal outcomes complicated by psychosis among pregnant women in the United States

Qiu-Yue Zhong[1]*[iD], Bizu Gelaye[1], Gregory L. Fricchione[2], Paul Avillach[1,3,4], Elizabeth W. Karlson[5] and Michelle A. Williams[1]

Abstract

Background: Adverse obstetric and neonatal outcomes among women with psychosis, particularly affective psychosis, has rarely been studied at the population level. We aimed to assess the risk of adverse obstetric and neonatal outcomes among women with psychosis (schizophrenia, affective psychosis, and other psychoses).

Methods: From the 2007 – 2012 National (Nationwide) Inpatient Sample, 23,507,597 delivery hospitalizations were identified. From the same hospitalization, *International Classification of Diseases* diagnosis codes were used to identify maternal psychosis and outcomes. Adjusted odds ratios (aOR) and 95% confidence intervals (CI) were obtained using logistic regression.

Results: The prevalence of psychosis at delivery was 698.76 per 100,000 hospitalizations. After adjusting for sociodemographic characteristics, smoking, alcohol/substance abuse, and pregnancy-related hypertension, women with psychosis were at a heightened risk for cesarean delivery (aOR = 1.26; 95% CI: 1.23 - 1.29), induced labor (aOR = 1.05; 95% CI: 1.02 - 1.09), antepartum hemorrhage (aOR = 1.22; 95% CI: 1.14 - 1.31), placental abruption (aOR = 1.22; 95% CI: 1.13 - 1.32), postpartum hemorrhage (aOR = 1.18; 95% CI: 1.10 - 1.27), premature delivery (aOR = 1.40; 95% CI: 1.36 - 1.46), stillbirth (aOR = 1.37; 95% CI: 1.23 - 1.53), premature rupture of membranes (aOR = 1.22; 95% CI: 1.15 - 1.29), fetal abnormalities (aOR = 1.49; 95% CI: 1.38 - 1.61), poor fetal growth (aOR = 1.26; 95% CI: 1.19 - 1.34), and fetal distress (aOR = 1.14; 95% CI: 1.10 - 1.18). Maternal death during hospitalizations (aOR = 1.00; 95% CI: 0.30 - 3.31) and excessive fetal growth (aOR = 1.06; 95% CI: 0.98 - 1.14) were not statistically significantly associated with psychosis.

Conclusions: Pregnant women with psychosis have elevated risk of several adverse obstetric and neonatal outcomes. Efforts to identify and manage pregnancies complicated by psychosis may contribute to improved outcomes.

Keywords: Psychosis, Schizophrenia, Affective psychosis, National (Nationwide) Inpatient Sample (NIS), Obstetric and neonatal outcomes

Background

Psychosis is often used as a generic description of severe mental illness characterized by delusions, hallucinations, disorganized thinking and speech, and other associated cognitive and behavioral impairments interfering with the ability to meet the ordinary demands of life [1, 2]. Psychosis is comorbid with a number of mental disorders including, but not limited to, schizophrenia, schizoaffective disorders, bipolar disorders, and major depressive disorders [3]. Immediately before and after birth, due to changes in medications, sleep deprivation, alterations in hormone levels [4, 5], and the physiological demands of pregnancy which may temporarily unmask subclinical disease [6], women may be at higher risk for psychosis, resulting in substantial distress and long-term implications for the wellbeing of mothers, families, and society [5]. Knowledge concerning the adverse obstetric and neonatal outcomes among pregnant women with psychosis is necessary to provide recommendations for optimal prenatal care [7].

* Correspondence: qyzhong@mail.harvard.edu
[1]Department of Epidemiology, Harvard T.H. Chan School of Public Health, Boston, 677 Huntington Avenue, Room Kresge 502A, Boston, MA 02115, USA

However, adverse obstetric and neonatal outcomes among pregnant women with psychosis have rarely been studied at the population level, and the evidence base in many areas remains poor [5, 8]. Early studies on this topic are based on small sample sizes with limited statistical power [7]. In addition, few studies have adequately accounted for confounders [5, 7]. Furthermore, the majority of previous studies have focused on schizophrenia, and little is known about the effects of affective psychosis (bipolar or major depressive disorders with psychotic symptoms) in pregnancy [9–12].

Therefore, in this study, we sought to assess the risk of adverse obstetric and neonatal outcomes for US pregnant women with prevalent psychosis, including schizophrenia, affective psychosis, and other psychoses, at the time of delivery in a population-based sample of delivery-related hospitalizations.

Methods
Database
The National (Nationwide) Inpatient Sample (NIS) of the Healthcare Cost and Utilization Project (HCUP), sponsored by the Agency for Healthcare Research and Quality (AHRQ), is the largest publicly available all-payer (including Medicare, Medicaid, other non-federal payers, and patients who are uninsured) inpatient health care database in the United States [13]. Approximately 1000 hospitals that represent all types of health facilities are selected for the NIS. Five hospital characteristics — geographic region, ownership, location, teaching status, and bed size — are used for stratification to create a representative sample of US hospitalizations [13]. Before 2012, a 20% stratified random sample of hospitals within the stratum defined by the aforementioned five hospital characteristics was drawn by the AHRQ [13–15]. All discharges from sampled hospitals were included. Beginning with 2012, the NIS was redesigned to improve national estimates, and within each stratum, a 20% stratified random sample of discharges from all HCUP-participating hospitals was drawn by the AHRQ [13–15]. Discharge-level sampling weights based on the sampling scheme are available to obtain national estimates [16, 17]. Approximately seven million unweighted discharges and 35 million weighted discharges nationally are recorded each year [16, 17]. The NIS does not allow linkage of patient's records. This study is exempt from review by institutional review boards given the data are publicly available and do not contain personal identifiers. Our study conforms to the Data Use Agreement for the Nationwide Databases from the HCUP.

Study population
Our analysis included pregnant women aged 12-55 years who were hospitalized for delivery during 2007-2012. The identification of delivery hospitalizations was predicated upon delivery-related *International Classification of Diseases*, Ninth Revision, Clinical Modification (ICD-9-CM) diagnosis and procedure codes and Diagnosis-Related Group (DRG) codes [18–20] (Additional file 1: Table S1).

Variable specification
Exposure
We used the ICD-9-CM diagnosis codes from the same delivery hospitalization to identify psychosis diagnoses. We included women with any (primary or secondary) discharge diagnosis codes for psychosis in the following groups: schizophrenia (ICD-9-CM: 295.**); affective psychosis (ICD-9-CM: 296.**), and other psychoses (ICD-9-CM: 297.** - 298.**) [21–24]. In a validation study, the set of diagnosis codes has demonstrated adequate sensitivity (91%) and positive predictive value (91%) [22].

Obstetric and neonatal outcomes
Maternal death during hospitalization was directly extracted from the NIS. Obstetric and neonatal outcomes included in this analysis were: cesarean delivery, length of stay (in days and in percentages with stays longer than 6 days) among cesarean and vaginal deliveries, induction of labor (applies to induction by cervical dilation and medical induction of labor), antepartum hemorrhage, placental abruption, postpartum hemorrhage, spontaneous delivery earlier than 37-week gestation, stillbirth, premature rupture of membranes, excessive fetal growth (applies to large-for-dates), poor fetal growth (applies to placental insufficiency and small-for-gestational-age), fetal distress (applies to fetal metabolic acidemia), and fetal abnormality affecting management of mother (including conditions in the fetus that affecting management of mother: central nervous system malformation, chromosomal abnormality, hereditary disease in family possibly affecting fetus, suspected damage to fetus from viral disease/other disease in the mother, suspected damage to fetus from drugs or radiation, decreased fetal movements, and other known or suspected fetal abnormality, not elsewhere classified) (Additional file 1: Table S2).

Covariates
Covariates including age, race/ethnicity, median household income quartiles for patient zip code, expected primary payer indicating patients' insurance payer, length of stay, and total charges were coded in the NIS. Median household income quartiles for patient zip code provided a quartile classification estimating income of residents based on the year of data collection. Other characteristics (ever smoking, alcohol/substance abuse, non-psychotic depression, pregnancy-related hypertension, pregestational diabetes, preexisting hypertension, infection, and previous cesarean delivery) were abstracted from the same delivery

hospitalization record (primary or secondary discharge diagnostic codes) using ICD-9-CM diagnosis codes listed in Additional file 1: Table S2. Hospital characteristics were obtained directly from the NIS, including hospital region, location, bed size, and teaching status.

Statistical analyses

Using weights provided by the datasets, we reported national estimates representing discharges from all US community hospitals. We compared the distributions of sociodemographic, baseline, and hospital characteristics between women with and without psychosis by performing Wald Chi-square and t-tests. We calculated odds ratios (ORs) and 95% confidence intervals (CIs) using logistic regression. We fit three consecutive models: 1) unadjusted model; 2) minimally adjusted model with adjustment for *a priori* confounders including maternal age (continuous), race/ethnicity, median household income quartiles, hospital region (Northeast, Midwest, South, West), hospital location (rural or urban), and year as potential confounders; and 3) fully adjusted model with additional adjustment for *a priori* confounders including ever smoking, alcohol/substance abuse, and pregnancy-induced hypertension. We reported adjusted odds ratios (aORs) derived from multivariable logistic regression models. All variables had <5% missing data except for race/ethnicity. We created missing indicator variables to address missing data for race/ethnicity and median household income quartiles. Total hospitalization charges were adjusted for inflation to reflect 2012 US dollars [25].

All analyses were conducted using SAS 9.4 (SAS Institute, Cary, NC, USA) and SAS-callable SUDAAN software (version 11.0.1, RTI International, Research Triangle, NC, USA). Statistical significance was set at two-sided $P<0.05$. Some computations were run on the Odyssey cluster supported by the Faculty of Arts & Sciences Division of Science, Research Computing Group at Harvard University.

Sensitivity Analyses

To evaluate the individual effect of schizophrenia (ICD-9-CM: 295.**) and affective psychosis (ICD-9-CM: 296.**) on adverse obstetric and neonatal outcomes, we conducted two sensitivity analyses among women with schizophrenia or women with affective psychosis. The reference group in these two analyses was identical to our main analysis, i.e., women without any psychosis. Considering the small sample size, we did not perform this analysis among women with other psychoses.

Given that multiple birth was associated with a myriad of complications such as preterm labor and fetal growth restriction [26], we first restricted our analyses to singletons. In a separate analysis, we also adjusted for multiple

birth in multivariable regression analyses of all pregnancies including multifetal pregnancies.

Results

A total of 23,507,597 delivery hospitalizations were included in this study after applying the NIS sampling weights. Among the delivery hospitalizations, 164,261 hospitalizations had a diagnosis of psychosis. The prevalence of psychosis at delivery was 698.76 per 100,000 hospitalizations. More than 90% (92.98%) of our study population were women with a diagnosis of affective psychosis (schizophrenia: $n = 14,125$; affective psychosis: $n = 152,727$; and other psychoses: $n = 2,387$). The prevalence of schizophrenia, affective psychosis, and other psychoses at delivery were 60.09, 649.69, and 10.15 per 100,000 hospitalizations, respectively.

The sociodemographic characteristics are presented in Table 1. Women with psychosis (mean age = 26.58 years) were younger as compared to women without psychosis (mean age = 27.68 years). More than 40% of women with psychosis (42.02%) were in the age group of 12-24 years while only 33.27% of women without psychosis were in this age group. Regarding race/ethnicity, as compared to women without psychosis, women with psychosis were more likely to be White (56.22% vs. 43.99%) or Black (14.97% vs. 11.81%) and less likely to be Hispanic (8.66% vs. 19.48%) or Asian or Pacific Islander (1.07% vs. 4.46%). Approximately one-third of women with psychosis (33.88%) were in the lowest quartile of median household income. The majority of women with psychosis had their medical care paid by Medicare or Medicaid (69.22%). Nearly half of women (50.13%) without psychosis had private insurance as the expected primary payer while this proportion was 25.77% among women with psychosis. Approximately 28.87% of women with psychosis had diagnosis codes for smoking while only 5.05% of women without psychosis had these diagnosis codes. Compared with women without psychosis, women with psychosis were more likely to have alcohol/substance abuse (15.67% vs. 1.46%), non-psychotic depression (16.06% vs. 1.87%), pregnancy-related hypertension (10.55% vs. 7.97%), pre-gestational diabetes (2.81% vs. 0.93%), preexisting hypertension (4.66% vs. 1.99%), infection (7.42% vs. 4.69%), and previous cesarean delivery (17.70% vs. 16.30%).

Table 2 shows the hospital characteristics. As compared with women without psychosis, women with psychosis at delivery were more likely to reside in the Northeast (19.98% vs. 16.13%) and Midwest region (25.55% vs. 21.33%). No statistically significant difference was found for hospital location (rural or urban) or bed size (small, medium, or large) between women with and without psychosis. A larger proportion of

Table 1 Baseline characteristics of women with and without psychosis at delivery hospitalizations (N=23,507,597)

Characteristics	Women					P-value
	With psychosis (N = 164,261)		Without psychosis (N = 23,343,336)			
	n	%	n	%		
Age, mean (SD), year	26.58 (1.89)		27.68 (1.73)			<0.0001
Age categories, year						
12-18	11,707	7.13	1,230,611	5.27		<0.0001
19-24	57,315	34.89	6,536,844	28.00		
25-29	43,579	26.53	6,569,694	28.14		
30-34	31,906	19.42	5,595,824	23.97		
35-39	15,497	9.43	2,758,774	11.82		
40-55	4,258	2.59	651,590	2.79		
Race						
White	92,341	56.22	10,269,706	43.99		<0.0001
Black	24,594	14.97	2,756,003	11.81		
Hispanic	14,217	8.66	4,546,581	19.48		
Asian or Pacific Islander	1,761	1.07	1,041,542	4.46		
Native American	1,118	0.68	176,796	0.76		
Other	4,115	2.51	979,229	4.19		
Missing	26,115	15.90	3,573,478	15.31		
Median household income quartiles						
Quartile 1 (poorest)	55,646	33.88	6,240,956	26.74		<0.0001
Quartile 2	43,865	26.70	5,759,232	24.67		
Quartile 3	36,093	21.97	5,646,070	24.19		
Quartile 4 (wealthiest)	24,844	15.13	5,248,090	22.48		
Missing	3,812	2.32	448,988	1.92		
Expected primary payer						
Medicare	13,505	8.22	150,033	0.64		<0.0001
Medicaid	100,197	61.00	10,016,502	42.91		
Private insurance	42,336	25.77	11,702,370	50.13		
Self-pay	3,387	2.06	735,501	3.15		
No charge	169	0.10	49,118	0.21		
Other	4,446	2.71	647,978	2.78		
Missing	221	0.13	41,835	0.18		
Smoking	47,428	28.87	1,179,021	5.05		<0.0001
Alcohol/substance abuse	25,747	15.67	340,451	1.46		<0.0001
Non-psychotic depression	26,388	16.06	436,901	1.87		<0.0001
Pregnancy-related hypertension	17325	10.55	1859437	7.97		<0.0001
Pregestational diabetes	4,609	2.81	217,748	0.93		<0.0001
Preexisting hypertension	7,659	4.66	463,822	1.99		<0.0001
Infection	12,187	7.42	1,095,394	4.69		<0.0001
Previous cesarean delivery	29,066	17.70	3,804,658	16.30		<0.0001

Individual cell counts may not add up to the global cell counts because of rounding and the differences arising from variance computations when using the discharge weights.
Percentages may not add up to 100% due to rounding or missing data.
Abbreviations: *SD* standard deviation

Table 2 Characteristics of hospitals where women with and without psychosis-hospitalizations being hospitalized (N=23,507,597)

Characteristics	Women					P-value
	With psychosis (N = 164,261)		Without psychosis (N = 23,343,336)			
	n	%	n	%		
Region						
Northeast	32,827	19.98	3,764,982	16.13		<0.0001
Midwest	41,969	25.55	4,979,708	21.33		
South	57,647	35.10	8,867,733	37.99		
West	31,818	19.37	5,730,913	24.55		
Location						
Rural	18,856	11.48	2,592,608	11.11		0.64
Urban	143,867	87.58	20,544,262	88.01		
Bed size						
Small	18,298	11.14	2,503,608	10.73		0.09
Medium	38,645	23.53	6,067,531	25.99		
Large	105,781	64.40	14,565,733	62.40		
Teaching hospital	90,599	55.16	10,902,764	46.71		<0.0001

Individual cell counts may not add up to the global cell counts because of rounding and the differences arising from variance computations when using the discharge weights
Percentages may not add up to 100% due to rounding or missing data

women with psychosis were admitted in a teaching hospital (55.16% vs. 46.71%).

The frequencies and ORs for obstetric and neonatal outcomes among women with and without psychosis is presented in Table 3. In the fully adjusted models, women with psychosis were more likely to undergo a cesarean delivery (aOR = 1.26; 95% CI: 1.23 - 1.29) and induction of labor (aOR = 1.05; 95% CI: 1.02 - 1.09). The mean length of stay was longer for women with psychosis than for women without psychosis (vaginal delivery: 3.08 days vs. 2.53 days; cesarean delivery: 4.29 days vs. 3.55 days). Women with psychosis were more likely than women without psychosis to experience antepartum hemorrhage (aOR = 1.22; 95% CI: 1.14 - 1.31), placental abruption (aOR = 1.22; 95% CI: 1.13 - 1.32), postpartum hemorrhage (aOR = 1.18; 95% CI: 1.10 - 1.27), premature delivery (aOR = 1.40; 95% CI: 1.36 - 1.46), stillbirth (aOR = 1.37; 95% CI: 1.23 - 1.53), premature rupture of membranes (aOR = 1.22; 95% CI: 1.15 - 1.29), and fetal abnormalities (aOR = 1.49; 95% CI: 1.38 - 1.61). No significant association was observed between psychosis and maternal death during hospitalizations (aOR = 1.00; 95% CI: 0.30 - 3.31). Offspring of women with psychosis were more likely to experience poor fetal growth (aOR = 1.26; 95% CI: 1.19 - 1.34) and fetal distress (aOR = 1.14; 95% CI: 1.10 - 1.18) as compared to offspring of women without psychosis. However, there was no evidence of a statistically significant association between psychosis and excessive fetal growth (aOR = 1.06; 95% CI: 0.98 - 1.14). Apart from the aforementioned obstetric and neonatal outcomes, women with psychosis had larger total charges ($16,332 vs. $13,710 US dollars).

In our sensitivity analysis for women with schizophrenia (Table 4), the unadjusted odds ratios were higher for the majority of the outcomes as compared to the analysis that included all women. After further adjustment for smoking, alcohol/substance abuse, and pregnancy-related hypertension, schizophrenia was statistically significantly associated with cesarean delivery (aOR = 1.16; 95% CI: 1.08 - 1.25), hospital stays of more than 6 days (cesarean delivery: aOR = 3.01; 95% CI: 1.11 - 8.13; vaginal delivery: aOR = 2.33; 95% CI: 1.86 - 2.93), placental abruption (aOR = 1.34; 95% CI: 1.06 - 1.68), premature delivery (aOR = 1.42; 95% CI: 1.26 - 1.59), premature rupture of membranes (aOR = 1.31; 95% CI: 1.12 - 1.53), fetal distress (aOR = 1.13; 95% CI: 1.03 - 1.25), and fetal abnormalities (aOR = 1.34; 95% CI: 1.08 - 1.66). However, no statistically significant associations were found of schizophrenia with death during hospitalizations (aOR = 2.23; 95% CI: 0.30 - 16.80), induction of labor (aOR = 0.98; 95% CI: 0.89 - 1.09), antepartum hemorrhage (aOR = 1.18; 95% CI: 0.96 - 1.46), postpartum hemorrhage (aOR = 1.09; 95% CI: 0.89 - 1.34), stillbirth (aOR = 1.28; 95% CI: 0.94 - 1.74), excessive fetal growth (aOR = 0.87; 95% CI: 0.66 - 1.14), or poor fetal growth (aOR = 1.10; 95% CI: 0.91 - 1.33).

Compared with the main analysis (Table 3), the results were largely similar in the sensitivity analysis for women with affective psychosis (Table 5) except for excessive fetal growth. Infants born to women with affective psychosis were at increased risk for excessive fetal

Table 3 Obstetric and neonatal outcomes among women with and without psychosis during delivery hospitalizations (N=23,507,597)

Obstetric and neonatal outcomes	Women				OR (95% CI)		
	With psychosis (N = 164,261)		Without psychosis (N = 23,343,336)		Unadjusted	Adjusted[a]	Adjusted[b]
	n	%	n	%			
Death during hospitalizations	19	0.01	1,468	0.01	1.82 (0.67, 4.92)	1.31 (0.42, 4.14)	1.00 (0.30, 3.31)
Cesarean delivery	62,496	38.05	7,718,434	33.06	1.24 (1.21, 1.28)	1.31 (1.28, 1.35)	1.26 (1.23, 1.29)
Length of stay, mean (SE), day							
Vaginal birth	3.08 (0.10)		2.53 (0.01)		NA	NA	NA
Cesarean delivery	4.29 (0.07)		3.55 (0.02)		NA	NA	NA
Length of stay >6 day							
Vaginal birth	243	0.15	9,526	0.04	4.12 (3.02, 5.63)	4.03 (2.94, 5.52)	3.19 (2.56, 4.50)
Cesarean delivery	4,800	2.92	245,416	1.05	2.53 (2.35, 2.74)	2.46 (2.27, 2.66)	2.14 (1.98, 2.32)
Induction of labor	32,876	20.01	4,247,666	18.20	1.13 (1.09, 1.17)	1.05 (1.02, 1.09)	1.05 (1.02, 1.09)
Antepartum hemorrhage	4,138	2.52	356,821	1.53	1.67 (1.55, 1.79)	1.67 (1.55, 1.79)	1.22 (1.14, 1.31)
Placental abruption	3,127	1.90	246,768	1.06	1.82 (1.68, 1.97)	1.75 (1.62, 1.90)	1.22 (1.13, 1.32)
Postpartum hemorrhage	5,460	3.32	654,043	2.80	1.19 (1.11, 1.28)	1.22 (1.13, 1.31)	1.18 (1.10, 1.27)
Spontaneous delivery <37-week gestation	20,059	12.21	1,692,651	7.25	1.78 (1.71, 1.85)	1.75 (1.68, 1.82)	1.40 (1.36, 1.46)
Stillbirth	1,811	1.10	153,045	0.66	1.69 (1.52, 1.88)	1.64 (1.47, 1.82)	1.37 (1.23, 1.53)
Premature rupture of membranes	8,318	5.06	904,679	3.88	1.32 (1.25, 1.40)	1.31 (1.24, 1.39)	1.22 (1.15, 1.29)
Excessive fetal growth	3,807	2.32	609,142	2.61	0.89 (0.82, 0.96)	0.91 (0.85, 0.98)	1.06 (0.98, 1.14)
Poor fetal growth	6,668	4.06	507,269	2.17	1.91 (1.79, 2.03)	1.75 (1.65, 1.86)	1.26 (1.19, 1.34)
Fetal distress	28,282	17.22	3,342,430	14.32	1.25 (1.20, 1.29)	1.21 (1.17, 1.26)	1.14 (1.10, 1.18)
Fetal abnormalities	4,380	2.67	337,978	1.45	1.87 (1.73, 2.01)	1.83 (1.70, 1.97)	1.49 (1.38, 1.61)

Abbreviations: *SE* standard error, *OR* odds ratio, *CI* confidence interval
[a]Adjusted for maternal age (continuous), race, median household income quartiles, hospital location, hospital region, and year
[b]Further adjusted for ever smoking, alcohol/substance abuse, and pregnancy-related hypertension

growth (aOR = 1.08; 95% CI: 1.00 - 1.16). The proportion of multiple birth among women with and without psychosis was 1.87% and 1.83%, respectively. Our two methods (restricting to singletons or controlling for multiple birth) in an attempt to explore the effect of multiple birth did not materially alter the reported effect estimates (Additional file 1: Table S3, Table S4).

Discussion

Using a nationally representative inpatient health care database, we observed that psychosis was associated with adverse outcomes including cesarean delivery, longer length of hospital stays, induction of labor, antepartum hemorrhage, placental abruption, postpartum hemorrhage, preterm delivery, and premature rupture of membranes. Infants born to mothers with psychosis were at higher risk of stillbirth, poor fetal growth, fetal distress, and fetal abnormalities. Similar results were seen among women with affective psychosis. Newborns of women with affective psychosis were also at greater risk for excessive fetal growth. After adjusting for potential confounders including smoking, alcohol/substance abuse, and pregnancy-related hypertension, schizophrenia

was statistically significantly associated with cesarean delivery, hospital stays of more than 6 days, placental abruption, premature delivery, premature rupture of membranes, fetal distress, and fetal abnormalities. Schizophrenia, however, was not associated with increased risk of induction of labor and postpartum hemorrhage.

Schizophrenia presents a higher risk for several adverse obstetric and neonatal outcomes, although the evidence is inconclusive. A meta-analysis [27] of 14 early case-control studies found that offspring of mothers with schizophrenia had elevated risk of low birthweight, stillbirth, and fetal or neonatal deaths although the effect size was small (mean correlation = 0.115). Similarly, Bennedsen's review [7] suggested that childbearing women with schizophrenia had an increased risk of low birthweight and intrauterine growth retardation. A more recent meta-analysis indicated an almost twofold higher risk of stillbirth or fetal death among offspring of women with schizophrenia [10]. Several population-based studies have produced more clear-cut evidence. In Denmark, Bennedsen et al. [28, 29] found a significantly increased risk for preterm birth (relative risk [RR] = 1.46; 95% CI: 1.19 - 1.79), low birth

Table 4 Obstetric and neonatal outcomes among women with and without schizophrenia during delivery hospitalizations (*N*=23,357,461)

Obstetric and neonatal outcomes	Women				OR (95% CI)		
	With schizophrenia (*N* = 14,125)		Without psychosis (*N* = 23,343,336)		Unadjusted	Adjusted[a]	Adjusted[b]
	n	%	n	%			
Death during hospitalizations	≤10 [c]	0.04	1,468	0.01	5.15 (0.73, 36.61)	3.21 (0.45, 23.11)	2.23 (0.30, 16.80)
Cesarean delivery	5,544	39.25	7,718,434	33.06	1.31 (1.22, 1.41)	1.22 (1.13, 1.31)	1.16 (1.08, 1.25)
Length of stay, mean (SE), day							
Vaginal birth	3.55 (0.48)		2.53 (0.01)		NA	NA	NA
Cesarean delivery	4.66 (0.19)		3.55 (0.02)		NA	NA	NA
Length of stay >6 day							
Vaginal birth	25	0.18	9,526	0.04	4.73 (1.93, 11.59)	3.86 (1.58, 9.41)	3.01 (1.11, 8.13)
Cesarean delivery	547	3.87	245,416	1.05	3.34 (2.70, 4.12)	2.71 (2.19, 3.36)	2.33 (1.86, 2.93)
Induction of labor	2,444	17.30	4,247,666	18.20	0.93 (0.85, 1.03)	0.97 (0.88, 1.07)	0.98 (0.89, 1.09)
Antepartum hemorrhage	422	2.99	356,821	1.53	1.98 (1.61, 2.44)	1.74 (1.41, 2.15)	1.18 (0.96, 1.46)
Placental abruption	355	2.51	246,768	1.06	2.43 (1.93, 3.04)	2.08 (1.66, 2.62)	1.34 (1.06, 1.68)
Postpartum hemorrhage	446	3.16	654,043	2.80	1.14 (0.93, 1.39)	1.13 (0.93, 1.39)	1.09 (0.89, 1.34)
Spontaneous delivery <37-week gestation	2,022	14.32	1,692,651	7.25	2.14 (1.92, 2.39)	1.85 (1.65, 2.06)	1.42 (1.26, 1.59)
Stillbirth	192	1.36	153,045	0.66	2.09 (1.54, 2.83)	1.62 (1.19, 2.19)	1.28 (0.94, 1.74)
Premature rupture of membranes	803	5.68	904,679	3.88	1.50 (1.28, 1.76)	1.44 (1.24, 1.69)	1.31 (1.12, 1.53)
Excessive fetal growth	237	1.68	609,142	2.61	0.64 (0.49, 0.84)	0.72 (0.55, 0.95)	0.87 (0.66, 1.14)
Poor fetal growth	560	3.96	507,269	2.17	1.86 (1.54, 2.24)	1.61 (1.33, 1.94)	1.10 (0.91, 1.33)
Fetal distress	2,590	18.34	3,342,430	14.32	1.34 (1.22, 1.49)	1.22 (1.11, 1.35)	1.13 (1.03, 1.25)
Fetal abnormalities	373	2.64	337,978	1.45	1.85 (1.50, 2.28)	1.75 (1.41, 2.16)	1.34 (1.08, 1.66)

Abbreviations: *SE* standard error, *OR* odds ratio, *CI* confidence interval
[a]Adjusted for maternal age (continuous), race, median household income quartiles, hospital location, hospital region, and year
[b]Further adjusted for ever smoking, alcohol/substance abuse, and pregnancy-related hypertension
[c]HCUP privacy protection requirements do not allow the reporting of data where there are less than or equal to 10 individual records in a given cell

weight (RR = 1.57; 95% CI: 1.36 - 1.82), and small-for-gestational age (RR = 1.34, 95% CI: 1.17 - 1.53) among women with schizophrenia. Children of women with schizophrenia had a marginally, statistically significant increase in the risk of congenital malformations. No significant increased risk of stillbirth or neonatal death was reported. However, the authors did not account for socioeconomic status, smoking, substance abuse, and psychotropic medication use in their analysis. Nilsson et al. [30] observed significantly increased risk of preterm delivery (aOR = 1.4; 95% CI: 1.2 - 1.7) and low birthweight (aOR = 1.3; 95% CI: 1.1 - 1.6), and the risk was particularly high in women admitted to hospital for schizophrenia during pregnancy. Controlling for smoking and other maternal factors (single motherhood, maternal age, parity, education, country of birth, and pregnancy-induced hypertensive diseases) reduced the risk estimates markedly. Jablensky et al. [12] found that Australian women with schizophrenia were significantly more likely to have placenta abruption (aOR = 3.17; 95% CI: 1.55 - 6.49) and to give birth to infants in the lowest weight/

growth decile (aOR = 1.38; 95% CI: 1.00 - 1.90) after adjusting for maternal age, marital status, parity, aboriginality, and infant sex. No significant association was found for stillbirth, neonatal death, or fetal abnormalities although adjusted models were not present. Lin et al using a population-based dataset [31] in Taiwan found that women with schizophrenia had increased risk of delivery babies with low birthweight and small-for-gestational-age, irrespective of antipsychotics use during pregnancy after adjusting for maternal and paternal socioeconomic status, parity, hypertension, diabetes, and infant sex. Within a universal healthcare system in Canada, Vigod et al. [11] reported that infants born to women with schizophrenia were at higher risk of preterm birth (aOR = 1.75; 95% CI: 1.46 - 2.08), small-for-gestational-age (aOR = 1.49; 95% CI: 1.19 - 1.86), large-for-gestational-age (aOR = 1.53; 95% CI: 1.17 - 1.99), placental abruption (aOR = 1.98, 95% CI: 1.33 - 2.96), induction of labor (aOR = 1.35, 95% CI: 1.20 - 1.52), and cesarean delivery (aOR = 1.45, 95% CI: 1.29 - 1.62) with adjustment for maternal age, income quintile,

Table 5 Obstetric and neonatal outcomes among women with and without affective-psychosis during delivery hospitalizations (*N*=23,507,597)

Obstetric and neonatal outcomes	Women				OR (95% CI)		
	With affective-psychosis (N = 152,727)		Without psychosis (N = 23,343,336)		Unadjusted	Adjusted[a]	Adjusted[b]
	n	%	n	%			
Death during hospitalizations	≤10 [c]	0.01	1,468	0.01	1.96 (0.72, 5.29)	1.49 (0.47, 4.66)	1.13 (0.34, 3.74)
Cesarean delivery	58,057	38.01	7,718,434	33.06	1.24 (1.21, 1.28)	1.33 (1.29, 1.36)	1.27 (1.24, 1.30)
Length of stay, mean (SE), day							
Vaginal birth	3.09 (0.10)		2.53 (0.01)		NA	NA	NA
Cesarean delivery	4.28 (0.07)		3.55 (0.02)		NA	NA	NA
Length of stay >6 day							
Vaginal birth	219	0.14	9,526	0.04	4.00 (2.87, 5.58)	3.98 (2.84, 5.56)	3.10 (2.15, 4.47)
Cesarean delivery	4,329	2.83	245,416	1.05	2.45 (2.26, 2.66)	2.41 (2.22, 2.62)	2.11 (1.94, 2.29)
Induction of labor	31,099	20.36	4,247,666	18.20	1.14 (1.10, 1.18)	1.06 (1.02, 1.10)	1.05 (1.02, 1.09)
Antepartum hemorrhage	3,807	2.49	356,821	1.53	1.65 (1.53, 1.77)	1.67 (1.55, 1.79)	1.22 (1.14, 1.31)
Placental abruption	2,835	1.86	246,768	1.06	1.76 (1.69, 1.84)	1.72 (1.58, 1.87)	1.20 (1.11, 1.31)
Postpartum hemorrhage	5,039	3.30	654,043	2.80	1.18 (1.10, 1.27)	1.21 (1.12, 1.30)	1.17 (1.09, 1.26)
Spontaneous delivery <37-week gestation	18,506	12.12	1,692,651	7.25	1.78 (1.71, 1.85)	1.75 (1.68, 1.82)	1.41 (1.36, 1.46)
Stillbirth	1,627	1.07	153,045	0.66	1.63 (1.46, 1.82)	1.61 (1.44, 1.80)	1.35 (1.20, 1.51)
Premature rupture of membranes	7,701	5.04	904,679	3.88	1.32 (1.24, 1.40)	1.31 (1.23, 1.39)	1.22 (1.14, 1.29)
Excessive fetal growth	3,628	2.38	609,142	2.61	0.91 (0.84, 0.98)	0.93 (0.86, 1.01)	1.08 (1.00, 1.16)
Poor fetal growth	6,229	4.08	507,269	2.17	1.92 (1.80, 2.04)	1.76 (1.66, 1.87)	1.27 (1.19, 1.35)
Fetal distress	26,240	17.18	3,342,430	14.32	1.24 (1.19, 1.29)	1.21 (1.17, 1.26)	1.14 (1.10, 1.18)
Fetal abnormalities	4,067	2.66	337,978	1.45	1.86 (1.72, 2.02)	1.83 (1.69, 1.98)	1.49 (1.38, 1.61)

Abbreviations: *SE* standard error, *OR* odds ratio, *CI* confidence interval
[a]Adjusted for maternal age (continuous), race, median household income quartiles, hospital location, hospital region, and year
[b]Further adjusted for ever smoking, alcohol/substance abuse, and pregnancy-related hypertension
[c]HCUP privacy protection requirements do not allow the reporting of data where there are less than or equal to 10 individual records in a given cell

parity, infant sex, and pre-existing diabetes and hypertension. The findings from our study confirmed that women with schizophrenia are at higher risk of preterm delivery as indicated by previous studies. However, with a considerably large sample size, we found no evidence of statistically significant associations of schizophrenia with poor fetal growth or stillbirth after adjustment for confounders including maternal smoking status.

Little is known about the effects of affective psychosis on pregnancy outcomes [9]. Using a national population cohort in Sweden, MacCabe et al. found that infants born to mothers with affective psychosis had an increased risk of low birth weight (OR = 2.22; 95% CI: 1.31 - 3.76), small-for-gestational-age (OR = 2.36; 95% CI: 1.34 - 4.16), and preterm birth (OR = 2.67; 95% CI: 1.71 - 4.17). The increased risk could not be accounted for by maternal sociodemographic characteristics, parity, smoking, and pregnancy-related hypertension. Jablensky et al. [12]

investigated maternal affective psychosis (bipolar disorder and unipolar depression) as separate exposure categories. After adjustment for confounders, women with bipolar disorder were at higher risk for antepartum hemorrhage (aOR = 1.60; 95% CI: 1.11 - 2.32) while women with unipolar depression had increased risk of fetal distress (aOR = 1.27; 95% CI: 1.03 - 1.56). No significant association (unadjusted) was found for stillbirth, neonatal death, or fetal abnormalities among women with bipolar disorder or unipolar depression. In the current study, significantly increased risk was found for all outcomes except for death during hospitalizations. MacCabe et al. have demonstrated that the risk for adverse outcomes was greatest in mothers receiving hospital treatment for affective psychosis during pregnancy compared to women with a lifetime history of affective psychosis or women who were admitted for affective psychosis any time before birth [9]. The fact that diagnosis codes for psychosis and obstetric and neonatal outcomes were extracted from the same delivery hospitalizations might explain these statistically robust associations. A modest statistically significant increased risk for excessive fetal growth (aOR = 1.08; 95% CI: 1.00 - 1.16) was found in our study for women with affective psychosis. Neither of these two studies [9, 12] assessed the association of affective psychosis with excessive fetal growth. However, a recent study suggests that there might be an association between schizophrenia and excessive fetal growth [11]. A higher risk of large-for-gestational-age has been found in mothers with schizophrenia [11], which might be due to *in utero* exposure to atypical antipsychotics [32] and the predisposition of women with schizophrenia to metabolic syndrome and metabolic abnormalities such as preconception diabetes or gestational diabetes [11, 33–36].This finding concerning excessive fetal growth among offspring of women with affective psychosis deserves to be investigated in future research, and possible mechanisms should be explored. Further, there may be merits to studying whether maternal psychosis is associated with increased long-term risk of metabolic syndrome in offspring.

An elevated risk for fetal abnormalities was observed for women with psychosis, schizophrenia, and affective psychosis in our analyses. The increased risk of fetal abnormalities among offspring of women with schizophrenia has been speculated to be related to the use of antipsychotics medications during pregnancy [28]. However, several reviews [37, 38] have not implicated any specific antipsychotic medication as teratogen [5]. The absence of information pertaining to maternal use of medication in the NIS prohibited our evaluation of the independent and joint associations of psychosis and medication use/withdrawal on obstetric and neonatal outcomes.

A combination of socioeconomic, behavioral, genetic factors and comorbid medical conditions, and environmental factors may explain the higher risk of adverse obstetric and neonatal outcomes among women with psychosis [8, 10]. Women with psychosis tend to live in poor socioeconomic conditions, lack social support, and have unwanted pregnancies [7, 11, 28]. They are known to have worse health behaviors, such as smoking, substance abuse, poor diet, and lack of exercise [7, 8]. In addition, psychosis has been shown to impair a patient's ability to seek appropriate medical care, recognize physical symptoms or warning signs, and be compliant with treatment [8]. Women with psychotic disorders are less likely to seek prenatal care [39] and may avoid psychiatric care during pregnancy [8, 39]. Investigators have also speculated that women with psychosis are at increased genetic risk for developing adverse obstetric and neonatal outcomes considering its high heritability and possible neurodevelopmental origins *in utero* [7, 11, 40, 41]. Furthermore, patients with psychosis, specifically those exposed to antipsychotics, have significantly higher rates of metabolic complications such as hypertension and diabetes

[8, 39]. These metabolic complications could also be present in pregnancy, manifesting in higher rates of pregnancy related hypertensive disorders and gestational diabetes [8, 11, 34]. Infection and inflammation also have a critical role in psychosis [42], which has been shown to be associated with various adverse obstetric and neonatal outcomes [43–45]. Although the causal mechanisms are not well-established, some posit that environmental factors, such as seasonality which relates to sun-derived vitamin D, might be another potential explanation for the observed associations. The main source of vitamin D is sunlight-induced synthesis in the skin [46]. Therefore, vitamin D shows a natural fluctuation throughout the year (i.e., seasonality), with maternal vitamin D insufficiency more likely to occur during winter due to the reduced winter photoperiod in regions with less winter sunlight [47–52]. Vitamin D deficiency has been linked with psychosis [48, 50, 53–56]. In addition, vitamin D regulates placental development and function, and can influence critical components of early brain development, suggesting that maternal vitamin D deficiency may be associated with adverse outcomes of pregnancy including miscarriage, preeclampsia, and preterm birth [57, 58].

In our analysis, women with psychosis were in poorer socioeconomic conditions and had a higher prevalence of smoking, alcohol/substance abuse, pregnancy-related hypertension, preexisting hypertension, pregestational diabetes, and infection. We have shown that poor socioeconomic conditions, worse health behaviors, and comorbid medical conditions were very likely to be responsible for the increased risk of adverse pregnancy outcomes among women with schizophrenia and, to a lesser degree, among women with affective psychosis [12]. However, the increased risk for adverse obstetric and neonatal outcomes was not fully explained by these factors, especially for women with affective psychosis. Future studies are needed to consider other genetic and environmental factors. Special attention should be paid to women with affective psychosis, an understudied population with increased risk of many adverse obstetric and neonatal outcomes that were not accounted for by socioeconomic and behavioral factors.

The major strengths of our study included the considerably large sample size and adjustment for important covariates including smoking, alcohol abuse, substance abuse, and pregnancy-related hypertension. The large sample size not only represented the general US pregnant population at delivery but also provided ample statistical power. We also presented separate results for affective psychosis. However, several limitations are noteworthy. The cross-sectional design limited our ability to establish causal relation and temporality between psychosis and adverse obstetric and neonatal outcomes. Although adverse pregnancy outcomes, such as perinatal death, congenital malformations, preterm birth, might be triggering factors of psychosis [24], these adverse outcomes were not likely to cause incident psychosis in our dataset considering that new-onset psychosis in pregnancy was exceptionally rare [59] and the mean length of delivery hospital stay in this study population was three days. In addition, we had no information on the time of disease onset and disease severity during pregnancy. Previous studies have suggested that the time of disease onset and case ascertainment in relation to childbirth is critical [12, 30]. Women admitted to hospital for schizophrenia during pregnancy were at particularly high risk for adverse obstetric and neonatal outcomes as compared to those who developed schizophrenia before pregnancy [12, 30]. We were not able to replicate this finding, which could be important to understand the cause of reproductive pathology in women with psychosis [12]. Also, some important reproductive characteristics were not included in the NIS dataset, including parity and gestational age. Furthermore, we used the ICD-9-CM codes to identify psychosis, obstetric and neonatal outcomes, and covariates. These diagnosis codes, which were coded for administrative and billing purposes, may not capture the quality of data desired for research purpose. For example, lifetime smoking status was defined by a set of diagnosis codes that applied to tobacco use disorder and personal history of tobacco use, which was very likely to be underreported. A lack of exact data on smoking could lead to residual confounding. Besides, the ICD-9-CM codes used to identify psychosis included psychosis in remission (1.39%), which may result in an underestimation of the associations between psychosis and adverse outcomes.

Conclusion

In conclusion, we observed that women with psychosis had elevated risk of adverse obstetric and neonatal outcomes. Therefore, it is important to raise awareness among clinicians of the increased risk of adverse obstetric and neonatal outcomes among these women. Coordinated antepartum care involving obstetric and psychiatric services providers may optimally manage maternal psychotic symptoms and contribute to improved obstetric and neonatal outcomes among this high-risk group of patients [8]. Special attention should be paid to women with affective psychosis. Women with affective psychosis have increased risk of several adverse obstetric and neonatal outcomes that are not accounted for by socioeconomic and behavioral factors. Future research on other genetic and environmental factors is warranted to elucidate the mechanisms underlying these associations. Behavioral health and medical interventions that target modifiable risk factors, such as smoking, hypertension, and diabetes, may be indicated for pregnant women with schizophrenia [11].

Additional file

Additional file 1: Table S1. International Classification of Diseases, Ninth Revision, Clinical Modification (ICD-9-CM) diagnosis and procedure codes, Diagnosis-Related Group (DRG) codes used to determine delivery-related hospitalizations. **Table S2.** International Classification of Diseases, Ninth Revision, Clinical Modification (ICD-9-CM) diagnosis and procedure codes used to determine selected baseline characteristics and obstetric and neonatal outcomes. **Table S3.** Obstetric and neonatal outcomes among women with and without psychosis during delivery hospitalizations (N=23,507,597). **Table S4.** Obstetric and neonatal outcomes among women with and without psychosis during singleton delivery hospitalizations (N = 23,076,251).

Abbreviations

AHRQ: Agency for Healthcare Research and Quality; aOR: Adjusted odds ratios; CI: 95% confidence intervals; DRG: Diagnosis-Related Group; HCUP: Healthcare Cost and Utilization Project; ICD-9-CM: *International Classification of Diseases*, Ninth Revision, Clinical Modification; NIS: National (Nationwide) Inpatient Sample; OR: Odds ratios

Acknowledgements

We thank the Research Computing Group at the Faculty of Art and Sciences of Harvard University, for continuous support with computational resources.

Funding

This research was supported by awards from the National Institutes of Health (the National Institute on Minority Health and Health Disparities: T37-MD001449; and the National Center for Research Resources (NCRR), the National Center for Advancing Translational Sciences (NCATS): 8UL1TR 000170-09). The NIH had no further role in study design; in the collection, analysis and interpretation of data; in the writing of the manuscript; and in the decision to submit the paper for publication.

Authors' contributions

QYZ, BG, and MAW contributed to the study concept, design, data retrieval, data analysis, data interpretation and presentation, manuscript construction and presentation. QYZ, BG, GLF, PA, EWK, and MAW contributed to the study design, data interpretation and presentation, and manuscript construct and presentation. All authors approved the final manuscript.

Competing interests

The authors declare that they have no competing interests.

Author details

[1]Department of Epidemiology, Harvard T.H. Chan School of Public Health, Boston, 677 Huntington Avenue, Room Kresge 502A, Boston, MA 02115, USA. [2]Division of Psychiatry and Medicine, Pierce Division of Global Psychiatry, Massachusetts General Hospital, Boston, Massachusetts, USA. [3]Department of Biomedical Informatics, Harvard Medical School, Boston, Massachusetts, USA. [4]Children's Hospital Informatics Program, Boston Children's Hospital, Boston, Massachusetts, USA. [5]Division of Rheumatology, Allergy and Immunology, Brigham and Women's Hospital, Boston, Massachusetts, USA.

References

1. Gaebel W, Zielasek J. Focus on psychosis. Dialogues Clin. Neurosci. 2015;17: 9–18.
2. Fergusson DM, Poulton R, Smith PF, Boden JM. Cannabis and psychosis. BMJ. 2006;332:172–5.

3.   Psychosis Endophenotypes International Consortium, Wellcome Trust Case-Control Consortium 2, Bramon E, Pirinen M, Strange A, Lin K, et al. A genome-wide association analysis of a broad psychosis phenotype identifies three loci for further investigation. Biol. Psychiatry. 2014;75:386–97.

4.   DeVylder J, Koyanagi A. Pregnant and peripartum women are not at increased risk for psychotic experiences at the population level: Evidence from 46 countries. Schizophr. Res. 2016;174:202–3.

5.   Jones I, Chandra PS, Dazzan P, Howard LM. Bipolar disorder, affective psychosis, and schizophrenia in pregnancy and the post-partum period. Lancet. 2014;384:1789–99.

6.   Williams D. Pregnancy: a stress test for life. Curr. Opin. Obstet. Gynecol. 2003;15:465–71.

7.   Bennedsen BE. Adverse pregnancy outcome in schizophrenic women: occurrence and risk factors. Schizophr. Res. 1998;33:1–26.

8.   Gold KJ, Marcus SM. Effect of maternal mental illness on pregnancy outcomes. Expert Rev. Obstet. Gynecol. Taylor & Francis. 2008;3:391–401.

9.   MacCabe JH, Martinsson L, Lichtenstein P, Nilsson E, Cnattingius S, Murray RM, et al. Adverse pregnancy outcomes in mothers with affective psychosis. Bipolar Disord. 2007;9:305–9.

10. Webb R, Abel K, Pickles A, Appleby L. Mortality in offspring of parents with psychotic disorders: a critical review and meta-analysis. Am. J. Psychiatry. 2005;162:1045–56.

11. Vigod SN, Kurdyak PA, Dennis CL. Maternal and newborn outcomes among women with schizophrenia: a retrospective population-based cohort study. BJOG. 2014;121:566–74.

12. Jablensky AV, Morgan V, Zubrick SR, Bower C, Yellachich L-A. Pregnancy, delivery, and neonatal complications in a population cohort of women with schizophrenia and major affective disorders. Am. J. Psychiatry. 2005;162:79–91.

13. Introduction to the HCUP national inpatient sample (NIS) [Internet]. Healthcare Cost and Utilization Project (HCUP). 2015 [cited 2016 Feb 1]. Available from: https://www.hcup-us.ahrq.gov/db/nation/nis/nisarchive.jsp. Accessed 1 Feb 2016.

14. Healthcare Cost and Utilization Project (HCUP) KID Notes [Internet]. [cited 2017 Jun 9]. Available from: https://www.hcup-us.ahrq.gov/db/vars/zipinc_qrtl/kidnote.jsp

15. Nationwide Inpatient Sample redesign report [Internet]. Healthcare Cost and Utilization Project (HCUP). 2015 [cited 2016 Feb 1]. Available from: https://www.hcup-us.ahrq.gov/db/nation/nis/reports/NISRedesignFinalReport040914.pdf

16. NIS Trend Weights [Internet]. Healthcare Cost and Utilization Project (HCUP). 2015 [cited 2016 Feb 1]. Available from: https://www.hcup-us.ahrq.gov/db/nation/nis/trendwghts.jsp

17. HCUP Methods Series Calculating National Inpatient Sample (NIS) Variances for Data Years 2012 and Later [Internet]. Healthcare Cost and Utilization Project (HCUP). 2015 [cited 2016 Feb 1]. Available from: https://www.hcup-us.ahrq.gov/reports/methods/2015_09.jsp

18. Bryant A, Mhyre JM, Leffert LR, Hoban RA, Yakoob MY, Bateman BT. The association of maternal race and ethnicity and the risk of postpartum hemorrhage. Anesth. Analg. 2012;115:1127–36.

19. Hornbrook MC, Whitlock EP, Berg CJ, Callaghan WM, Bachman DJ, Gold R, et al. Development of an algorithm to identify pregnancy episodes in an integrated health care delivery system. Health Serv. Res. 2007;42:908–27.

20. Kuklina EV, Whiteman MK, Hillis SD, Jamieson DJ, Meikle SF, Posner SF, et al. An enhanced method for identifying obstetric deliveries: implications for estimating maternal morbidity. Matern. Child Health J. 2008;12:469–77.

21. Selten JP, van der Graaf Y, van Duursen R, Gispen-de Wied CC, Kahn RS. Psychotic illness after prenatal exposure to the 1953 Dutch Flood Disaster. Schizophr. Res. 1999;35:243–5.

22. Nazareth I, King M, Haines A, Rangel L, Myers S. Accuracy of diagnosis of psychosis on general practice computer system. BMJ. 1993;307:32–4.

23. Marcelis M, Navarro-Mateu F, Murray R, Selten J-P, Van Os J. Urbanization and psychosis: a study of 1942–1978 birth cohorts in The Netherlands. Psychol. Med. Cambridge University Press. 1998;28:871–9.

24. Valdimarsdóttir U, Hultman CM, Harlow B, Cnattingius S, Sparén P. Psychotic illness in first-time mothers with no previous psychiatric hospitalizations: a population-based study. PLoS Med. 2009;6:e13.

25. Consumer Price Index, 1913-|Federal Reserve Bank of Minneapolis [Internet]. [cited 2017 Nov 26]. Available from: https://www.minneapolisfed.org/

community/teaching-aids/cpi-calculator-information/consumer-price-index-and-inflation-rates-1913. Accessed 26 Nov 2017.

26. Garite TJ, Clark RH, Elliott JP, Thorp JA. Twins and triplets: the effect of plurality and growth on neonatal outcome compared with singleton infants. Am. J. Obstet. Gynecol. 2004;191:700–7.

27. Sacker A, Done DJ, Crow TJ. Obstetric complications in children born to parents with schizophrenia: a meta-analysis of case–control studies. Psychol. Med. Cambridge University Press. 1996;26:279–87.

28. Bennedsen BE, Mortensen PB, Olesen AV, Henriksen TB. Congenital malformations, stillbirths, and infant deaths among children of women with schizophrenia. Arch. Gen. Psychiatry. 2001;58:674–9.

29. Bennedsen BE, Mortensen PB, Olesen AV, Henriksen TB. Preterm birth and intra-uterine growth retardation among children of women with schizophrenia. Br. J. Psychiatry. 1999;175:239–45.

30. Nilsson E, Lichtenstein P, Cnattingius S, Murray RM, Hultman CM. Women with schizophrenia: pregnancy outcome and infant death among their offspring. Schizophr. Res. 2002;58:221–9.

31. Lin H-C, Chen I-J, Chen Y-H, Lee H-C, Wu F-J. Maternal schizophrenia and pregnancy outcome: Does the use of antipsychotics make a difference? Schizophr. Res. 2010;116:55–60.

32. Newham JJ, Thomas SH, MacRitchie K, McElhatton PR, McAllister-Williams RH. Birth weight of infants after maternal exposure to typical and atypical antipsychotics: prospective comparison study. Br. J. Psychiatry. 2008;192:333–7.

33. Mitchell AJ, Vancampfort D, Sweers K, van Winkel R, Yu W, De Hert M. Prevalence of metabolic syndrome and metabolic abnormalities in schizophrenia and related disorders–a systematic review and meta-analysis. Schizophr. Bull. 2013;39:306–18.

34. Bodén R, Lundgren M, Brandt L, Reutfors J, Kieler H. Antipsychotics during pregnancy: relation to fetal and maternal metabolic effects. Arch. Gen. Psychiatry. 2012;69:715–21.

35. Ahlsson F, Lundgren M, Tuvemo T, Gustafsson J, Haglund B. Gestational diabetes and offspring body disproportion. Acta Paediatr. 2010;99:89–93.

36. Baird JD. Some aspects of carbohydrate metabolism in pregnancy with special reference to the energy metabolism and hormonal status of the infant of the diabetic woman and the diabetogenic effect of pregnancy. J. Endocrinol. 1969;44:139–72.

37. Gentile S. Antipsychotic therapy during early and late pregnancy. A systematic review. Schizophr. Bull. 2010;36:518–44.

38. Galbally M, Snellen M, Power J. Antipsychotic drugs in pregnancy: a review of their maternal and fetal effects. Ther Adv Drug Saf. 2014;5:100–9.

39. Howard LM. Fertility and pregnancy in women with psychotic disorders. Eur. J. Obstet. Gynecol. Reprod. Biol. 2005;119:3–10.

40. Mittal VA, Ellman LM, Cannon TD. Gene-environment interaction and covariation in schizophrenia: the role of obstetric complications. Schizophr. Bull. 2008;34:1083–94.

41. Suvisaari JM, Taxell-Lassas V, Pankakoski M, Haukka JK, Lönnqvist JK, Häkkinen LT. Obstetric complications as risk factors for schizophrenia spectrum psychoses in offspring of mothers with psychotic disorder. Schizophr. Bull. 2013;39:1056–66.

42. Yolken RH, Torrey EF. Are some cases of psychosis caused by microbial agents? A review of the evidence. Mol. Psychiatry. 2008;13:470–9.

43. Gibbs RS. The relationship between infections and adverse pregnancy outcomes: an overview. Ann. Periodontol. 2001;6:153–63.

44. Liu B, Roberts CL, Clarke M, Jorm L, Hunt J, Ward J. Chlamydia and gonorrhoea infections and the risk of adverse obstetric outcomes: a retrospective cohort study. Sex. Transm. Infect. 2013;89:672–8.

45. Ellis J, Williams H, Graves W, Lindsay MK. Human immunodeficiency virus infection is a risk factor for adverse perinatal outcome. Am. J. Obstet. Gynecol. 2002;186:903–6.

46. Boyle VT, Thorstensen EB, Mourath D, Jones MB, McCowan LME, Kenny LC, et al. The relationship between 25-hydroxyvitamin D concentration in early pregnancy and pregnancy outcomes in a large, prospective cohort. Br J Nutr. 2016;116:1409–15.

47. McGrath J. Hypothesis: is low prenatal vitamin D a risk-modifying factor for schizophrenia? Schizophr Res. 1999;40:173–7.

48. Bruins J, Jörg F, van den Heuvel ER, Bartels-Velthuis AA, Corpeleijn E, Muskiet FAJ, et al. The relation of vitamin D, metabolic risk and negative symptom

severity in people with psychotic disorders. Schizophr. Res [Internet]. 2017; Available from: http://dx.doi.org/10.1016/j.schres.2017.08.059.

49. Rosecrans R, Dohnal JC. Seasonal vitamin D changes and the impact on health risk assessment. Clin Biochem. 2014;47:670–2.

50. Byrne EM, Psychiatric Genetics Consortium Major Depressive Disorder Working Group, Raheja UK, Stephens SH, Heath AC, Madden PAF, et al. Seasonality shows evidence for polygenic architecture and genetic correlation with schizophrenia and bipolar disorder. J Clin Psychiatry. 2015; 76:128–34.

51. Chirumbolo S, Bjørklund G, Sboarina A, Vella A. The Role of Vitamin D in the Immune System as a Pro-survival Molecule. Clin Ther. 2017;39:894–916.

52. Daglar K, Tokmak A, Kirbas A, Guzel AI, Erkenekli K, Yucel A, et al. Maternal serum vitamin D levels in pregnancies complicated by neural tube defects. J Matern Fetal Neonatal Med. 2016;29:298–302.

53. Eyles DW, Burne THJ, McGrath JJ. Vitamin D, effects on brain development, adult brain function and the links between low levels of vitamin D and neuropsychiatric disease. Front Neuroendocrinol. 2013;34:47–64.

54. Crews M, Lally J, Gardner-Sood P, Howes O, Bonaccorso S, Smith S, et al. Vitamin D deficiency in first episode psychosis: a case-control study. Schizophr Res. 2013;150:533–7.

55. Schneider B, Weber B, Frensch A, Stein J, Fritz J. Vitamin D in schizophrenia, major depression and alcoholism. J Neural Transm. 2000;107:839–42.

56. Belvederi Murri M, Respino M, Masotti M, Innamorati M, Mondelli V, Pariante C, et al. Vitamin D and psychosis: mini meta-analysis. Schizophr. Res. 2013; 150:235–9.

57. Bodnar LM, Simhan HN, Powers RW, Frank MP, Cooperstein E, Roberts JM. High prevalence of vitamin D insufficiency in black and white pregnant women residing in the northern United States and their neonates. J Nutr. 2007;137:447–52.

58. Evans KN, Bulmer JN, Kilby MD, Hewison M. Vitamin D and placental-decidual function. J Soc Gynecol Investig. 2004;11:263–71.

59   Wilson MP, Nordstrom K, Shah AA, Vilke GM. Psychiatric Emergencies in Pregnant Women. Emerg Med Clin North Am. 2015;33:841–51.

7

The experience of women with an eating disorder in the perinatal period: a meta-ethnographic study

Sarah Fogarty[1]* ⓘ, Rakime Elmir[2,3], Phillipa Hay[4] and Virginia Schmied[3]

Abstract

Background: Pregnancy is a time of enormous body transformation. For those with an eating disorder during pregnancy this time of transformation can be distressing and damaging to both the mother and the child. In this meta-ethnographic study, we aimed to examine the experiences of women with an Eating Disorder in the perinatal period; that is during pregnancy and two years following birth.

Method: A meta-ethnographic framework was used in this review. After a systematic online search of the literature using the keywords such as pregnancy, eating disorders, anorexia, bulimia, binge eating disorder, perinatal, postnatal and post-partum, 11 papers, involving 94 women, were included in the review.

Results: A qualitative synthesis of the papers identified 2 key themes. The key theme that emerged during pregnancy was: navigating a 'new' eating disorder. The key that emerged in the perinatal period was return to the 'old' eating disorder.

Conclusion: Following a tumultuous pregnancy experience, many described returning to their pre-pregnancy eating behaviors and thoughts. These experiences highlight the emotional difficulty experienced having an eating disorder whilst pregnant but they also point to opportunities for intervention and a continued acceptance of body image changes. More research is needed on the experiences of targeted treatment interventions specific for pregnant and postpartum women with an eating disorder and the effectiveness of putative treatment interventions during this period.

Keywords: Pregnancy, Eating disorders, Anorexia nervosa, Bulimia nervosa, Perinatal, Midwives, Qualitative research, Meta-synthesis, Women

Background

Eating disorders are associated with the highest mortality and morbidity of any mental illness and it is estimated that around 10% of the general population is affected by eating disorders and related behaviors [1, 2]. The most common and well-recognised eating disorders are anorexia nervosa, bulimia nervosa, and binge eating disorder (BED) [3]. For individuals with anorexia nervosa, the state of self-starvation commonly gives a sense of achievement, self-worth and control [3]. Depression and anxiety disorders are common co-morbidities of anorexia nervosa which can make treatment and recovery more difficult [4–6].

Bulimia nervosa and BED both involve binge eating (un-controlled episodes of overeating) and in bulimia nervosa these are followed by compensatory behaviours such as purging (self-induced vomiting, diuretics or laxatives) or excessive exercise [3]. Due to the menstrual dysfunction that can occur with eating disorders, it was originally considered rare for pregnancy to occur in this population [7, 8]. A growing body of evidence has contradicted this belief and provided confirmation that not only can pregnancy occur during an eating disorder but that it is more common than previously thought [9, 10].

Pregnancy is a time of enormous body transformation. Body and body weight dissatisfaction can affect pregnant women with or without an eating disorder [11]. Women with an eating disorder or a past history of an eating

* Correspondence: doctorfogarty@gmail.com
[1]School of Medicine, Western Sydney University, Locked Bag 1797, Penrith, NSW 2751, Australia
Full list of author information is available at the end of the article

disorder are more vulnerable to heightened body image concerns and the adjustments of an enlarging abdomen and other physical and hormonal changes over which they have no control [12]. There is no uniform behaviour that occurs when a woman with an eating disorder discovers she is pregnant. For some women, their concern for their unborn child motivates a complete cessation of eating disorder behaviours during pregnancy [13–16], yet for other women, the most they can manage is a reduction of disordered eating behaviours [8, 16, 17] and for some their eating disorder stays the same, gets worse or improves for example, from binge-purging to just binging alone [16, 18]. The importance of improving eating disorder behaviour in pregnancy has been highlighted by the link to eating disorders and poor maternal and neonatal outcomes including miscarriages, significant morbidity and increased mortality, pre-eclampsia, and low birth weight [8, 19, 20]. Eating disorders have also been linked to poor health outcomes for pregnant and postpartum women including depressive symptoms during pregnancy, postnatal depression, and poor infant attachment or maternal bonding [21–25].

Lack of disclosure of an eating disorder by women in pregnancy has been reported [26] potentially increasing adverse health outcomes if women do not receive treatment, or assistance to address the eating behaviour symptoms and/or pathology. The need for health professionals providing antenatal care to be more aware of eating disorders in pregnancy and have the capacity and resources to adequately address and treat pregnant women with an eating disorder was reported in a recent qualitative review [13]. It is important to investigate the experiences of women in order to understand how to assist women to reduce disordered eating behaviours during pregnancy, and improve their access to appropriate community, medical and psychological support during the perinatal period. In this perinatal period, research has found that for some individuals their eating disorder symptoms either worsened or returned to their pre-pregnancy levels [8, 11, 25]. This was commonly motivated by the desire to return to a pre-pregnancy weight and shape [24, 27–29]. Returning to eating disorder behaviours in the postpartum period may result in a shorter duration of breastfeeding and may impact on the interaction the mother has with her baby and her relationship with her partner [5, 25, 30]. A recent review on women's' experiences of pregnancy and eating disorders found that women experienced turmoil related to fear and guilt about their changing soma and the sense of self, wanting to be a good mother and concern about how others would perceive their behaviour during their pregnancy, however this review did not explore the period following birth [13]. Thus there is need not only to conceptualize the experiences of pregnancy for those

with an eating disorder in the antenatal period, but also during the immediate postpartum period and up to the infant age of two years.

There has been an increase in the number of in-depth qualitative studies of women's experiences of eating disorders in pregnancy and following birth. This offers a timely opportunity to undertake a synthesis of these studies. This meta-ethnographic study aimed to explore the experience of women with an eating disorder or past history of an eating disorder during the perinatal period.

Methods

A meta-ethnographic framework outlined by Noblit and Hare was used to synthesise the findings reported in included papers as this approach is "well suited to producing new theories and conceptual models" [31]. Meta-ethnography is an interpretive approach combining findings of qualitative studies. This method provides a more comprehensive analysis of the original research findings and provides new insights to the research while simultaneously preserving the authentic meaning of primary data [32]. In this approach there are seven steps to guide the synthesis, see Table 1 [33]. The authors followed the enhancing of transparency in reporting the synthesis of qualitative research (ENTREQ) in reporting this meta-ethnographic study [34]. An ENTREQ checklist is available in the Supporting Information Additional file 1.

A comprehensive, pre-planned search strategy was used to seek all available studies. This meta-ethnographic study considered studies and literature that investigated the experiences of women with an eating disorder or past history of an eating disorder during the perinatal period

Table 1 The 7 steps of the Noblit and Hare meta-ethnographic method [33]

Steps		
Step 1	Getting started	These steps involve defining the search criteria and parameters, conducting the search, including, quality assessment and excluding studies [33].
Step 2	Confirming the initial interest	
Step 3	Reading studies	
Step 4	Extracting date from included studies	This step involves extracting data from the included studies and 'determining how studies are related' and identifying common themes, and concepts [33].
Step 5	Translating Studies	This step involves 'comparing first and/or second order themes against each other [33]
Step 6	Synthesising translations	This step creates new third order themes from first and second order concepts.
Step 7	Expressing the synthesis	This step the authors expressing the synthesis implications in relation to clinical practice, policy, treatment, program development and/or research [33].

(the perinatal period is defined as from conception to two years post birth). Eating disorders included Anorexia Nervosa Bulimia Nervosa, BED, PICA, Avoidant/Restrictive Food Intake Disorder or Other Specified or Unspecified Feeding or Eating Disorder (OSFED or UFED) [35]. OSFED/UFED replaces the former Eating Disorder Not Otherwise Specified category) [35].

This meta-ethnographic study did not review publications or literature assessing the side effects or outcome of pregnancy on those with an eating disorder or the outcomes for the children. Literature published after 1980 was considered for inclusion in the study. It was important to the authors that the accounts of women's' experiences with pregnancy and eating disorders was inclusive. Purely quantitative studies were excluded, as the purpose of meta-ethnographic studies is to synthesize qualitative research findings. The research on the challenges of having an eating disorder during pregnancy was first reported in the late 1980's. Research published in the languages English, Portuguese or Spanish were also considered for inclusion, as the authors had access to translational services in Portuguese and Spanish.

The meta-ethnographic study considered qualitative papers and mixed methods studies that reported rich qualitative data. This meta-ethnography also considered case studies reporting the experiences of individual women.

The first three steps involved in the meta-ethnographic framework outlined by Noblit and Hare [31] involved defining the search criteria and parameters, the search itself, including, quality assessment and excluding studies. Relevant publications were identified using a systematic online search of CINAHL Plus with Full Text (EBSCOhost, EBSCO), Scopus (Pubmed), Dissertation and Theses, Google Scholar and Google up to the date of 14th March 2016. The keywords **"pregnancy"** AND **"eating disorders"**) as well as (**"pregnancy"** AND **"anorexia"**), (**"pregnancy"** AND **"bulimia"**), (**"pregnancy"** AND **"EDNOS"**), (**"pregnancy"** AND **"PICA"**), (**"pregnancy"** AND **"UFED"**), (**"pregnancy"** AND **"OSFED"**), (**"pregnancy"** AND **"binge eating disorder"**), (**"prenatal"** AND **"eating disorders"**), (**"postnatal"** AND **"eating disorders"**), (**"antenatal"** AND **"eating disorders"**), (**"antepartum"** AND **"eating disorders"**), (**"perinatal"** AND **"eating disorders"**), and (**"post-partum"** AND **"eating disorders"**), were used. The Scopus search used 'All Fields' and retrieved 1798 results and a further 7 results were retrieved from Dissertation and Theses and a manual search of the reference sections of the identified studies (see Fig. 1). The aim of the search was to obtain sufficient articles to reach 'conceptual saturation' from both published and unpublished studies [31]. Author SF undertook identification of the studies. Figure 1 shows the selection of included studies. 1798 publications were initially identified, of which 736 duplicates were removed. Relevant studies were then selected using a two-stage screening procedure.

First stage screening

The first stage of screening involved eliminating abstracts/publications that did not meet the meta-ethnographic study inclusion criteria based on titles. SF then assessed all literature for possible retrieval of the full text article based on the study inclusion criteria. This first stage of screening generated 25 relevant papers.

Second stage screening

The 25 articles were read in full by the authors, 12 articles were included and 12 were excluded. There was one instance where two papers used the same data; Burton et al. 2014 [36] and Burton et al. 2015 [20]. In this case, the later of the two papers was used in the review as this represented the most comprehensive dataset. Two papers reported from the same research project; Stringer et al. [37] and Tierney et al. 2011 [8], are treated together within the review. Two articles sampled non-eating disorder participants [38, 39] and one included a combined sample of non-disordered eating participants and participants with disordered eating [40]. Two articles were review articles [13, 41] and two were not qualitative papers [42, 43]. Four papers were excluded as the participants' interviews had occurred past 24 months following birth [25, 44–46]. All authors were involved in the second stage screening and all authors agreed on the final papers to be included and excluded.

Quality appraisal

There is no consensus on which quality assessment tool should be employed for qualitative synthesis and no agreement on how quality assessment tools should be used or applied. There is also a debate about whether quality appraisal should form part of a meta-ethnography at all [32]. The authors used a standardised critical appraisal instrument called Critical Appraisal Skills Programme (CASP) [47] to assess the range of quality of the publications selected for inclusion in the study. The CASP is a qualitative assessment tool that provides an indication of the trustworthiness and relevance of findings ("Critical Appraisal Skills Program (CASP) Qualitative Research Checklist 31. 5.13,"). The CASP was completed independently and any disagreements that arose between the reviewers regarding inclusion were resolved through discussion. As per the instructions, the CASP was not scored [47]. Similar to Atkins et al., a decision was made that no study that meet the basic criteria for inclusion would be excluded as the CASP provides a description of the range of quality found in papers and major gaps in reporting, if any, not a

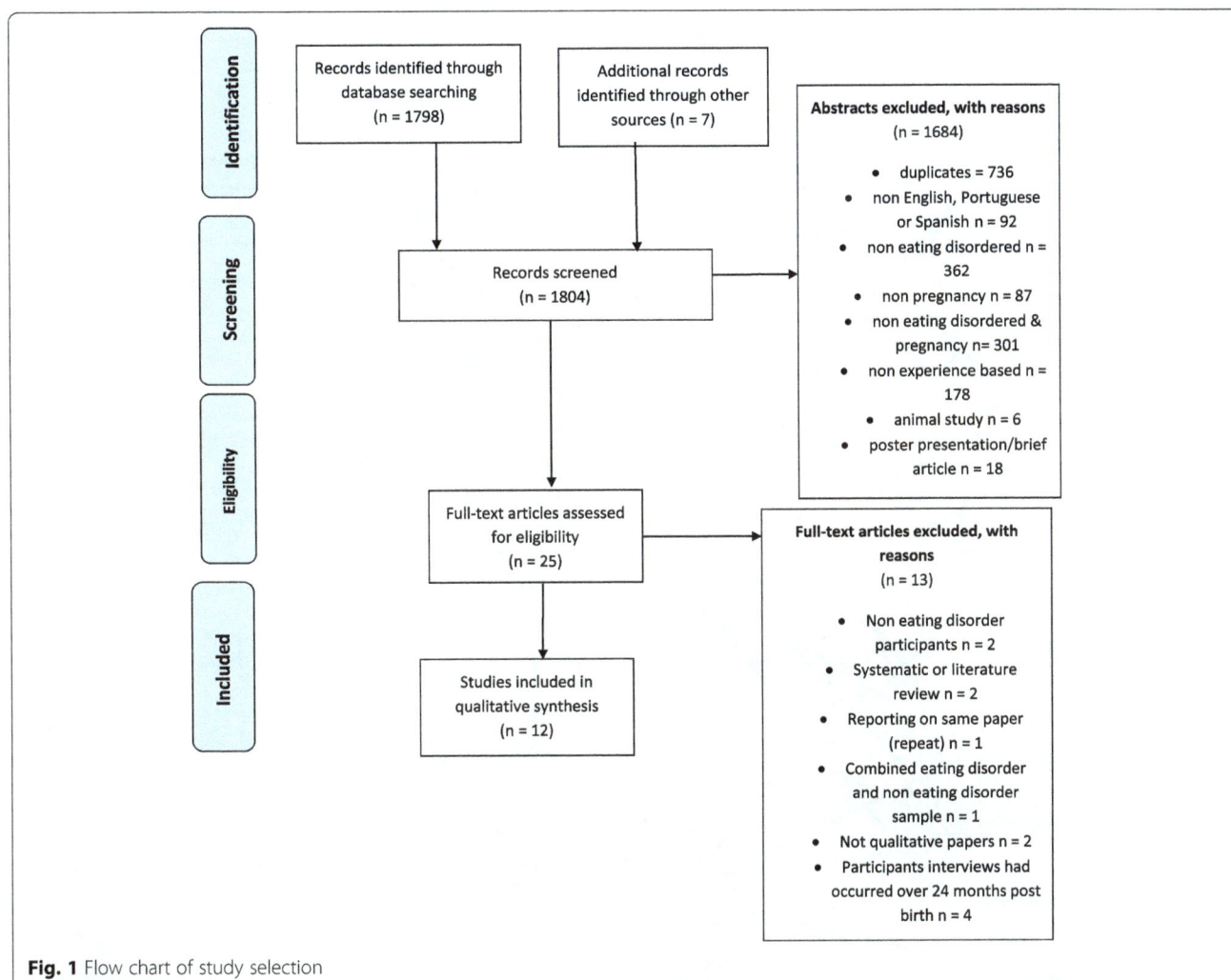

Fig. 1 Flow chart of study selection

reproducible guidelines on how to accurately assess good quality studies or when to include or exclude papers.

Data extraction

Data extracted included specific details about the participants, study methods, and specific objectives. Step four involved extracting data from the included studies and 'determining how studies are related'. Authors SF and RE read and re-read the included papers to identify common themes and concepts. The themes reported by authors in each of the included qualitative studies, were extracted as first and second order data. The discussion section of the papers was also read to identify any further key themes or concepts extracted as second order data. The case studies did not present findings in terms of succinct themes. In these cases author SF read the case study results and discussion, and undertook a thematic analysis of the data to include in the review. Authors SF, RE and VS confirmed the first and/or second order data and themes.

Data synthesis

Step five was 'translating studies' which compared first and/or second order data against each other. Step six was 'synthesising translations'. The authors created new third order themes from first and second order concepts [33]. The authors used both reciprocal and refutational translation to note similarities and differences in findings. The majority of the concepts reflected similar findings and themes across the included studies. There were no papers that refuted the findings of another study. This continual process of comparison and development of themes enabled the development of third order themes. The final synthesis included a line of argument that summarized the key findings from the different stages of the antenatal and postnatal periods. See Fig. 2. These findings were presented as a series of themes supported by quotes from the original papers. Again all authors were involved in the step five and six. Step seven was 'expressing the synthesis' where the authors reported the implications of the findings of this synthesis

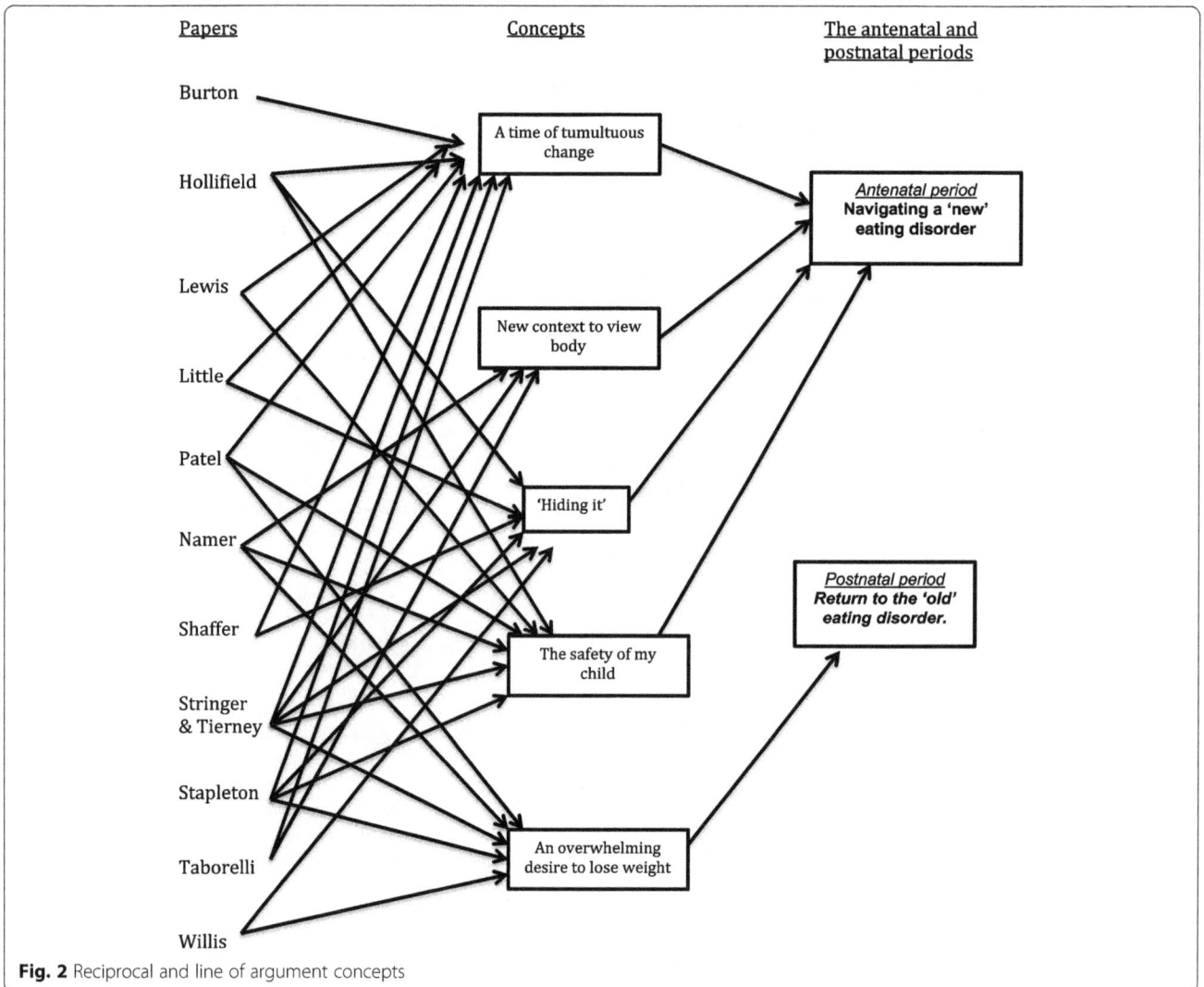

Fig. 2 Reciprocal and line of argument concepts

for clinical practice, policy, treatment, program development and/or research. The process of synthesis was inductive.

Results
Study characteristics
Detailed characteristics such as the populations, study methods, and specific objectives are described in Table 2. The majority of the studies were from the United States (12 studies) and the United Kingdom (9 studies) with the remaining studies being from Australia and South Africa. All studies were published between 1986 and 2015. Sample sizes ranged from 3 to 20 (median 6) across all studies. The total number of women involved across all included studies was 94. The age range for participants in the studies ranged from 21 to 45 years. Twenty-two women were pregnant at the time of the interview and 72 had given birth. The types of eating

disorders examined in the study included 22 with Anorexia Nervosa, 17 with Bulimia Nervosa, 10 with Bulimia Nervosa, BED or Eating Disorder Not Otherwise Specified, 34 with an Eating Disorder (type not specified), and 11 with Anorexia Nervosa or Bulimia Nervosa.

Quality of included studies
The majority of the studies included in the synthesis were of good quality; however, no studies meet all the CASP criteria. Through our critical appraisal we identified several areas where the reporting and methodology was good including study aims, justification of methodology, participant inclusion, data collection, analysis process, and study findings. Areas identified that were not as well reported included a lack of data about those that chose not to take place in the study and limited data on the critical examination undertaken or the role of researchers in the analysis (see Table 2). The case-studies

Table 2 Characteristics of included papers/literature

Author (Year)	Country Setting	Participants N, age, ED features	Study aim/objective	Study design/methodology & transparency	Rigour of analysis and reporting
Journal Articles					
Burton et al. 2015 [20]	Perth, Australia.	20 women, aged between 21 and 40, with an eating disorder diagnosis and who had birthed within the last 12 months. 8 had Anorexia Nervosa(AN), 4 had Bulimia Nervosa (BN), BED or Eating Disorder Not Otherwise Specified (EDNOS). Other 12 not accounted for re eating disorder (ED) diagnosis. All had given birth.	*Aim:* To address a gap in current literature of how pregnant women with eating disorders make meaning of their experience.	*Study design:* Semi-structured in-depth interview. *Methodology:* Used purposive sampling. *Data Collection:* Taped interview, which was then transcribed. *Data analysis:* Colaizzi's method.	Nothing about those who chose not to take place in the study. Limited data on the critical examination undertaken or the researchers role in the analysis.
Patel et al. 2005 [27]	United Kingdom.	6 mothers, mean age (range 29–42) with either Diagnostic and Statistical Manual of Mental Disease IV (DSM-IV) BN or EDNOS and 9 mothers, mean age 33.6 (range 28–43) at risk for an eating disorder (high concerns about body weight and shape but little behavioural disturbance). Comparison group: 6 mothers, mean age 32.5 (range 28–36), with low body shape and weight concerns. All had given birth.	*Aim:* To examine how three groups of women with different levels of eating disorder psychology, perceived and coped with changes in eating and body shape and weight following pregnancy and the birth of a baby.	*Study design:* In-depth interview. *Methodology:* Used purposive sampling. *Data Collection:* Interview, which was then transcribed. *Data analysis:* Thematic content analysis.	Nothing about those who chose not to take place in the study. Limited data on the critical examination undertaken or the researchers role in the analysis. Nothing in the reporting about receiving ethical approval.
Shaffer et al. 2008 [28]	USA	10 women with a self-reported history of an eating disorder during pregnancy, age range 26–39. 6 were pregnant at time of data collection. 4 had given birth.	*Aim:* To explore the experiences of women who have an eating disorder prior to, or during pregnancy.	*Study design:* In-depth interview. *Methodology:* Used purposive sampling. *Data Collection:* Interview, which was audiotaped then transcribed. *Data analysis:* Manen's Thematic content analysis.	Nothing about those who chose not to take place in the study.
Stapleton et al. 2008 [29]	United Kingdom.	16 women who self-reported as having an eating disorder, age range 23–44 years. 5 were pregnant at time of data collection. 11 had given birth.	*Aim:* To examine participants' motivation for, and understandings of, infant-feeding decisions and practices.	*Study design:* In-depth interview. *Methodology:* Used purposive sampling. *Data Collection:* Interview, which was audiotaped then transcribed. *Data analysis:* Feminist and ethnographic approach.	Limited data on the critical examination undertaken or the researchers role in the analysis
Taborelli et al. 2015 [30]	United Kingdom.	12 women with severe eating disorders during pregnancy (8 with Anorexia Nervosa Binge-purge (AN-BP) and 4 with BN), age range 23–39. All had given birth.	*Aim:* To examine in depth the individuals' experience of transition from pregnancy to motherhood, among women with current eating disorders, focusing on differences between first and subsequent pregnancies.	*Study design:* In-depth interview. *Methodology:* Used purposive sampling. *Data Collection:* Interview, which was audiotaped then transcribed. *Data analysis:* Interpretative phenomenological analysis.	No information on dropouts during the data collection. Limited data on the critical examination undertaken or the researchers role in the analysis
Stringer et al. 2010 [37] and Tierney et al. 2011 [8]	United Kingdom.	8 women with self reported AN or BN, mean age 29.4 years.	*Aim:* To examine in depth the experiences of pregnant women with an ED and during the early years of the child's life.	*Study design:* Semi-structured interview. *Methodology:* Used purposive sampling.	Limited data on the critical examination undertaken or the researchers role in the analysis

Table 2 Characteristics of included papers/literature *(Continued)*

Author (Year)	Country Setting	Participants N, age, ED features	Study aim/objective	Study design/methodology & transparency	Rigour of analysis and reporting
		3 were pregnant at time of data collection. 5 had given birth.		*Data Collection:* Interview, which was audiotaped then transcribed. *Data analysis:* Framework analysis.	
Willis & Rand 1988 [55]	USA.	4 women who meet the criteria (DSM-III) for BN. All women had given birth.	*Aim:* To describe pregnancy outcome in four bulimic women.	*Study design:* Interview. *Methodology:* Used purposive sampling. *Data Collection:* Interview. *Data analysis:* Unclear.	Age of women not reported. Limited information on how data was collected and no information on how the data was analysed.
Case Studies					
Hollifield & Hobdy 1990 [18]	USA.	3 women with DSM diagnosis of BN, aged 23–31, from an eating disorder therapy group who became pregnant. All pregnant at time of interview.	Aim: To present the experiences of three pregnant women with BN whose experience of pregnancy did not match the current literature.	*Study design:* Case studies. *Data Collection:* Semi-structured interview.	No information on the duration or the type of questions asked during the interview.
Lewis & le Grange 1994 [53]	South Africa.	6 mothers aged 27–45 years, with a DSM-IV diagnosis of BN. All had given birth.	*Aim:* To investigate retrospectively i) The emotional experience of pregnancy by women suffering from BN, and ii) Whether pregnancy has an ameliorating, neutral or exacerbating effect on bulimic symptoms during, and/or following, pregnancy.	*Study design:* Case studies. *Data Collection:* Semi-structured interview.	
Little & Lowkes 2000 [52]	USA	3 women with anorexic-bulimic symptoms aged 28–36 years. Two had given birth and one was 9 months pregnant.	*Aim:* Not stated.	*Study design:* Case studies. *Data Collection:* Semi-structured interview.	Not stated what eating disorder the participants were suffering from. The aim of the study not clearly stated.
Namer et al. 1986 [50]	USA	6 women, mean age 28.7 years, with AN. Four were pregnant at time of data collection. Two had given birth.	*Aim:* To learn more about the psychological as well as physiological aspects of pregnancy, birth and the post-partum period in AN.	*Study design:* Case studies. *Data Collection:* Semi-structured interview.	

were also generally well reported; however, as expected, there was less description about interview duration, interview questions, sampling method and the role of the researchers in the analysis (17, 46–48). Similar to other authors, the CASP assessment was limited by the papers written report and the word limits of the journals they were published in, which often did not allow for elaboration of the research process [32, 48].

The experience of pregnancy and the postnatal period for women with an eating disorder

Themes related to pregnancy and the two-year period following birth in the 12 articles are summarized in Tables 3 and 4 respectively. The themes resulting from the reciprocal translation and line of argument across studies are summarized in Table 5. The themes in table three were broken up into time periods: during the pregnancy, during and post pregnancy and the post partum period.

Findings

The findings relate to women's' experience of the physical changes to their bodies, their management of an eating disorder during the perinatal period, and concern about the health of their child. The main theme that emerged for women with an eating disorder during pregnancy was navigating a 'new' eating disorder. The key theme that emerged for women with an eating disorder post pregnancy was return to the 'old' eating disorder.

Navigating a 'new' eating disorder

The experience of having an eating disorder whilst pregnant was not like their pre-pregnancy eating disorder. The eating disorder during pregnancy was 'new' and

Table 3 First and second order themes related to the experience of pregnancy for those with an eating disorder as reported in the primary paper

Publication	Theme 1	Theme 2	Theme 3	Theme 4	Theme 5	Theme 6
Journal Publications						
Burton et al. 2015 [20]	"The battle" between the eating disorder, your body and the baby.	"Going around on the treadmill" – dealing with the eating disorder and the pregnancy and doing the same thing all the time; exhaustion.	"Recreational show ride"- highs and lows and feeling of being out of control.	"Walking the tightrope"- Staying in control and stopping from falling.	"Teetering on the edge"- Feeling like about to fall off into the unknown.	"Uninvited visitor from the past" – Known but unwanted visitor (ED) returning.
Patel et al. 2005 [27]	Loss of pre-pregnancy self - Concerns about pregnancy weight gain - Fear of not losing pregnancy weight	Life transitions - Using weight to control their lives - Physical changes in pregnancy reawakened weight and body concerns	Relationship with family members - Lack of comfort with reliance on help from partners.	Role within wider society - Experiencing the world as hostile and critical in relation to their new maternal selves especially when their was distress about their changed bodies.		
Shaffer et al. 2008 [28]	A constant mental battle to prevent losing control - Struggle to accept weight gain and size - Struggle to accept the pregnancy - Fear of control over their changing bodies.	A distorted body image - Difficulty looking in the mirror - Use of restrictive eating, compulsive exercise, laxative use or binging and purging and controlling weight, a compensation for low self-esteem.	Hiding their experience - Lied about eating behaviours and exercise - Used pregnancy symptoms e.g. nausea to explain/hide behaviours. - Most didn't tell their physicians or midwives.	Scale-induced trauma at prenatal visits - Routine weigh-ins at prenatal ap-pointments traumatic. - Fear and anxiety regarding weight gain and being weighted.		
Stapleton et al. 2008 [54]	Fighting to control the urge to restrict or binge-purge.	Lack of disclosure of their eating disorder to maternity health professionals				
Taborelli et al. 2015 [49]	Approaching pregnancy: Not expecting to be pregnant	Early pregnancy A difficult transition a) Highly anxiety provoking b) Loss of control over their body Making space for the baby The sacrifice of the eating disorder identity.	Middle to late pregnancy Assuming the pregnancy identity. - a new body to love.			
Stringer et al. 2010 [37] and Tierneyet al. 2011 [8]	Transforming body and eating behaviours - Concern about body shape - First trimester difficult ("seen as fat" rather than pregnant)	Uncertainties about child's shape - Not wanting their children to be obese - Not wanting them to obsess about food	Emotional regulation - Use of SIV in pregnancy to regulate emotion.	Professional awareness - Lack of empathy (from healthcare professionals)	Type of care - Early Support - High risk surveillance	

Table 3 First and second order themes related to the experience of pregnancy for those with an eating disorder as reported in the primary paper *(Continued)*

Publication	Theme 1	Theme 2	Theme 3	Theme 4	Theme 5	Theme 6
	- Less stress about body shape when obviously pregnant- not "fat" Concern about weight gain during pregnancy.			- Information deficits -Language used		
Willis & Rand 1988 [55]	Decrease in binge/ vomiting behaviours during pregnancy.	SIV occurred during pregnancy.	Mixed reporting of eating disorders to obstetric/ maternal health care providers.			
Case Studies						
Hollifield & Hobdy 1990 [18]	Hiding the Eating disorder from obstetricians and other health care personal.	Lied about specific behaviours to their spouse/therapists/ family/friends.	Experienced tremendous fears regarding health and wellbeing of their unborn child.	Profound shame and guilt in relation to their inability to refrain from bulimic practices while pregnant.	Rationalisation of behaviours.	
Lewis & le Grange 1994 [53]	Fear of losing control of their eating and weight during pregnancy.	Fear of damaging their unborn child as a result of their unhealthy eating behaviours.	Fear not enough to stop them from engaging in bulimic behavior.	Anxiety about their ability to cope when their baby was born.	Anxiety about the health of their unborn child.	
Little & Lowkes 2000 [52]	Hiding the Eating disorder.	Difficulty giving up the eating disorder behavior.				
Namer et al. 1986 [50]	Positive benefits- a) Being able to fall pregnant made them feel 'normal' and 'better' b) Pregnancy pleased their husbands Being 'forced' to take care of a baby made it easier to take care of themselves	Change in body image- a) Change in focus from stomach to weight and size of thighs as stomach considered to be the baby. Reliance on husband to provide perspective about their changing bodies and weight gain	Change in eating habits- a) Ability to eat 3–4 meals a day and not skip meals Increased variety in foods, eating foods not eaten in years	Effects on marital relationship- a) Husbands pleased with them but arguments about food intake and distress about their insecurity with their appearances.	Mood states and cognitive concerns during pregnancy- a) Concern about baby's health b) Irritability/ Anxiety/ Depression especially during first pounds of weight gain c) Fear body wouldn't return to pre- pregnancy weight d) Later months of pregnancy diminution of anorexic thinking.	Strong desire not to pass on food obsession to their child.

involved times of tumultuous change including feeling grotesque, a struggle over their changing body weight and shape, new feelings of losing control, and a tug-of-war over their desires to both stop and continue their eating disorder behaviours. Some women also experienced their body in a new and positive context experiencing a positive change in body image and eating habits, and discovering a new body to love especially middle to late pregnancy. Women also encountered new reasons for hiding their eating disorder and new challenges around keeping their child safe. Overall these changes express the difficulty that women with an eating disorder can encounter during pregnancy and the depth to which these feelings, struggles and battles consume and

Table 4 First and second order themes related to the experience of post-pregnancy for those with an eating disorder as reported in the primary papers

Publication	Theme 1	Theme 2	Theme 3	Theme 4
Journal Publications				
Namer et al. 1986 [50]	All lost pregnancy related weight gain, some weighted less. All concerned and struggling with their weight. Post pregnancy weight loss "allowed" and given permission to lose weight therefore it was hard to control weight loss.	No longer eating 3–4 meals or quantity of food eaten during pregnancy.	All returned to anorexic thinking within several weeks of giving birth.	Anxiety about breastfeeding. Anxiety about not eating enough to breastfeed. No desire to breastfeed as wanted to be able to lose weight.
Patel et al. 2005 [27]	Loss of pre-pregnancy self - Fear of not losing pregnancy weight. - Distress about changes and lack of return to pre-pregnancy weight.	Feeding relationship with infant - Anxiety and discomfort (need to eat to provide milk). - Using breast-feeding to lose weight.	Relationship with family members - Comments about post pregnancy body by partner viewed as derogatory or critical.	
Shaffer et al. 2008 [28]	Post-partum panic and fear - Concern, fear, worry or panic about their bodies post birth	Preconception with body image	Worsening of eating disorder symptoms after birth.	
Stapleton et al. 2008 [54]	Benefits for not breastfeeding - Choice not to breastfeed to be able to engage in eating disorder behavior.	Perceived positives for breastfeeding - Breastfeeding was motivated by the belief it would help with weight loss. - Increase in caloric expenditure from breast feeding allowed consumption of additional food (used as a compensatory mechanism instead of purging) - Feeling that breastfeeding assuages some of the guilt eating disorder women felt about potential damage done to the child because of the mothers eating disorder.	Bottle-feeding - Desire to bottle-feed to ensure child's nutritional needs are met.	Distress about post pregnancy shape and weight. Resumption of eating disorder behaviours post pregnancy.
Taborelli et al. 2015 [49]	Loss of the pre-pregnancy body identity, loss of pregnant identity. - Distress at post birth body shape Urge to lose weight increases and is compelling post-birth.	Subsequent pregnancies Less dissonance between eating disorders and pregnancy in subsequent pregnancies.		
Tierney et al. 2011 [8]	Fear of failure - Unable to breast feed due to poor mild supply	Emotional regulation - Return to exercise quickly post birth to help regulate negative emotions		
Willis & Rand 1988 [55]	Majority returned to their pregnancy binge/vomiting levels	Extreme distress about post partum body shape prompted relapse.		
Case Studies				
Little & Lowkes 2000 [52]	Increase of eating disorder behaviours postpartum.			

Table 5 Third order themes: Translation of themes related to pregnancy across the 12 primary studies

Relates to:	Themes	Paper origin
During the pregnancy	A time of tumultuous change 1) 'I feel grotesque': an ongoing struggle 2) feelings of loss of control, 3) a tug-of-war.	Burton 2015 Patel 2005 Shaffer 2008 Stapleton 2008 Taborelli 2015 Stringer 2010 and Tierney 2011 Hollifield 1990 Lewis 1994 Little 2000
	New context to view body 1) Experiencing a positive change in eating habits, and 2) a new body to love	Namer 1986 Taborelli 2015 Tierney 2011
	'Hiding it'	Shaffer et al. 2008 Stapleton 2008 Stringer 2010 Willis 1988 Hollifield 1990 Little 2000
	The safety of my child	Namer 1986 Patel 2005 Stringer 2010 and Tierney 2011 Hollifield 1990 Lewis 1994 Stapleton 2008
Post pregnancy-mother	An overwhelming desire to lose weight	Namer 1986 Patel 2005 Stapleton 2008 Taborelli 2015 Tierney 2011 Willis 1988 Little 2000

construct the pregnancy experiences of women with an eating disorder.

'Feeling grotesque': An ongoing struggle

A cornerstone to an eating disorder is body dissatisfaction, drive for thinness and the effect of weight and shape on self-image and self-esteem [3]. Pregnancy is a time of changing body shape and weight and women in these studies grappled with these changes and felt disgust and dissatisfaction about their changing bodies and they were constantly monitoring their weight gain [8, 27, 49, 50].

> "I was weighing myself lots....it was very difficult the first 3 months....when I became pregnant I hated it (long pause); first because I felt fat, and then because my clothes stopped fitting. It just makes you feel worse. I felt just absolutely grotesque" [49] p 6.

For some women, as their body changed, their thighs and their bottom became more of a focus of body dissatisfaction and disgust and they struggled to look at

themselves in the mirror with one participant saying *"when I look in the mirror and I see that my butt has gotten bigger, or that I have cellulite for the first time again since I was seventeen and my butt and thighs... those are my bad days"* [28] p 26.

Women felt stressed and anxious over their changing body weight and shape during the pregnancy and experienced a struggle with the weight gained. They often perceived this weight change as "getting fat" or: "feeling fat" rather than the outcomes of pregnancy. Women felt this particularly in early pregnancy as they initially gained weight.

> "...my boobs changed first and automatically I thought 'oh God I'm getting fat'. It was the first three months, you know, when your body starts changing but not enough to look pregnant. So you look like you're getting fatter rather than being pregnant. So that bit was difficult, emotionally" [37] p 8.

Some of the participants in the study experienced 'panic', 'distress and 'hatred' for their bodies [8, 49, 50] and struggled as "they were the heaviest they had ever been" [8] p 1228. This struggle with gaining weight was not the 'tug-of-war' oscillation and competition between two strong feelings i.e. managing the eating disorder and the needs of the unborn child, but rather a constant ongoing, daily struggle and a warring down from dealing with the affects of an increasing changing weight and shape.

> "Those ever present annoying voices in my head that were telling me I was fat were a constant battle for me....It was a constant struggle after that to try and have some control over my body and my weight....". [20] p 128.

Feelings of loss of control

Women with an eating disorder during pregnancy experienced a loss of control. A feature of eating disorders is the provision of a sense of control for the sufferer [51]. In the case of pregnancy the capacity to regulate emotions with the usual methods of exercise, food, purging, binging and or restrictions is constrained and if no other method of control is available then a feeling of being out of control can ensue. Women experienced this lack of capacity to regulate emotions as a struggle where they were eventually overwhelmed/worn down by the consistent chatter of their inner eating disorder voices, and their sense of control was swept away.

> "I knew my body would change and I would have to cope with that, but when it began to do so I was not prepared for the struggle that I would go through in

having to battle with the day-to-day changes, which I did not like. I got fatter and fatter and I had to battle with the voices telling me that I had lost control and that I would be fat forever" [20] p 129.

"Control was a big thing because I felt like I could always control my weight and I guess I lost that control in a way because I did gain weight, which was the very opposite of what I wanted to be doing or several years before I got pregnant. It was scary to be out of control of my body and my weight" [28] p 25.

Tug of war

Women experienced a 'tug-of-war' struggle to manage the needs of the eating disorder and the unborn child, with the two desires often conflicting during the course of the pregnancy. This struggle was experienced as a tug-of-war, with participants being strong at both ends of their convictions. Participants intensely desired both outcomes: their eating disorder behavior and 'healthy' eating for a healthy baby. Whilst participants oscillated between opposing desires, their convictions were strong and resolute. The outcome of this struggle appeared to be a fine-tuning of the two competing behaviors and needs; the eating disorder behaviors and the meeting the needs of their unborn child, which often resulted in a change in eating behaviors rather than a total relinquishing their eating disordered behavior [8, 18].

"...I struggled you know, dealing with the weight gain, kind of between not likening it and being uncomfortable with it but also knowing that it needed to happen to have healthy babies, so it was kind of a constant struggle" [28] p25.

"I was terribly anorexic for a while in the beginning of the pregnancy. I was so afraid to get fat. I knew I had to, it was an awful conflict" [52] p 303.

The affirmative 'new' experiences of their eating disorder while pregnant included experiencing a positive change in body image and eating habits, and a new body to love especially middle to late pregnancy. Some women experienced a time of positive change in their eating disorder behaviors and acceptance, liking and even loving their obviously pregnant bodies and new shape.

Experiencing a positive change in eating habits

In contrast to the struggles mentioned in above, pregnancy was also often a time of positive change in eating habits. Women were prompted to make changes

to their eating disorder behaviors by being responsible for the well-being of another dependent person. This generally included moderation or a decrease in severity of eating behaviors, and for a small number of women, a complete cessation of eating disorder behaviors. Some women were able to view these changes as positive and necessary, and in a different context to weight gain for medical or eating disorder treatment purposes [8, 49, 52]. It also became apparent that the rigid rules that individuals with an eating disorder set around certain foods, such as fat, diary, carbohydrates for example, could be relaxed during pregnancy.

"I didn't want to gain too much weight, so I still restricted but I ate healthier foods like nonfat yoghurt and vegetables" [52] p 302.

"I was a total freak about my diet and about fat intake and about exercising before I got pregnant, and it continued somewhat during my pregnancy, but again, I had to let myself gain weight" [28] p 25.

A new body to love

As the pregnancy progressed some women with an eating disorder were better able to like and even love their bodies as it became clearer to both themselves and others that they were obviously pregnant not 'fat' [8]. The influence of body shape and weight on self-evaluation is a feature of eating disorders [35], and thus weight gain and or being 'fat' is often viewed as particularly repulsive and displeasing. The context of being pregnant, not 'fat', could be experienced positively by liking or even loving their expanding body, in a way that weight gain experienced in their eating disorder did not [8, 27, 49].

"I didn't gain any weight for the first five months and then my doctor got really worried so I began to eat and I gained xx pounds in the last three months. I actually loved gaining weight, I really did" [52] p 302.

"I didn't mind how I looked when I was pregnant... I was more comfortable because you have a reason, people will see you pregnant and they won't think 'oh my god she's really fat' they just think she's just pregnant" [49] p 8

For some women pregnancy provided an opportunity to experience their stomach/abdomen in a positive way such as one participant who *"loved her bump because it was solid and round"* [8] p 1228 and another participant who felt her *"stomach is beautiful....nice and smooth.....I am the happiest I have ever been with my body"* [8] *p 1228.*

'Hiding it'

Women were hesitant to disclose their eating behaviors and eating disorder history to others including maternity care providers (midwives, maternity nurses, nurse-midwives and or obstetricians) and or significant others (friends, partner, husband). This practice ranged from actively hiding their eating disorder and eating behaviors to just not sharing their eating disorder history, as they were never asked.

"With my first no one asked and I didn't tell. I was ashamed" [52] *p 305.*

"I never shared it with my husband. He thought I had completely stopped purging. I pretty much had stopped it, but there were times I would indulge in a craving knowing that I could get away with throwing up by just saying that I was nauseous and it just came up" [28] *p 26.*

The lack of disclosure of their eating disorder to healthcare providers had the potential to add to their distress especially when being weighed at antenatal visits.

"It was always a trauma. It's very hard. I wish you weren't facing the scale and they didn't let you see your weight. I was stressed every time I had to go to the doctor and be weighted to see how much I'd gained because I was very, very rigid so that I wouldn't gain what I thought was too much weight." [28] *p 27.*

The safety of my child

Research has shown a link to eating disorders and poor maternal and neonatal outcomes including miscarriages, significant morbidity and increased mortality, pre-eclampsia, low birth weight, and poor infant attachment/bonding [8, 19–25]. Women in these studies were very aware of the capacity of their behaviors to influence the health of their unborn child [8, 18, 27, 50, 53, 54] and they were concerned and worried that their eating behaviours may lead to serious damage to their child during the pregnancy [8, 18, 20, 36, 50, 53].

"The pregnancy was like a rollercoaster ride. It caught my breath at times and made me feel really scared.....Was it going to conclude safely or would my baby be damaged with the fallout from the ride?" [20] *p 129.*

"I am not doing it (eating more) for myself, you understand, but have to do it so that the baby will be O.K." [50] *p 842.*

Women commonly expressed their general concerns about their child's health rather than citing a specific outcome. The included studies did not provide enough information to determine if the mothers were aware of specific risks related to eating disorders and maternal health or just generalised risks.

Return to the 'old' eating disorder

The main theme that emerged for women with an eating disorder following the birth was a return to the 'old' eating disorder. During this time women experienced an overwhelming desire to lose weight and a pull to return to the old and comfortable eating disorder behaviours. The overwhelming desire to lose weight involved not only how women experienced their weight and shape after giving birth but it also influenced their feeding choices for their newborn. This led to a distressing and precarious time where women with an eating disorder were highly vulnerable to returning to eating disorder behavior and symptomology.

Women with an eating disorder experienced anxiety and distress about their post pregnancy weight and shape and capacity to lose their pregnancy weight [27, 50, 55]. The postpartum body shape and weight were perceived as repulsive and upsetting, and there was accompanying anxiety and distress [28, 29, 49]. There was also a strong desire and need to lose the pregnancy weight and return to their post pregnancy shape and weight [27, 49]. The majority of the women quickly returned to their pre-pregnancy eating disorder behaviors and thoughts. It was apparent that the changes that had occurred during pregnancy, such as the reduction of eating behaviors, liking their body, disappeared once the baby was born and or after breastfeeding stopped.

I think the harder part is after you've had they baby and coming to terms with that [sic] new body, you know, when you still look like you're pregnant. I probably had more instances of binging and purging right after the baby was born because of the lack of sleep and also the feeling that, well, the baby's not inside of me anymore, you know, I'm not really hurting the baby if I binge and purge [28] *p 27.*

I joined a dieting group for a week... I didn't lose anything so I left...I weighed myself all the time waiting for a miracle... I have the intention of doing it (taking appetite suppressants) again as soon as I stop breastfeeding. The only way I know how to control this voice inside of me telling me to eat, eat, eat is when I take those pills [27] *p 354.*

In the postnatal period, women's decisions around infant feeding were influenced by their overwhelming desire to lose the pregnancy weight and the effect this may have on their weight and shape [27, 50, 52, 54]. Some women chose to breastfeed because they perceived they would lose weight faster such as *"I think it (breastfeeding) was partly about me behaving selfishly. It was knowing that it brought your figure back more quickly so I kept putting off weaning him because I know the weight was still dropping off me"* [54] *p 111.* For others breastfeeding was avoided so that eating disorder behaviors could resume e.g. exercise, restricting, and or purging.

I couldn't breastfeed. I just couldn't. I was desperate to get rid of the weight [54] *p 110.*

As soon as I could walk after I had her, I started doing exercises again... I just wanted to get the fat off. I was going to the gym 2 or 3 hours a day in the morning at 3.30 in the morning until 5.30 in the morning or 2 in the morning until 5. Just to get the fat off. I didn't even attempt to breastfeed; I was so focused on losing the weight [52] *p 303.*

Discussion

The present research is to our knowledge the first meta-ethnographic study exploring the perinatal period for women with eating disorders or a history of an eating disorder. The findings from this study relate to women's' experience of the physical changes to their bodies, their management of an eating disorder during the perinatal period, and concern about the health of their child. Pregnancy was experienced as a time of tumultuous change with stress and anxiety over body weight and shape changes, 'a tug-of-war' battle' managing the needs of the eating disorder and the unborn child, feelings of loss of control. For some women they experienced a positive change in body image and eating habits, and found a new way to love their body, especially middle to late pregnancy. The main theme that emerged for women with an eating disorder during pregnancy was navigating a 'new' eating disorder. The key theme that emerged for women with an eating disorder post pregnancy was return to the 'old' eating disorder.

While Tierney et al. reported similar findings of an internal turmoil [13] they did not report on the potential for positive experiences. In this meta-ethnographic study we found some women experienced a new context to view their body and talked of a new body to love once

they were more obviously pregnant and a motivation to alter eating habits [13]. Tierney and colleagues mention: "pregnancy is an optimum moment for women to consider their behaviours and make lasting changes to eating and weight control practices" [13] p. 547, they do not provide evidence of where these opportunities to intervene may occur.

Our ethnographic study findings indicate a number of possible opportune times for intervention. These include during the stage where women experience more acceptance of their body, when their desire is strong not to harm the health of their child, and during the tug-of-war, where the desire to meet the needs of their unborn child is greater than the desire of the eating disorder. In addition to using these opportunities to intervene, there is also the opportunity to work with women to promote a continuation of greater body acceptance and change post pregnancy. While rare in our sample of women, other studies have shown that some women, due to their concern for their unborn child, experience a complete cessation of eating disorder behaviours during pregnancy [14–16]. Taking advantage of the desire of women with an eating disorder to care for their unborn child could be explored through the development of a program that aims to support women to understand the specific risks eating disorder pose to their child and to highlight the positive effects in terms of child development and a stronger sense of connectedness with their mother that the baby might experience from these changes. In addition, it is hypothesized that treatment aimed at capitalizing on this opportunity to intervene and influence post pregnancy behaviors may need to be more intensive than pre-pregnancy treatment given the changing nature of the body during pregnancy and treatments may need to focus more on interventions that provide resources for self-nurturing, reducing anxiety and coping with stress, including a focus on the mother-infant relationship [56].

The time after pregnancy is experienced as a defining moment, it is during this time that women can return or rebound to pre-pregnancy eating disorder levels or more dangerously, experience greater eating disorder behaviors. The changes experienced during pregnancy, which are commonly motivated by the needs of their unborn child [29, 49, 50, 52], are replaced by distress and disgust with their new shape and weight, and the opportunity to return to their pre-pregnancy eating behaviors without the fear of directly effecting their child [27–29, 49]. Whilst positive changes in eating disorder have been experienced during pregnancy [49, 52, 57] these changes are generally not sustained post pregnancy [27–29, 49, 50]. Thus it is imperative to ensure that any mental health intervention/treatment for pregnant women with an eating disorder continues into the postpartum period and the possible 'red flag times' within these two periods to better understand how to enhance support and treatment options for pregnant and postpartum women with an eating disorder. Ideally, maternity care providers would also provide continuity of care for women with an eating disorder in the perinatal period, supporting the mother in her transition to motherhood and linking her with services and referral pathways to meet her complex health care needs. Further research is needed to determine the best practice for ensuring continuity of care among women with eating disorders.

Eating disorders are often a secretive disease [58] and this seems to extend into pregnancy with a finding of a lack of disclosure or hiding of eating behaviors to maternity care providers and or significant others. This behavior of hiding the eating disorder, whilst having common features with non-pregnant eating disorder individuals, seems to be distinguished in pregnancy by the motivation of discomfort from receiving inappropriate care and also the shame of having an eating disorder while pregnant although more qualitative research is needed to determine the exact differences. The findings of this meta-ethnographic study revealed the reasons for the lack of disclosure included not being asked by maternity care providers, discomfort disclosing their eating disorder, and a lack of appropriate care, specific for their eating disorder, when they did disclose their eating disorder [18, 28, 29, 55]. The reason for lack of disclosure and barriers to accessing health care treatment for eating disorders is similar among pregnancy and non-pregnant women. These include the severity of the health threat, the perception of the individuals' eating disorder health, feelings of shame, stigma and the clinicians understanding and capacity to recognize an eating disorder [59]. While women with an eating disorder who are not pregnant may choose not to disclose and seek any medical treatment, pregnant women with an eating disorder are often already seeking care through a maternity care provider and may have frequent visits with a maternity care provider thus providing multiple potential opportunities for disclosure. As such, maternity care providers are in a unique position to provide an environment where pregnant individuals would feel comfortable disclosing their eating disorder. Maternity care providers could also help identify potential eating disorder behaviors, explain how serious eating disorders are especially during pregnancy and provide understanding and support [59]. Improving the eating disorder health literacy of maternal health care providers to be able to provide these services is an integral part of improving disclosure of an eating disorder during pregnancy and utilizing this opportunity to intervene [60].

The lack of disclosure or hiding of an eating disorder during pregnancy also raises a number of implications for antenatal care including screening and screening

tools, assessment and support during the antenatal period. There has been a growing emphasis to identify women at risk for emotional and mental health conditions in the perinatal period [61]. In many States in Australia and overseas, the knowledge of the impact of previous or current social and or mental health problems has led to the implementation of psychosocial assessment and depression screening as part of routine clinical practice of midwives and child and family health nurses [62]. However, this study identifies a need to better prepare and train health professionals, such as midwives, child and family health nurses and doctors, for this work and thus support them to be able to offer empathetic and sensitive care to women who are disclosing personal information [62]. The aim of identifying women with risk factors for poor perinatal health including those with an eating disorder is to be able to offer early intervention, support services and appropriate individualized care [13, 61]. The ongoing care by maternity care providers of a woman who has been identified with an eating disorder requires additional skills to screening and assessing. It has been identified that maternity care providers may not have the skills, knowledge, or work resources to manage pregnant women with an eating disorder [13] and their specific needs such as sensitivity when being weighed and managing individuals fears about their changing shape. There is a need, despite the challenges of time and other work demands, to provide the resources for training and eating disorder awareness to maternity care providers.

There is substantial research on the effects of eating disorders on the health of the mother and the unborn baby including miscarriages, significant morbidity and increased mortality, pre-eclampsia, and low birth weight [8, 19, 20] and a growing body of research investigating the experiences of those with an eating disorder during pregnancy [8, 20, 28, 29, 49] however there is one notable aspect of research that is missing and that is research on the efficacy of treatment interventions specifically during the pregnancy period. A brief search of research databases by the authors did not find any studies that address current best-practice interventions for eating disorder treatment or any other adjunct therapies assessing treatment efficacy for those with an eating disorder during pregnancy. While there may be some published research studies available, more research is needed on the effectiveness of a specific perinatal treatment for those with an eating disorder. The publication of well-presented casa studies and case-series that highlight treatment approaches that may be beneficial is required and these studies may provide the foundations for much needed larger efficacy/effectiveness research studies. In addition there was no qualitative research on how treatment was experienced during pregnancy and the aspects of treatment that were helpful and those that were not beneficial. Specific pregnancy related treatment is needed during the perinatal to maximize the opportunity to intervene and make lasting changes, and treatment must address both the turmoil experienced and new and effective ways to manage stress and feeling out of control. Future research into psychological approaches that focus on reinforcing the positive changes during pregnancy, and strategies addressing how these might be carried over once the baby is born is needed. In addition, given the distressing and precarious time that is experienced post pregnancy, qualitative research into a treatment or intervention that specifically aimed to provide support, education and treatment during the postpartum period is warranted.

Strengths and weaknesses

The meta-ethnographic study undertaken did not lead to a loss of contextualised data about the lived experience of women with an eating disorder during the perinatal period as the context and integrity of the original data was the backbone to the themes. The process of undertaking the meta-ethnographic study highlighted important areas for future research. Understanding more deeply about other factors that may influence the experiences of perinatal women with an eating disorder such as their relationship with the baby's father, if the pregnancy was planned (or unplanned), if they were first-time mothers, social support received, life stressors, and or if they felt unwell during their pregnancy. The current body of qualitative literature on perinatal women with an eating disorder has limited reporting on if the pregnancies were planned (or unplanned) and they do not generally report on other possible contributing factors. Six papers reported if the pregnancy was planned [8, 18, 49, 50, 53, 55] with 19 of 39 participants having planned their pregnancies. These papers did not report on the impact a planned or unplanned pregnancy had on the perspective or experiences of having an eating disorder during the perinatal period.

Limitations of this study were the inclusion of papers that specifically investigated women with only Anorexia Nervosa or Bulimia Nervosa or papers that investigated eating disorders in general. There were no studies that specifically investigated the experiences of those with BED thus the review findings may not be applicable for those with BED. The meta-ethnographic study limited participation to those interviewed within 24 months of giving birth and papers in English, Spanish and Portuguese,

which meant that some papers and themes might have been not identified. The authors acknowledge that the number of studies included (including only 6 studies on the post-natal period) is not large however the role of meta-ethnography is not to summaries the entire body of knowledge but to focus on conceptual insight and "including too many studies might make conceptual analysis 'unwieldy' or make it difficult to maintain insight" [63]. The authors feel that the number of papers included were sufficient to produce conceptual insight.

Clinical implications

An avenue for addressing maternal care for those with an eating disorder is to target maternity care providers at hospitals with an interest in eating disorders and to provide training, support and a pathway of care specifically to these individuals. Eating disorder treatment providers could then refer pregnant eating disorder patients to these trained maternity care providers (and visa versa) and they could be included in part of the eating disorder multi-disciplinary team, all of whom are working with the same aims and goals for the pregnant woman (59). Pregnant women may see multiple health providers during their pregnancy, such as midwives and doctors, meaning the individual might experience a lack on continuity of antenatal eating disorder care. The importance of the appropriate practitioner in the management and recovery from an eating disorder has been well highlighted (60, 61) and the above mentioned treatment option of specific eating disorder pregnancy related treatment would also provide continuity of care for the pregnant woman with an eating disorder.

There is a need for more training for health professionals such as midwives, child and family health nurses and doctors to screen, and then provide appropriate ongoing support and care, for pregnant women with an eating disorder.

Conclusion

This meta-ethnographic review provides insight into the experience of having an eating disorder during the perinatal period and highlighted the 'new' and tumultuous nature of this. It also drew attention to the difficulties experienced in the post-partum period with a drive for weight loss and a return to pre-pregnancy eating behaviors and thoughts. These experiences highlight the turmoil and crisis of having an eating disorder whilst pregnant but they also highlight the opportunities for intervention and a continued acceptance of body image changes. There are several clinical implications regarding the care of pregnant and postpartum women particularly around opportune times to intervene include during the stage where women experience more acceptance of their body, when their desire is strong not to harm the health of their child, and during the "tug-of-war", where the desire to meet the needs of their unborn child is greater than the desire of the eating disorder. Further research is needed on effective treatment and management interventions during the perinatal period and the need to educate health care providers who are able to provide care for women with an eating disorder in the perinatal period.

Abbreviations

AN: Anorexia nervosa; AN-BP: Anorexia nervosa binge-purge; BED: Binge eating disorder; BN: Bulimia nervosa; CASP: Critical appraisal skills program; DSM: Diagnostic and statistical manual of mental disease; ED: Eating disorder; EDNOS: Eating disorder not otherwise specified; OSFED: Other specified; UFED: Unspecified feeding or eating disorder

Acknowledgements

This review is part of an Early Career Research grant to RE funded by Western Sydney University.

Funding

This review is part of an Early Career Research grant to RE funded by Western Sydney University.

Authors' contributions

Authors SF, RE, VS and PH were involved in the conception, methodology, reviewing, and editing of this paper. Author SF completed the initial searching of the data and was a major contributor in writing the first draft of the manuscript. Authors SF, RE, VS and PH read and approved the final manuscript.

Competing interests

Professor Hay receives sessional fees and lecture fees from the Australian Medical Council, Therapeutic Guidelines publication, and New South Wales Institute of Psychiatry and royalties from Hogrefe and Huber, McGraw Hill Education, and Blackwell Scientific Publications. Other authors declare that they have no competing interests.

Author details

[1]School of Medicine, Western Sydney University, Locked Bag 1797, Penrith, NSW 2751, Australia. [2]Affiliate Ingham Institute for Applied Medical Research, Centre for Applied Nursing Research (CANR), Liverpool, NSW 2170, Australia. [3]School of Nursing and Midwifery, Western Sydney University, Locked Bag 1797, Penrith, NSW 2751, Australia. [4]School of Medicine and Centre for Health Research, Western Sydney University, Locked Bag 1797, Penrith, NSW 2751, Australia.

References

1. Hay P, Girosi F, Mond J. Prevalence and sociodemographic correlates of DSM-5 eating disorders in the Australian population. J Eat Dis. 2015;3(April 25):19.
2. Hudson JI, et al. The prevalence and correlates of eating disorders in the National Comorbidity Survey Replication. Biol Psychiatry. 2007;61(3):348–58.
3. American Psychiatric Association. Diagnostic and statistical manual of mental disorders, DSM 5. Washington DC: American Psychiatric Publishing; 2013.
4. Swinbourne JM, Touyz SW. The co-morbidity of eating disorders and anxiety disorders: a review. Eur Eat Disord Rev. 2007;15:253–24.
5. Augustyn-Lawton S. Eating disorders: information for teens. 2nd ed. Detroit: Omnigraphics; 2009.
6. Costin C. The eating disorder sourcebook. New York: McGraw-Hill; 2007.
7. Glassman JN, et al. Menstrual dysfunction in bulimia. Ann Clin Psychiatry. 1991;3:161–5.
8. Tierney S, et al. Treading the tightrope between motherhood and an eating disorder: a qualitative study. Int J Nurs Stud. 2011;48(10):1223–33.
9. Easter A, et al. Recognising the symptoms: how common are eating disorders in pregnancy? Eur Eat Disord Rev. 2013;21(4):340–4.
10. Cardwell MS. Eating disorders and pregnancy. Obstet Gynecol Surv. 2013; 68(4):312–23.
11. Coker E, Abraham S. Body weight dissatisfaction before, during and after pregnancy: a comparison of women with and without eating disorders. Eat Weight Disord. 2015;20(1):71–9.
12. Koubaa S, Hällström T, Hirschberg AL. Early maternal adjustment in women with eating disorders. Int J Eat Disord. 2008;41:405–10.
13. Tierney S, McGlone C, Furber C. What can qualitative studies tell us about the experiences of women who are pregnant that have an eating disorder? Midwifery. 2013;29(5):542–9.
14. Lacey J, Smith G. Bulimia nervosa. The impact of pregnancy on mother and baby. Br J Psychiatry. 1987;150:777–81.
15. Ramchandani D, Whedon B. The effects of pregnancy on bulimia. Int J Eat Disord. 1988;7:845–8.
16. Bulik CM, et al. Patterns of remission, continuation and incidence of broadly defined eating disorders during early pregnancy in the Norwegian mother and child cohort study (MoBa). Psychol Med. 2007;37(08):1109–18.
17. Crow SJ, et al. Eating disorder symptoms in pregnancy: a prospective study. Int J Eat Disord. 2008;41(3):277–9.
18. Hollifield J, Hobdy J. The course of pregnancy complicated by bulimia. Psychother Theory Res Pract Train. 1990;27(2):249–55.
19. Micali N, Treasure J, Simonoff E. Eating disorders symptoms in pregnancy: a longitudinal study of women with recent and past eating disorders and obesity. J Psychosom Res. 2007;63(3):297–303.
20. Burton T, Hands B, Bulsara C. Metaphors used by women with eating disorders to describe their experience of being pregnant. Evidence Based Midwifery. 2015;13(4):126–31.
21. Mazzeo SE, et al. Associations among postpartum depression, eating disorders, and perfectionism in a population-based sample of adult women. Int J Eat Disord. 2006;39(3):202–11.
22. Abraham S, Taylor A, Conti J. Postnatal depression, eating, exercise, and vomiting before and during pregnancy. Int J Eat Disord. 2001;29(4):482–7.
23. Welch SL, Doll HA, Fairburn CG. Life events and the onet of bulimia nervosa: a controlled study. Psychol Med. 1997;27:515–22.
24. Ward VB. Eating disroders in pregnancy. Br Med J. 2008;336:93–6.
25. Morgan JF, Lacey JH, Sedgwick PM. Impact of pregnancy on bulimia nervosa. Br J Psychiatry. 1999;174:135–40.
26. Franko DL, Walton BE. Pregnancy and eating disorders: a review and clinical implications. Int J Eat Disord. 1993;13(1):41–8.
27. Patel P, et al. Concerns about body shape and weight in the *postpartum period and their relation to women's self-identification*. J Reprod Infant Psychol. 2005;23(4):347–64. 18p
28. Shaffer SE, Hunter LP, Anderson G. The experiences of pregnancy for women with a history of anorexia or bulimia nervosa. Canadian Journal of Midwifery Research and Practice. 2008;7:17–30.
29. Stapleton, H., Women with eating disorders: a study of their perceptions of childbearing and maternity services. International Nursing Link-Up, 2001; 7(20): p. 7–7 1p.
30. Larrson G, Anderson-Ellstron A. Experiences of pregnancy related body shape changes and of breastfeeding in women with a history of eating disorders. Eur Eat Disord Rev. 2003;11:116–24.
31. France EF, et al. A methodological systematic review of what's wrong with meta-ethnography reporting. BBMC Med Res. 2014;14(19):1–16.
32. Atkins S, et al. Conducting a meta-ethnography of qualitative literature: lessons learnt. BMC Med Res Methodol. 2008;8(1):21.
33. Noblit G, Hare R. Meta-ethnogaphy: synthesizinf qualitative research: a case of the tail waggin the dog? Newbury Park: Sage; 1988.

34. Tong A, et al. Enhancing transparency in reporting the synthesis of qualitative research: ENTREQ. BMC Med Res Methodol. 2012;12:181.

35. American Psychiatric Association. The diagnostic and statistical manual of mental disorders, vol. 2013. 5th ed. Washington: American Psychiatric Publishing; 2013.

36. Burton T. Walking a tightrope: women's experiences of having an eating disorder while pregnant. Aust Nurs Midwifery J. 2014;21(9):45.

37. Stringer E, et al. Pregnancy, motherhood and eating disorders: a qualitative study describing women's views of maternity care. Evidence Based Midwifery. 2010;8(4):112–21. 10p

38. Robb-Todter GE. Women's experience of weight and shape changes during pregnancy (Doctoral dissertation). University Of Vlirginia; 1996.

39. Stein A, Fairburn CG. Eating habits and attitudes in the postpartum period. Psychosom Med. 1996;58(4):321–5.

40. Abraham S, King W, Llewellyn-Jones D. Attitudes to body weight, weight gain and eating behavior in pregnancy. J Psychosom Obstet Gynaecol. 1994;15(4):189–95.

41. Gomez E. Eating Disorders and Pregnancy: A Theoretical Understanding of the Experience of Pregnancy for Women with Eating Disorders (Doctoral dissertation). ProQuest: Wright Institute; 2007.

42. Ambroz JR. Eating disorders and pregnancy. Midwifery Today Childbirth Educ. 1996;40:24–5.

43. Abraham SF, et al. Anorexia nervosa, pregnancy and XO/XX mosaicism. Med J Aust. 1981;1(11):582–3.

44. Seamans J. Experiences of pregnancy for women with eating disroders: A qualitative investigation (Doctoral dissertation). Lancaster University; 2004.

45. Hill BC. Eating Disorders and Pregnancy (Masters dissertation). University of Alberta; 1997.

46. Cooper D. Eating Disorders in Pregnancy (Masters dissertation). California State Univeristy; 1995.

47. Critical Appraisal Skills Program (CASP) Qualitative Research Checklist 31. 5.13. [cited 2014 22nd September]; Available from: http://www.casp-uk.net.

48. Jones ML. Application of systematic review methods to qualitative research: practical issues. J Adv Nurs. 2004;48(3):271–8.

49. Taborelli E, et al. Transition to motherhood in women with eating disorders: a qualitative study. Psychol Psychother. 2015; [Epub ahead of print]

50. Namer S, Melman KN, Yager J. Pregnancy in Restriter-type anorexia nervosa: a study of six women. Int J Eat Disord. 1986;5(5):837–45.

51. Hale A, Rieger E, Russell J. A qualitative investigation into the relationship between stress and eating disordered behaviours in patients with anorexia nervosa. J Eat Disord. 2014;2(1):1–1.

52. Little L, Lowkes E. Critical issues in the care of pregnant women with eating disorders and the impact on their children. J Midwifery Womens Health. 2000;45(4):301–7.

53. Lewis L, le Grange D. The experience and impact of pregnancy in bulimia nervosa: a series of case studies. Eur Eat Disord Rev. 1994;2(2):93–105.

54. Stapleton H, Fielder A, Kirkham M. Breast or bottle? Eating disordered childbearing women and infant-feeding decisions. Matern Child Nutr. 2008; 4(2):106–20.

55. Willis DC, Rand CS. Pregnancy in bulimic women. Obstet Gynecol. 1988; 71(5):708–10.

56. Myors KA, et al. Engaging women at risk for poor perinatal mental health outcomes: a mixed-methods study. Int J Ment Health Nurs. 2015;24(3):241–52.

57. Coker EL, Mitchell-Wong LA, Abraham SF. Is pregnancy a trigger for recovery from an eating disorder? Acta Obstet Gynecol Scand. 2013;92(12):1407–13.

58. Vandereycken W, Van Humbeeck I. Denial and concealment of eating disorders: a retrospective survey. Eur Eat Disorders Rev. 2008;16:109–14.

59. Thompson C, Park S. Barriers to access and utilization of eating disorder treatment among women. Archives of Women's Mental Health. 2016;19(5):753–60.

60. Mond JM. Eating disorders "mental health literacy": an introduction. J Ment Health. 2014;23(2):51–4.

61. Rollans M, et al. We just ask some questions…' the process of antenatal psychosocial assessment by midwives. In: Midwifery; 2012.

62. Rollans M, et al. Digging over that old ground: an Australian perspective of women's experience of psychosocial assessment and depression screening in pregnancy and following birth. BMC Womens Health. 2013;13(1):18.

63. Toye F, et al. Meta-ethnography 25 years on: challenges and insights for synthesising a large number of qualitative studies. BMC Med Res Methodol. 2014;14(1):80.

8

Development of a melting-curve based multiplex real-time PCR assay for simultaneous detection of *Streptococcus agalactiae* and genes encoding resistance to macrolides and lincosamides

Eliane Saori Otaguiri[1], Ana Elisa Belotto Morguette[1], Alexandre Tadachi Morey[1], Eliandro Reis Tavares[1], Gilselena Kerbauy[2], Rosângela S. L. de Almeida Torres[3], Mauricio Chaves Júnior[4], Maria Cristina Bronharo Tognim[5], Viviane Monteiro Góes[6], Marco Aurélio Krieger[6], Marcia Regina Eches Perugini[7], Lucy Megumi Yamauchi[1] and Sueli Fumie Yamada-Ogatta[1,8]*

Abstract

Background: *Streptococcus agalactiae* or Group B *Streptococcus* (GBS) remains the leading cause of infections in newborns worldwilde. Prenatal GBS screening of pregnant women for vaginal-rectal colonization is recommended in many countries to manage appropriate intrapartum antimicrobial prophylaxis for those identified as carriers. In this study, a novel melting-curve based multiplex real-time PCR assay for the simultaneous detection of GBS and macrolide and lincosamide resistance markers was developed. The usefulness of the assay was evaluated for rapid and accurate prenatal GBS screening.

Methods: One hundred two pregnant women who were at 35–37 weeks of gestation were enrolled in this study. The analytical performance of the multiplex real-time PCR was first tested using a panel of reference and clinical bacterial and fungal strains. To test the clinical performance, vaginal-rectal swabs were obtained from pregnant women who were seen at the teaching hospital for regular prenatal care. The results of real-time were compared with those obtained from microbiological analyses.

Results: The real-time PCR assay showed 100% specificity and a limit of detection of 10^4 colony forming units equivalent per reaction. The prevalence of GBS colonization among the population studied was 15.7% (16/102) based on a positive culture and the real-time PCR results. Agreement between the two assays was found for 11 (68.75%) GBS colonized women. Using the culture-based results as a reference, the multiplex real-time PCR had a sensitivity of 91.7% (11/12, CI 59.7–99.6%), a specificity of 95.5% (86/90, CI 89.8–98.7%), a positive predictive value of 73.3% (11/15, CI 44.8–91.1%) and a negative predictive value of 98.9% (86/87, CI 92.9–99.9%).

(Continued on next page)

* Correspondence: ogatta@uel.br
[1]Departamento de Microbiologia, Centro de Ciências Biológicas,
Universidade Estadual de Londrina, Londrina, Paraná, Brazil
[8]Departamento de Microbiologia, Universidade Estadual de Londrina, Centro
de Ciências Biológicas, Rodovia Celso Garcia Cid, PR 445, km 380. CEP,
Londrina 86057-970, Brazil
Full list of author information is available at the end of the article

(Continued from previous page)

Conclusion: The multiplex real-time PCR is a rapid, affordable and sensitive assay for direct detection of GBS in vaginal-rectal swabs.

Keywords: *cfb* gene, *erm* and *mef* antimicrobial resistance markers, Group B *Streptococcus*, Melting curve, Pregnant women; vaginal-rectal swab

Background

Streptococcus agalactiae or Group B *Streptococcus* (GBS) is a leading cause of infections in newborns worldwide [1, 2]. Neonatal GBS diseases are associated with significant morbidity and mortality, and infants who survive may incur long-term disabilities [3, 4]. GBS can asymptomatically colonize the human gastrointestinal and/or genital tract [5–7]. During pregnancy, this colonization represents the most important risk factor for the development of invasive GBS diseases, most of which affect babies within the first week of life [8]. Maternal GBS transmission to the newborn may occur vertically by ascending infection or during passage through the birth canal [9].

Women can be transiently, intermittently or persistently colonized by GBS in their vaginal or anorectal mucosae [6]. Accordingly, the risk of maternal GBS transmission to the newborn and development of infection persists. The prevention strategy based on bacterium screening and intrapartum antimicrobial prophylaxis (IAP) in those pregnant women identified as carriers has led to a substantial reduction in the incidence of neonatal GBS diseases in various regions of the world [10]. Currently penicillin is recommended as first-line antibacterial for IAP, and clindamycin or erythromycin (second line) may be used in penicillin-allergic pregnant women at risk of anaphylaxis [8]. In general, GBS isolates remain susceptible to penicillin [5, 11] however isolates with reduced susceptibility to this antibacterial have been reported [12]. In contrast, resistance to clindamycin and erythromycin among GBS isolated from pregnant women is increasing in different regions of the world [5, 11, 13, 14]. The most common antimicrobial resistance mechanisms are post-transcriptional methylation of adenine residues present in 23S rRNA, which is mediated by *erm* class gene-encoded methylases [15, 16], and efflux of the antibiotic mediated by a membrane-bound protein encoded by *mef* genes [17]. The expression of *erm* genes usually results in cross-resistance to macrolides, lincosamides and streptogramin B, the MLS_B phenotype [18]. On the other hand, resistance encoded by *mef* genes (phenotype M) confers resistance only to 14- and 15-membered ring macrolides (erythromycin and azithromycin) [19].

Standard culture-based methods for GBS detection involve the inoculation of a vaginal-rectal swab specimen into selective enrichment broth medium. Following enrichment, the specimen is subcultured on blood agar plates or alternatively on chromogenic Granada agar for visual detection of beta-hemolytic or orange carotenoid pigment-producing colonies, respectively. The identification of presumptive GBS colonies is performed by phenotypic methods. Moreover, it is also recommended that GBS isolated from penicillin-allergic pregnant women at risk of anaphylaxis should be screened for antimicrobial susceptibility pattern [8]. Corroborating this, a study of Desai and colleagues [20] reported that 8.8% of GBS-positive pregnant women also had a penicillin allergy at delivery.

In general, these procedures may require up to 72 h for results, which does not impact pregnant women undergoing routine prenatal care. However, many cases of GBS diseases have been reported in newborns from mothers with negative prenatal bacterial screen [21, 22]. These false-negative results may be due to limitations of the current culture methods that cannot promptly detect either non-hemolytic nor non-pigment producing isolates [23]. In addition, a small proportion of pregnant women may become colonized with GBS in the period following prenatal screening and the onset of labor [24]. Another concern associated with culture-based strategies is the unavailability of results for pregnant women in premature labor or who have not had prenatal care [25].

There is a need for a rapid and sensitive test for detecting GBS-colonized pregnant women at the time of delivery, and determining GBS antibacterial resistance to manage appropriate IAP. The aim of this study was to develop a melting curve-based multiplex real-time polymerase chain reaction (PCR) assay for simultaneous detection of GBS and macrolide and lincosamide resistance markers. The assay targets the *cfb* gene used for specific identification of GBS and *erm* and *mef* genes. The *cfb* gene encodes an extracellular pore-forming protein [26] known as CAMP (acronym for Christie, Atkins and Munch-Peterson) factor [27], which has been widely used for phenotypic identification of GBS isolates [28]. Furthermore, most nucleic acid amplification tests (including commercially available ones) target *cfb* gene for detection of GBS vaginal-rectal colonization [29]. The potential usefulness of the assay was evaluated for prenatal GBS screening in vaginal-rectal swab specimens. The results of the multiplex real-time PCR assay were compared with those obtained with culture-based analyses.

Methods

Microbial strains

A panel of 37 microbial species (27 bacteria and 10 fungi, Table 1) was used to develop the assays. These included various streptococcal and closed-related species and other microbial components of the intestinal and genital microbiota. Two species of *Cryptococcus* were also included. Reference strains were kindly donated by Instituto Oswaldo Cruz (FIOCRUZ, Rio de Janeiro, Brazil) and Laboratório Central do Paraná (LACEN, Paraná, Brazil). LMC and HU strains were obtained from the bacterial collection of the Laboratório de Microbiologia Clínica of the Universidade Estadual de Londrina (UEL); LBBA strains were obtained from the Laboratório de Bacteriologia Básica e Aplicada of UEL. Bacterial and fungal species were cultivated at 37 °C for 24 h in tryptic soy broth (TSB, Oxoid) and Sabouraud dextrose broth (SDB, Himedia), respectively. Bacteria and fungi were kept at – 20 °C in TSB containing 20% glycerol and 5% sheep blood and SDB containing 20% glycerol, respectively.

DNA isolation from in vitro cultured microbial species

The Gentra Puregene Blood kit (Qiagen, Brazil) was used for DNA isolation, according to manufacturer's recommendations. All clinical and reference strains were cultivated in specific broth medium at 37 °C for 24 h. Microbial cultures were centrifuged at 10,000 x *g* for 5 min, and the pellets were washed twice with sterile 0. 15 M phosphate-buffered saline (PBS) pH 7.2 before DNA extraction.

Oligonucleotide primers and PCR design

The nucleotide sequences of *cfb* encoding genes from *S. agalactiae* deposited in the GenBank/EMBL databases were analyzed using the *BioEdit v.7.2.0* software. Specific primers were designed using a consensus sequence and the OligoAnalyzer 3.1 (http://www.idtdna.com/calc/analyzer) tool. Primers for genes [*erm*(A) subclass of *erm*(TR)], *erm*(B) and *mef*(A/E) encoding erythromycin and clindamycin resistance were as described previously [5]. Primers targeting the human tRNA processing ribonuclease P (*RNAseP*) gene [30, 31] and intergenic spacer

Table 1 Panel of microorganisms used to evaluate the multiplex real-time PCR specificity and sensitivity

Species	Source	Species	Source
Streptococcus agalactiae	ATCC 13813	*Escherichia coli*	ATCC 25922
Streptococcus agalactiae	LMC UEL 15	*Escherichia coli*	ATCC 35218
Streptococcus agalactiae	LMC UEL 65	*Klebsiella pneumoniae*	ATCC 700603
Streptococcus agalactiae	LMC UEL 66	*Proteus mirabilis*	HU-UEL
Streptococcus agalactiae serotype Ia	LMC UEL 43	*Providencia stuartii*	HU-UEL
Streptococcus agalactiae serotype II	LMC UEL 92	*Salmonella* sp.	HU-UEL
Streptococcus agalactiae serotype III	LMC UEL 59	*Shigella dysenteriae*	ATCC 13313
Streptococcus agalactiae serotype V	LMC UEL 73	*Enterococcus faecalis*	ATCC 29212
Streptococcus agalactiae serotype IX	LMC UEL 11	*Enterococcus faecium*	ATCC 6569
Streptococcus dysgalactiae subsp. *equisimilis* group G.	LACEN 6196	*Lactobacillus acidophilus*	ATCC 4356
Streptococcus dysgalactiae subsp. *equisimilis* group C	LACEN 53157	*Lactobacillus rhamnosus*	LBBA-UEL
Streptococcus mitis	ATCC 49456	*Lactococcus lactis* subsp. *lactis*	LBBA-UEL 22
Streptococcus mutans	ATCC 25175	*Lactococcus lactis* subsp. *cremoris*	LBBA-UEL 22–1
Streptococcus pneumoniae	ATCC 49619	*Leuconostoc mesenteroides*	LBBA-UEL 704
Streptococcus pyogenes	ATCC 19615	*Candida albicans*	ATCC 26790
Streptococcus sanguis	ATCC10557	*Candida bracarensis*	LMC UEL1217
Staphylococcus aureus	ATCC 25923	*Candida dubliniensis*	LMC UEL 947C
Staphylococcus epidermidis	ATCC 12228	*Candida glabrata*	LMC UEL 51B
Staphylococcus haemolyticus	ATCC 29668	*Candida metapsilosis*	LMC UEL 2263
Staphylococcus saprophyticus	HU-UEL	*Candida orthopsilosis*	LMC UEL 2259
Bacillus subtilis	ATCC 23857	*Candida parapsilosis*	ATCC 22019
Aeromonas sp.	HU-UEL	*Candida tropicalis*	ATCC 28707
Pseudomonas aeruginosa	ATCC 27853	*Cryptococcus gattii*	ATCC 56990
Citrobacter freundii	HU-UEL	*Cryptococcus neoformans*	ATCC 66031

ATCC American Type Culture Collection, *LMC* Laboratório de Microbiologia Clínica, *UEL* Universidade Estadual de Londrina, *LACEN* Laboratório Central do Estado do Paraná, *HU* Hospital Universitário de Londrina, *LBBA* Laboratório de Bacteriologia Básica e Aplicada

1 (IGS1) of ribosomal RNA (rDNA) gene cluster of the *Cryptococcus gattii* [32], an encapsulated yeast found in the environment, were included in this study to evaluate the quality of the DNA and potential PCR interfering substances, respectively.

The primer sequences and expected size of amplicons are shown in Table 2. All primers were used in conventional PCR in a final volume of 25 µL containing 20 mM Tris-HCl, pH 8.4, 5 mM KCl, 1.5 mM MgCl$_2$, 100 µM of each dNTP, 10 $p$mol of each forward and reverse primer, 2.5 U *Taq* DNA polymerase (Invitrogen, São Paulo, Brazil), and 2 µL of genomic DNA. The amplification reactions were performed in a Veriti 96-well Thermal Cycler (Applied Biosystems) with an initial denaturation at 95 °C for 1 min, followed by 35 cycles of 95 °C for 30 s, annealing at 67 °C for 1 min and an extension step at 72 °C for 45 s. Negative template control (NTC) reactions without any template DNA were carried out simultaneously. Amplicons were analyzed by 3% agarose gel electrophoresis after DNA staining with 0.5 µg/mL ethidium bromide. The identity of the amplicons was confirmed after determination of the nucleotide sequences with a 3730 xl DNA Analyzer (Applied Biosystems) using the Big Dye Terminator v.3.1 Cycle Sequencing Kit. Search for homologies in the GenBank/EMBL databases was carried out with the Blast algorithm.

Multiplex real-time PCR assay

All PCRs were performed on a Rotor-Gene Q 5-Plex (Qiagen, Germany), and the assay conditions were optimized for various parameters, including concentration of each primer set, annealing temperature and number of PCR cycles (data not shown). The optimized assay was performed in two separate tubes each containing a final volume of 25 µL: a) 2× High-Resolution Melt (HRM) PCR Master Mix (Qiagen, Brazil), 10 $p$mol of forward and reverse *erm*(B), *cfb* and IGS1 primer sets, 20 $p$mol of forward and reverse *mef*(A/E) primers, and 10 ng of recombinant plasmid pCR2.1/IGS1 [32]; b) 2× HRM PCR Master Mix and 10 $p$mol of forward and reverse *erm*(A) and human *RNAseP* primers. For both reaction mixtures, 6 µL of template DNA were added and the final volume was adjusted with deionized water. The cycling conditions included an initial denaturation step at 95 °C for 5 min, followed by 35 cycles of 95 °C for 10 s, annealing at 67 °C for 30 s and an extension step at 72 °C for 20 s. Melting curves were acquired using 0.05 °C steps with a hold of 60 s at each step from 75 to 85 °C. NTC reactions were carried out simultaneously. Data were analyzed using Rotor Gene software version.

Analytical specificity and sensitivity

Multiplex real-time PCR specificity was analyzed using 100 ng genomic DNA obtained from cultures of a panel of bacteria and fungi (Table 1). All amplification reactions were performed in duplicate in three independent experiments. In silico analysis was also carried out to determine the specificity of the *cfb* amplification reactions. Primer sequences targeting the *cfb* gene were compared with nucleotide sequences available in GenBank databases of the National Center for Biotechnology Information (NCBI, http://www.ncbi.nlm.nih.gov) using the Blast algorithm (*blastn*).

Multiplex real-time PCR sensitivity was determined empirically using macrolide and lincosamide resistant GBS strains (LMC UEL 15 *cfb*$^+$, *mef*(A/E)$^+$; LMC UEL

Table 2 Oligonucleotide primers of melting curve-based multiplex real-time PCR

Target[a]	Nucleotide sequence (5′ to 3′)	Amplicon size (bp)	Reference
cfb[b]	F: CACACATGCTGTTGGAGTTCAGTTGA	138	This study
	R: ACGAAGTCGACAGCATCACACGAAA		
erm(A)/(TR)	F: CCGGCAAGGAGAAGGTTATAATGA	190	Otaguiri et al. [5]
	R: GCATTCACCCGTTGACTCATTTCC		
erm(B)	F: GCTCTTGCACACTCAAGTCTCGAT	117	Otaguiri et al. [5]
	R: ACATCTGTGGTATGGCGGGTAAGT		
mef(A/E)	F: GCGATGGTCTTGTCTATGGCTTCA	225	Otaguiri et al. [5]
	R: AGCTGTTCCAATGCTACGGAT		
RNaseP	F: AGATTTGGACCTGCGAGCG	64	WHO [27]
	R: GAGCGGCTGTCTCCACAAGT		
IGS1	F: GTCATTTCAGCTGGCGCCATCGATAC	260	Tavares et al. [32]
	R: TTGCCGCATAACGCATCTTAGCCA		

[a]*cfb* gene encodes the CAMP factor; *erm* genes encode 23S rRNA methylases; *mef* gene encodes efflux pumps; *RNaseP* gene encodes human ribonuclease P; IGS1, intergenic spacer 1 of ribosomal RNA gene cluster of *Cryptococcus gattii*. [b]The nucleotide sequences of *Streptococcus agalactiae* genes deposited in the GenBank/EMBL databases were used for specific primer design

65 *cfb*[+], *erm*(A)[+]; LMC UEL 66 *cfb*[+], *erm*(B)[+]), according to published recommendations [33]. Three colonies forming unit (CFU) of each GBS strains were cultivated in TSB at 37 °C for 24 h. The bacterial cells were harvested by centrifugation (10,000 x *g* for 5 min), washed twice with sterile PBS and the cell density was adjusted to 9.0×10^8 (3.0 McFarland standard) using the DensiCHECK™ PLUS colorimeter (bioMérieux, Brazil) in 1.0 mL of the same buffer. DNA extraction was performed as above. Each strain was processed in duplicate on five consecutive days. Tenfold serial dilutions were prepared and 6 μL of DNA template of each dilution were included in amplification reactions. For each primer pair, a standard curve was generated from the Ct values as a function of log CFU and R^2 was calculated to evaluate the efficiency of the reaction. The slope of this line was used to determine the efficiency (E) according to the equation: $E = 10^{-1/\text{slope}} - 1$.

Performance of the multiplex real-time PCR assay in clinical samples in comparison to culture based analysis

The performance of real-time PCR in GBS isolates and clinical samples was compared with the results obtained from microbiological analyses. Thirty one GBS isolates recovered from the vaginal-rectal swab screening cultures of women seen at University Hospital of Londrina, Paraná, Brazil from March to September of 2012 [5] were analyzed by the multiplex real-time PCR assay. These isolates were taken from the bacterial collection of the Laboratory of Clinical Microbiology of Universidade Estadual de Londrina and were processed as described below. For direct analysis, a total of 102 pregnant women seen at the UniversityHospital of Londrina, Paraná, Brazil from June to December 2015, and October 2017 were enrolled in this study. The study protocol was approved by the Ethics Committee of the Universidade Estadual de Londrina (Document 193/12-CEP/UEL). Written informed consent was obtained from the women to participate in this study, agreeing with the publication of this report and any accompanying images. Two vaginal-rectal swabs of each woman were collected. Sampling was performed on the lower third of the vagina followed by the rectum using the COPAN Transystem Stuart collection device (COPAN Diagnostic, Italy).

One swab specimen was inoculated into a Granada Biphasic broth (BioMérieux, Brazil) and incubated at 37 °C for 24 h. After incubation, the sample was subcultured on Columbia blood agar base (Oxoid, Brazil) containing 5% sheep blood (Newprov, Brazil) at 37 °C for 24 h. Suggestive colonies of GBS were subjected to standard phenotypic identification based on colony morphology, Gram staining, catalase and CAMP tests. Concomitantly, tests for growth in 6.5% NaCl, bile-esculin reaction, sodium hippurate hydrolysis, and susceptibility

to bacitracin and sulfamethoxazole *plus* trimethoprim were also performed. Bacteria were kept at – 20 °C in TSB containing 20% glycerol and 5% sheep blood. The second swab was vortexed for 2 min in 1 mL of deionized sterile water, the suspension was centrifuged and the pellet was used for DNA extraction as described above. DNA was stored at – 20 °C until use.

GBS isolates were tested for penicillin, clindamycin and erythromycin susceptibility using the disk-diffusion method according to the recommendations of the Clinical Laboratory Standards Institute [34]. The phenotypes of erythromycin- and clindamycin-resistant GBSs were determined by the double-disk diffusion method as described by Seppala et al. [35].

Results
Assay design

In this study, a multiplex-PCR assay using real-time and melting curves was standardized for simultaneous detection of the genes *cfb*, *erm*(A), *erm*(B), and *mef*(A/B). The conditions of amplification for simultaneous detection of these genes were first standardized in conventional monoplex PCR using genomic DNA of GBS strains. All specific primer pairs generated amplicons with the expected size shown in Table 2 using an annealing temperature of 67 °C. The identity of each amplicon was further confirmed by sequencing and searching for nucleotide sequence homology in the GenBank/EMBL databases. After determining the optimal conditions for amplification, all primer pairs were combined in a conventional multiplex-PCR format and the results are shown in Fig. 1. For establishment of melting-curve based multiplex real-time PCR, equivalent melting temperatures (T_m) of each primer pair were initially detected in a monoplex real-time PCR assay. All primer pairs successfully amplified the corresponding genes generating a dissociation curve with a single peak, and the T_m values of all amplicons were as follows: 76.7 ± 0. 4 °C for *cfb*, 75.5 ± 0.5 °C for *erm*(A), 78.8 ± 0.7 °C for *erm*(B), 80.65 ± 0.55 °C for *mef*(A/E) (Fig. 2). In addition, T_m values of 82.8 ± 0.55 °C and 81.8 ± 0.21 °C were detected for *RNaseP* gene and IGS1 region, respectively (Additional file 1: Figure S1A-B). According to these data, the multiplex real-time PCR assay was performed with two tubes in one reaction. One tube corresponded to the targets *cfb*, *erm*(B), *mef*(A/E) genes, IGS1 region and recombinant plasmid pCR2.1/IGS1, and the other to the targets *erm*(A) and *RNaseP* genes.

Analytical performance

The specificity of multiplex real-time PCR was determined using genomic DNA from a panel of bacteria and fungi (Table 1), and amplification signals were detected for all GBS strains, including five different capsular

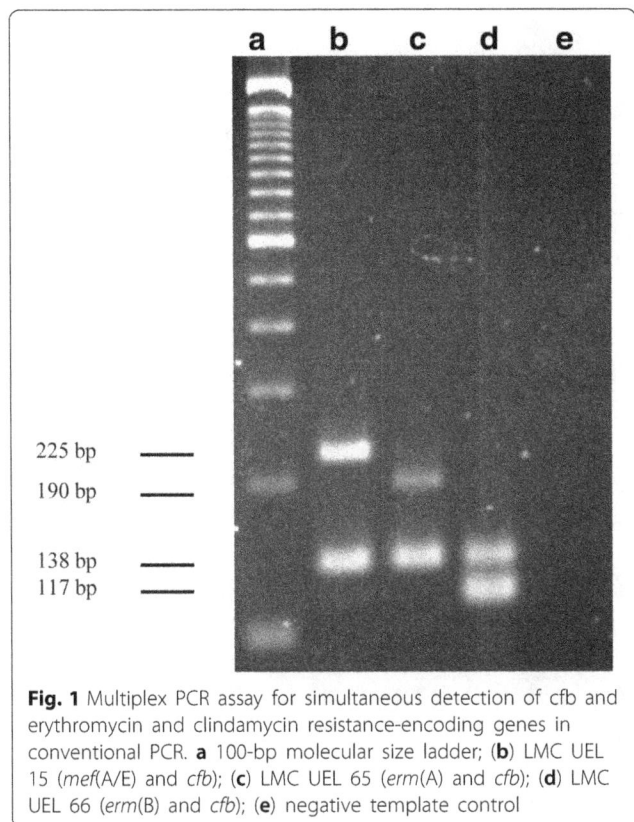

Fig. 1 Multiplex PCR assay for simultaneous detection of cfb and erythromycin and clindamycin resistance-encoding genes in conventional PCR. **a** 100-bp molecular size ladder; (**b**) LMC UEL 15 (*mef*(A/E) and *cfb*); (**c**) LMC UEL 65 (*erm*(A) and *cfb*); (**d**) LMC UEL 66 (*erm*(B) and *cfb*); (**e**) negative template control

serotypes. No cross-reactivity was observed between non-GBS strains. Primer specificity for the *cfb* gene was also evaluated in silico using the GenBank/EMBL database of the NCBI homepage, and no matches were found other than those with the corresponding gene of GBS.

The linearity and limits of detection (LOD) of the multiplex real-time PCR for the target DNAs were determined with tenfold serial dilutions (at a cell density of 10^7 to 10 CFU equivalents per reaction) of each genomic DNA from macrolide- and lincosamide-resistant GBS strains. Each concentration was analyzed in 6 replicates on five different days ($n = 30$). The LOD of the multiplex real-time PCR for the target DNAs was 10^4 CFU equivalents per reaction, and the reaction efficiencies calculated from the slope of the standard curve were within the range of 94 to 100% (Fig. 3).

To further verify the specific performance of the assay, genomic DNA extracted from 31 GBS isolates from the bacterial collection were analyzed by the multiplex real-time PCR. The results showed 100% concordance with those obtained previously by Otaguiri et al. [5]. All isolates were positive for *cfb* gene and the erythromycin and lincosamide resistance markers were detected in three isolates: one isolate each carried the *mef*(A/E); *erm*(B); and *erm*(A) and *erm*(B) genes.

Evaluation of real-time multiplex PCR in clinical samples

Performance of the multiplex real-time PCR assay was analyzed in vaginal-rectal swabs obtained from 102 pregnant women, and the results were compared to the standard culture-based method for GBS detection. *RNaseP* and IGS1 amplification signals were detected in all reactions, indicating no PCR inhibitors (Additional file 1: Figure S1A-B). NTC amplification signals were not detected in any specific PCR. The prevalence of GBS colonization among the population studied was 15.7% (16/102) based on a positive culture and the multiplex real-time PCR results. Agreement between the two assays was found for 11 (68.75%) GBS-colonized women. Four samples (25%) were positive by multiplex real-time PCR and negative by the culture method, and one (6.25%) was negative by multiplex real-time PCR and positive by the culture method.

Using the culture-based results as a reference, the multiplex real-time PCR had a sensitivity of 91.7% (11/ 12, CI 59.7–99.5%), a specificity of 95.5% (86/90, CI 88. 4–98.6%), a positive predictive value of 73.3% (11/15, CI 44.8–91.1%) and a negative predictive value of 98.9% (86/87, CI 92.9–99.9%) (Table 3).

All GBS isolates were susceptible to penicillin according to the disk-diffusion method. Regarding the erythromycin and clindamycin susceptibility profile, of the 11 GBS-positive isolates by the culture method, 10 were susceptible and one was resistant to both antibacterials according to the phenotypic methods. Of the four vaginal-rectal swabs testing positive for GBS by multiplex real-time PCR, one was negative for antimicrobial resistance markers, two tested positive for *erm*(B) and *mef*(A/E) genes, and the other tested positive for *mef*(A/E) genes.

For the comparison analysis, the GBS-colonized pregnant women whose *cfb* gene was not detected by multiplex real-time PCR or tested negative in culture approaches were excluded from the comparative analysis. The phenotypic results were in accordance with those obtained in real-time multiplex PCR for nine GBS-colonized pregnant women. No antimicrobial resistance marker was detected in seven susceptible isolates. One erythromycin/clindamycin-resistant isolate displayed the constitutive macrolide-lincosamide-streptogramin B (cMLS$_B$) phenotype, and carried the *erm*(A) and *erm*(B) genes. Whereas, one erythromycin-resistant isolate carried the *mef*(A/E) gene. In the discordant results, two pregnant women colonized with erythromycin/clindamycin susceptible isolates, one tested positive for *erm*(A) and *mef*(A/E) and the other for *erm*(B) genes by the multiplex real-time PCR assay (Table 4).

All GBS isolates were subjected to re-examination using genomic DNA extracted from axenic cultures and there was no difference between the concordant results. For the above mentioned two discrepant results, the

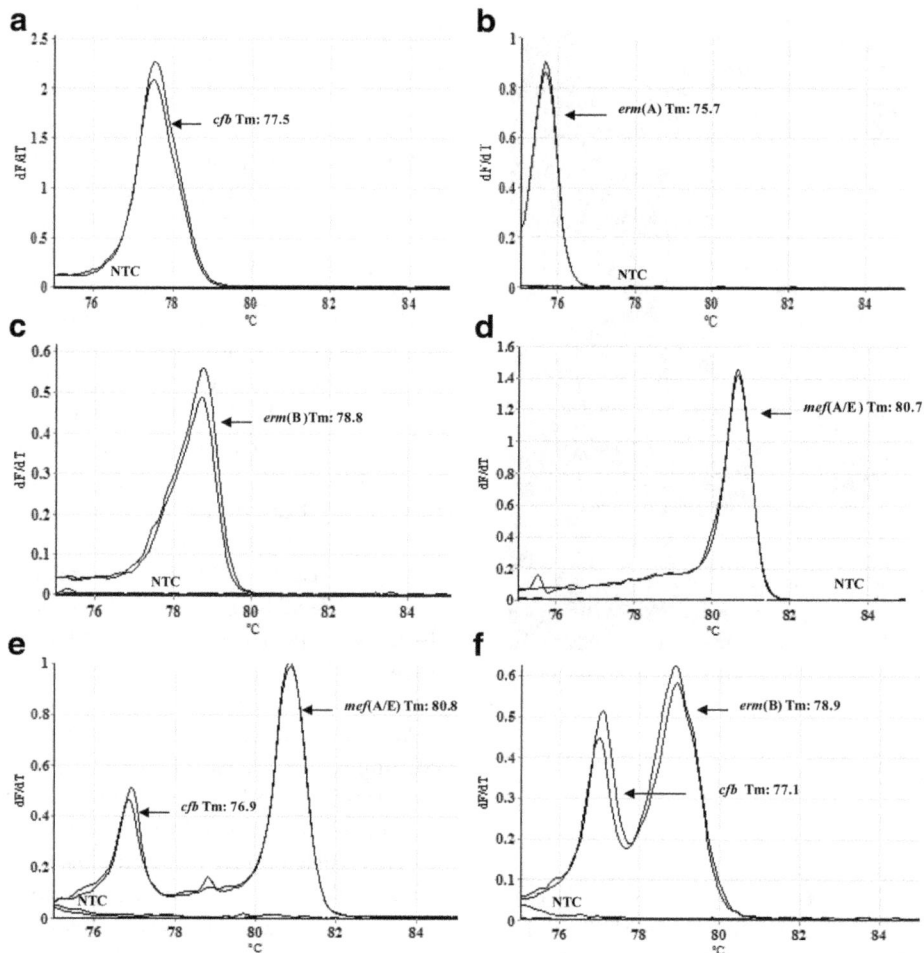

Fig. 2 Melting curve analysis showing the melting temperature peaks (Tm) of *Streptococcus agalactiae* with macrolide and lincosamide resistance genes and negative template controls (NTC). **a** LMC UEL 65 (*cfb*); (**b**) LMC UEL 65 [*erm*(A)]; (**c**) LMC UEL 66 [*erm*(B)]; (**d**) LMC UEL 15 [*mef*(A/E)]; (**e**) LMC UEL 15 [*cfb* and *mef*(A/E)]; (**f**) LMC UEL 66 [*cfb* and *erm*(B)]

erm(A), *erm*(B) and *mef*(A/E) genes were not detected by multiplex real-time PCR, confirming the phenotypic results, and indicating the presence of other bacteria carrying the detected genes in the vaginal-rectal swab sample.

Discussion

Real-time PCR is one of the rapid and feasible methods for maternal intrapartum GBS screening, and most of the in house and commercial tests are based on the utilization of probes [29, 36–41]. In this study, a sensitive melting curve-based multiplex real-time PCR was designed and evaluated for simultaneous detection of GBS and the most prevalent macrolide and lincosamide resistance markers. According to the literature, only the study of Dela Cruz et al. [42] reported an assay for simultaneous detection of GBS and antimicrobial resistance markers. These authors developed a probe-based real-time multiplex PCR for

detection of *cfb*, *erm*(TR), *erm*(B) and *mef*(A/E) genes in genomic DNA extracted from GBS cultures isolated from vaginal-rectal swabs, with a sensitivity of 93% and specificity of 90%.

The analytical and experimental data showed that the primers designed, in this study, to target the GBS *cfb* gene did not cross-react with another nucleotide sequence of different microbial species. One GBS-colonized pregnant woman was falsely identified as a non-GBS carrier by multiplex real-time PCR. In this case, the presence of PCR inhibitors was discarded since the amplification signals of the *RNaseP* and IGS1 controls were detected in the reaction. Thus, this result could be explained by the low bacterial load on the swab, which was below the LOD of the assay. Similarly, other real-time PCR-based assays for GBS detection have shown discrepant results when compared to culture-based approach [43], including those marketed tests [36].

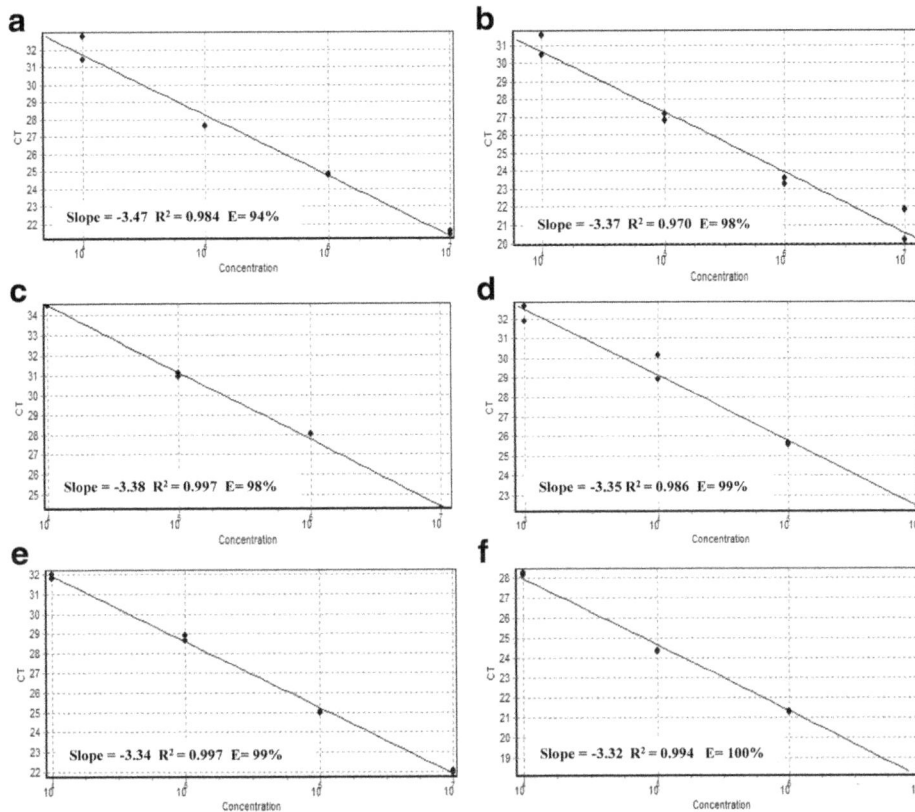

Fig. 3 Sensitivity of multiplex real-time PCR assays. **a** LMC UEL 65 (*cfb*); (**b**) LMC UEL 65 [*erm*(A)]; (C) LMC UEL 66 [*erm*(B)]; (**d**) LMC UEL 15 [*mef*(A/E)]; (**e**) LMC UEL 15 [*cfb* and *mef*(A/E)]; (**f**) LMC UEL 66 [*cfb* and *erm*(B)]. Amplification plot of 10-fold serial dilution corresponding to 10^4–10^7 CFU; standard curve represented by linear regression line for threshold cycle (Ct) versus sample log concentration. Slope, regression coefficient and efficiency of the real-time PCR method are noted (**a-f**)

Several real-time PCR-based assays have been developed in the last decades for GBS detection in vaginal-rectal swab from pregnant women [29, 36–41]. Most of these studies target the *cfb* gene for specific detection of GBS [8, 29, 37]. However, the following genes were also used for GBS detection by real-time PCR assays: those of the operon *dlt* [37, 38], which catalyze the

Table 3 Sensitivity, specificity, positive predictive value (PPV) and negative predictive value (NPV)

Multiplex real-time PCR	Culture[a]		Total
	Positive	Negative	
Positive	11	4	15
Negative	1	86	87
Total	12	90	102
Sensitivity (95% CI)[b]	91.7% (59.7–99.5%)		
Specificity (95% CI)[b]	95.5% (88.4–98.6%)		
PPV (95% CI)[b]	73.3% (44.8–91.1%)		
NPV (95% CI)[b]	98.9% (92.9–99.9%)		

[a]Standard routine culture of vaginal-rectal swab specimen collected from pregnant women at 35–37 weeks of gestation; [b]Values calculated with 95% confidence interval (CI) using the program available at http://faculty.vassar.edu/lowry/clin1.html

incorporation of D-alanine residues into GBS cell wall lipoteichoic acids [44]; *cyl*B [39], which encodes a transmembrane protein of ABC transporter required for the production of GBS hemolysin [45]; *ssr*A [40], encoding tmRNA involved in the degradation of truncated proteins [46]; and *sip* [41], encoding a surface immunogenic protein [47].

The timely direct detection of resistance genes in GBS from pregnant women will contribute to prompt and appropriate administration of antimicrobial during the intrapartum period. In addition, the IAP for prevention of GBS neonatal infections has raised worries about the selection of antimicrobial resistant and/or potentially more virulent microorganisms for newborns [10]. Since the *erm* genes are located mainly on mobile genetic elements such as plasmids and conjugative transposons [16, 48], selective pressure imposed by the antimicrobials may trigger horizontal DNA transfer between microbiota members, contributing to the spread of resistance. Thus, besides reliable GBS detection, the determination of its antimicrobial susceptibilities is important to implement effective IAP for all GBS-colonized pregnant women, thereby preventing inappropriate use of antimicrobials.

Table 4 Data from phenotypic characterization and multiplex real-time PCR of *Streptococcus agalactiae*

Isolates	Susceptibility phenotype		Real-time multiplex PCR			
	E[a]	DA[b]	*cfb*[c]	*erm*(A)[c]	*erm*(B)[c]	*mef*(A/E)[c]
LMC UEL 5	S	S	+	−	−	−
LMC UEL 21	S	S	+	−	−	−
LMC UEL 23	S	S	+	−	+	−
LMC UEL 27	S	S	+	−	−	−
LMC UEL 30	S	S	+	−	−	−
LMC UEL 34	S	S	+	−	−	−
LMC UEL 43	S	S	+	−	−	−
LMC UEL 43A	R	R	+	+	+	−
LMC UEL 57	S	S	+	+	−	+
LMC UEL 60	S	S	+	−	−	−
LMC UEL 68	S	S	−	−	−	−
LMC UEL 103	R	S	+	−	−	+
LMC UEL 28	CN	CN	+	−	−	−
LMC UEL 63	CN	CN	+	−	+	+
LMC UEL 95	CN	CN	+	−	−	+
LMC UEL 99	CN	CN	+	−	+	+

[a]E (erythromycin) and [b]DA (clindamycin) resistance phenotypes were determined by the double-disk diffusion method [34]. (S) Susceptible; (R) Resistant; (CN) Culture-Negative. [c]Target genes detected in vaginal-rectal swab specimens by multiplex real-time PCR. (+) Presence; (−) Absence

In this study, a good agreement was observed between culture- and PCR-based results for GBS positive result and the presence of erythromycin and clindamycin resistance encoded genes. However, two false-positive were detected by multiplex real-time PCR regarding the resistance markers. In fact, other bacterial species colonizing the urogenital and intestinal tracts that are known to harbor *erm* and *mef* genes [49] can be detected in a molecular assay. Taken together, the data indicate that these genes are not suitable for specific detection of GBS resistance markers in direct analysis of vaginal-rectal swabs. Despite this limitation, the assay for simultaneous detection of GBS and resistance markers could reduce the turnaround time (about 24–48 h) for both GBS identification and detection of its antimicrobial resistance after axenic cultivation compared to phenotypic methods. Moreover, in smaller laboratories with limited resources due to the equipment cost and the price of a single real-time PCR test, this assay could be used in a conventional multiplex-PCR format, which can be performed in one tube.

In general, nucleic acid amplification tests (NAAT) have been proven highly specific and with higher sensitive (reported sensitivity range of 86 to 100%) for detection of GBS vaginal-rectal colonization compared to the conventional culture-based test [8, 29, 36, 50]. This difference can be due to the presence of both non-viable cells or GBS antagonistic microorganisms [51]. In this study, the

number of vaginal-rectal swabs from pregnant women analyzed can limit generalization. More samples may provide better estimates with less uncertainty [33]. Despite this limitation, the clinical sensitivity and specificity of the multiplex real-time PCR assay were determined to be 91.7 and 95.1%, respectively, which was comparable to the results of previously reported studies based on probe approaches [29, 36–41].

Although a number of commercial kits are available, their utilization has not yet been universally implemented in hospitals, primarily due to costs and inability to determine the antimicrobial susceptibility profile if a NAAT shows positive. As stated before, most of the real-time PCR assays previously described (including those commercially available ones) use a specific probe for the target gene, besides oligonucleotide primers, which increases the costs [29, 36–41].

In this study, labor costs (the primers for resistance markers, equipment and personal were not included) for sample collection and processing of multiplex real-time PCR were estimated at US$3.47, compared with culture screening estimated cost of US$4.95 *per* swab. Furthermore, the assay provided a short turnaround time as full test, including DNA extraction, sample preparation and multiplex real-time PCR analysis, which can be performed in about 4 h. Another limitation of this study is that the time between vaginal-rectal swab collection and delivery was not analyzed and it was not possible to evaluate whether the result could be available in time for IAP. However, this assay provides reliable and faster results than culture that will help make appropriate decisions about the administration of antibiotics for neonates of women with unknown GBS colonization *status*.

Conclusion

The results presented here showed that the multiplex real-time PCR is a rapid, affordable and sensitive assay suitable for direct detection of GBS in vaginal-rectal swab. Accordingly, the present molecular assay has potential usefulness during the intrapartum period, mainly for women who did not have a prenatal screening result. In the present format, simultaneous detection of GBS and its erythromycin and lincosamide resistance markers should be applied after bacterium recover by cultivation.

Additional file

Additional file 1: Figure S1. Melting curve analysis showing the melting temperature peaks (Tm) of *RNaseP* (A) and IGS1 (B) controls. Primers targeting the human tRNA processing ribonuclease P (*RNaseP*) gene and intergenic spacer 1 (IGS1) of ribosomal RNA (rDNA) gene cluster of the *Cryptococcus gattii*, an encapsulated yeast found in the environment, were included in this study to evaluate the quality of the DNA and potential PCR interfering substances, respectively. The multiplex real-time PCR assay was performed with two tubes in one reaction using a Rotor-Gene Q 5-Plex equipment (Qiagen, Germany): a) 2× High-Resolution Melt (HRM) PCR Master Mix (Qiagen, Brazil), 10 *p*mol of forward and reverse *erm*(B), *cfb* and IGS1 primer sets, 20 *p*mol of forward and reverse *mef*(A/E) primers, and 10 ng of recombinant plasmid pCR2.1/IGS1 [32]; b) 2× HRM PCR Master Mix and 10 *p*mol of forward and reverse *erm*(A) and human *RNaseP* primers. The cycling conditions included an initial denaturation step at 95 °C for 5 min, followed by 35 cycles of 95 °C for 10 s, annealing at 67 °C for 30 s and an extension step at 72 °C for 20 s. Melting curves were acquired using 0.05 °C steps with a hold of 60 s at each step from 75 to 85 °C. NTC reactions were carried out simultaneously. Data were analyzed using Rotor Gene software version. (TIF 330 kb)

Abbreviations

ATCC: American Type Culture Collection; CAMP: acronym for Christie, Atkins and Munch-Peterson; CFU: Colonies Forming Unit; CI: Confidence Interval; GBS: Group B *Streptococcus*; HRM: High-Resolution Melt; IAPS: Intrapartum Antimicrobial Prophylaxis; LBBA: Laboratório de Bacteriologia Básica e Aplicada; LMC: Laboratório de Microbiologia Clínica; LOD: Limits of Detection; NAAT: Nucleic Acid Amplification Test; NTC: Negative Template Control; PCR: Polimerase Chain Reaction; UEL: Universidade Estadual de Londrina

Acknowledgements

We thank Dr. A. Leyva for English editing of the manuscript, and Ediel Clementino da Costa and Jussevania Pereira Santos for technical support. This work is part of the PhD thesis of E.S. Otaguiri.

Funding

This study was supported by grants from DECIT/SCTIE/MS/CNPq, Fundação Araucária e SESA-PR (Edital PPSUS: Gestão Compartilhada em Saúde/2011) and Coordenação de Aperfeiçoamento de Pessoal de Nível Superior (CAPES - PROAP and Chamada Pública 17/2014-AUXPE 3299/2014. Process 23038.007056/2014-77). E.S. Otaguiri and E.R. Tavares were supported by student scholarships from CAPES. A.E.B. Morguette was supported by a student scholarship from Conselho Nacional de Desenvolvimento Científico e Tecno-lógico-CNPq. S.F.Yamada-Ogatta was supported by a research fellowship from CNPq.

Authors' contributions

ESO: Contributed in all methodological activities and analysis and interpretation of data; AEBM, RSLAT and MREP: Performed the microbiological experiments and analyzed the data; ERT, VMG and ATM: Nucleotide sequence analysis, primer design, amplicon sequencing; GK: Collected the vaginal-rectal swabs of pregnant women; MCJ, MCBT and MAK: Interpretation of data and critical revision of the manuscript for important intellectual content. LMY and SFY-O: Conception, design, analysis and interpretation of data. All authors read and approved the final manuscript.

Competing interests

The authors declare that they have no competing interests.

Author details

[1]Departamento de Microbiologia, Centro de Ciências Biológicas, Universidade Estadual de Londrina, Londrina, Paraná, Brazil. [2]Departamento de Enfermagem, Universidade Estadual de Londrina, Londrina, Paraná, Brazil. [3]Laboratory of Bacteriology, Epidemiology Laboratory and Disease Control Division, Laboratório Central do Estado do Paraná – LACEN, Curitiba, PR, Brazil. [4]Departamento de Medicina, Hospital Universitário de Maringá, Universidade Estadual de Maringá, Maringá, Brazil. [5]Departamento de Ciências Básicas da Saúde, Universidade Estadual de Maringá, Maringá, Brazil. [6]Instituto Carlos Chagas, Fundação Instituto Oswaldo Cruz, Curitiba, Brazil. [7]Departamento de Patologia, Análises Clínicas e Toxicológicas, Centro de Ciências da Saúde, Universidade Estadual de Londrina, Londrina, Paraná, Brazil. [8]Departamento de Microbiologia, Universidade Estadual de Londrina, Centro de Ciências Biológicas, Rodovia Celso Garcia Cid, PR 445, km 380. CEP, Londrina 86057-970, Brazil.

References

1. Seale AC, Koech AC, Sheppard AE, Barsosio HE, Langat J, Anyango E, et al. Maternal colonization with *Streptococcus agalactiae*, and associated stillbirth and neonatal disease in coastal Kenya. Nat Microbiol. 2016;1:16067.
2. Cools P, Melin P. Group B *Streptococcus* and perinatal mortality. Res Microbiol. 2017; https://doi.org/10.1016/j.resmic.2017.04.002.
3. Likitnukul S, Pokato S, Nunthapisud P. Group B streptococcal sepsis and meningitis complicated with severe sensorineural hearing loss in a fourteen-year-old boy. Pediatr Infect Dis J. 1996;15:468–70.
4. Tibussek D, Sinclair A, Yau I, Teatero S, Fittipaldi N, Richardson SE, et al. Late-onset group B streptococcal meningitis has cerebrovascular complications. J Pediatr. 2015;166:1187–92.
5. Otaguiri ES, Morguette AEB, Tavares ER, dos Santos PM, Morey AT, Cardoso JD, et al. Commensal *Streptococcus agalactiae* isolated from patients seen at University Hospital of Londrina, Paraná, Brazil: capsular types, genotyping, antimicrobial susceptibility and virulence determinants. BMC Microbiol. 2013;13:297.
6. Kwatra G, Cunnington MC, Merrall E, Adrian PV, Ip M, Klugman KP, et al. Prevalence of maternal colonisation with group B *Streptococcus*: a systematic review and meta-analysis. Lancet Infect Dis. 2016;16(9):1076–84.
7. Slotved HC, Dayie NTKD, Banini JAN, Frimodt-Moller N. Carriage and serotype distribution of *Streptococcus agalactiae* in third trimester pregnancy in southern Ghana. BMC Pregnancy Childbirth. 2017;17:238.
8. Verani JR, McGee L, Schrag SJ. Prevention of perinatal group B streptococcal disease-revised guidelines from CDC, 2010. MMWR Recomm Rep. 2010;59:1–36.
9. Melin P. Neonatal group B streptococcal disease: from pathogenesis to preventive strategies. Clin Microbiol Infect. 2011;17:1294–303.
10. Verani JR, Schrag SJ. Group B streptococcal disease in infants: progress in prevention and continued challenges. Clin Perinatol. 2010;37:375–92.
11. Teatero S, Ferrieri P, Martin I, Demczuk W, McGeer A, Fittipaldi N. Serotype distribution, population structure, and antimicrobial resistance of group B *Streptococcus* strains recovered from colonized pregnant women. J Clin Microbiol. 2017;55:412–22.
12. Kimura K, Matsubara K, Yamamoto G, Shibayama K, Arakawa Y. Active screening of group B *streptococci* with reduced penicillin susceptibility and altered serotype distribution isolated from pregnant women in Kobe, Japan. Jpn J Infect Dis. 2013;66:158–60.

13. Bolukaoto JY, Monyama CM, Chukwu MO, Lekala SM, Nchabeleng M, Maloba MR, et al. Antibiotic resistance of *Streptococcus agalactiae* isolated from pregnant women in Garankuwa, South Africa. BMC Res Notes. 2015;8:364.

14. Barros RR, de Souza AF, Luiz FB. Polyclonal spread of *Streptococcus agalactiae* resistant to clindamycin among pregnant women in Brazil. J Antimicrob Chemother. 2016;71:2054–6.

15. Weisblum B. Inducible resistance to macrolides, lincosamides and streptogramin type B antibiotics: the resistance phenotype, its biological diversity, and structural elements that regulate expression-a review. J Antimicrob Chemother. 1985;16:63–90.

16. Da Cunha V, Davies MR, Douarre PE, Rosinski-Chupin I, Margarit I, Spinali S, et al. *Streptococcus agalactiae* clones infecting humans were selected and fixed through the extensive use of tetracycline. Nat Commun. 2014;5:4544.

17. Luna VA, Coates P, Eady EA, Cove JH, Nguyen TT, Roberts MC. A variety of gram-positive bacteria carry mobile *mef* genes. J Antimicrob Chemother. 1999;44:19–25.

18. Leclercq R. Mechanisms of resistance to macrolides and lincosamides: nature of the resistance elements and their clinical implications. Clin Infect Dis. 2002;34:482–92.

19. Clancy J, Petitpas J, Dib-Hajj F, Yuan W, Cronan M, Kamath AV, et al. Molecular cloning and functional analysis of a novel macrolide-resistance determinant, mefA, from *Streptococcus pyogenes*. Mol Microbiol. 1996;22:867–79.

20. Desai SH, Kaplan MS, Chen Q, Macy EM. Morbidity in pregnant women associated with unverified penicillin allergies, antibiotic use, and group B *Streptococcus* infections. Perm J. 2017; https://doi.org/10.7812/TPP/16-080.

21. Joubrel C, Tazi A, Six A, Dmytruk N, Touak G, Bidet P, et al. Group D streptococcus neonatal invasive infections, France 2007-2012. Clin Microbiol Infect. 2015;21:910–6.

22. Schrag SJ, Farley MM, Petit S, Reingold A, Weston EJ, Pondo T, et al. Epidemiology of invasive early-onset neonatal sepsis, 2005 to 2014. Pediatrics. 2016:138. pii: e20162013

23. Six A, Firon A, Plainvert C, Caplain C, Touak G, Dmytruk N, et al. Molecular characterization of nonhemolytic and nonpigmented group B Streptococci responsible for human invasive infections. J Clin Microbiol. 2016;54:75–82.

24. Tejada MB, Stan CM, Boulvain M, Renzi G, François P, Irion O, et al. Development of a rapid PCR assay for screening of maternal colonization by group B *Streptococcus* and neonatal invasive *Escherichia coli* during labor. Gynecol Obstet Investig. 2010;70:250–5.

25. Schrag SJ. The past and future of perinatal group B streptococcal disease prevention. Clin Infect Dis. 2004;39:1136–8.

26. Lang S, Palmer M. Characterization of *Streptococcus agalactiae* CAMP factor as a pore-forming toxin. J Biol Chem. 2003;278:38167–73.

27. Christie R, Atkins NE, Munch-Petersen EA. Note on a lytic phenomenon shown by group B *streptococci*. Aust J Exp Biol Med Sci. 1944;22:197–200.

28. Phillips EA, Tapsall JW, Smith DD. Rapid tube CAMP test for identification of *Streptococcus agalactiae* (Lancefield group B). J Clin Microbiol. 1980;12:135–7.

29. Emonet S, Schrenzel J, Tejada BM. Molecular-based screening for perinatal group B streptococcal infection: implications for prevention and therapy. Mol Diagn Ther. 2013;17:355–61.

30. World Health Organization (WHO). CDC protocol of real-time RTPCR for swine influenza A (H1N1). 2009. http://www.who.int/csr/resources/publications/swineflu/CDCrealtimeRTPCRprotocol_2009042

31. Altman S. The road to RNase P. Nat Struct Biol. 2000;7:827–8.

32. Tavares ER, Azevedo CS, Panagio LA, Pelisson M, Pinge-Filho P, Venancio EJ, et al. Accurate and sensitive real-time PCR assays using intergenic spacer 1 region to differentiate *Cryptococcus gattii sensu lato* and *Cryptococcus neoformans sensu lato*. Med Mycol. 2016;54:89–96.

33. Burd CE, Jeck WR, Liu Y, Sanoff HK, Wang Z, Sharpless NE. Expression of linear and novel circular forms of an INK4/ARF-associated non-coding RNA correlates with atherosclerosis risk. PLoS Genet. 2010;6:e1001233.

34. Clinical and Laboratory Standards Institute. Performance standards for antimicrobial susceptibility testing. Twentieth informational supplement. Document M100-S22. Wayne: PA; 2012. p. 2012.

35. Seppala H, Nissinen A, Yu Q, Huovinen P. Three different phenotypes of erythromycin-resistant *Streptococcus pyogenes* in Finland. J Antimicrob Chemother. 1993;32:885–91.

36. Couturier BA, Weight T, Elmer H, Schlaberg R. Antepartum screening for group B *Streptococcus* by three FDA-cleared molecular tests and effect of shortened enrichment culture on molecular detection rates. J Clin Microbiol. 2014;52:3429–32.

37. Morozumi M, Chiba N, Igarashi Y, Mitsuhashi N, Wajima T, Iwata S, et al. Direct identification of *Streptococcus agalactiae* and capsular type by real-time PCR in vaginal swabs from pregnant women. J Infect Chemother. 2015;21:34–8.

38. Furfaro LL, Chang BJ, Payne MS. A novel one-step real-time multiplex PCR assay to detect *Streptococcus agalactiae* presence and serotypes Ia, Ib, and III. Diagn Microbiol Infect Dis. 2017;89:7–12.

39. Winkler DS, Rocha A, Fabião CD, De Marco M, Proto-Siqueira R. Highly sensitive and efficient screening of *Streptococcus agalactiae* through improved real-time PCR protocols and optimized analytical parameters. Clin Lab. 2015;61:1581–4.

40. Wernecke M, Mullen C, Sharma V, Morrison J, Barry T, Maher M, et al. Evaluation of a novel real-time PCR test based on the ssrA gene for the identification of group B *streptococci* in vaginal swabs. BMC Infect Dis. 2009;4:148.

41. Bergseng H, Bevanger L, Rygg M, Bergh K. Real-time PCR targeting the *sip* gene for detection of group B *Streptococcus* colonization in pregnant women at delivery. J Med Microbiol. 2007;56:223–8.

42. Dela Cruz WP, Richardson JY, Broestler JM, Thornton JA, Danaher PJ. Rapid determination of macrolide and lincosamide resistance in group B *Streptococcus* isolated from vaginal-rectal swabs. Infect Dis Obstet Gynecol. 2007;46581

43. Park JS, Cho DH, Yang JH, Kim MY, Shin SM, Kim EC, et al. Usefulness of a rapid real-time PCR assay in prenatal screening for group B *Streptococcus* colonization. Ann Lab Med. 2013;33:39–44.

44. Poyart C, Lamy MC, Boumaila C, Fiedler F, Trieu-Cuot P. Regulation of D-alanyl-lipoteichoic acid biosynthesis in *Streptococcus agalactiae* involves a novel two-component regulatory system. J Bacteriol. 2001;183:6324–34.

45. Spellerberg B, Pohl B, Haase G, Martin S, Weber-Heynemann J, Lütticken R. Identification of genetic determinants for the hemolytic activity of *Streptococcus agalactiae* by ISS1 transposition. J Bacteriol. 1999;181:3212–9.

46. Keiler KC, Waller PR, Sauer RT. Role of a peptide tagging system in degradation of proteins synthesized from damaged messenger RNA. Science. 1996;271:990–3.

47. Brodeur BR, Boyer M, Charlebois I, Hamel J, Couture F, Rioux CR, et al. Martin D identification of group B streptococcal sip protein, which elicits cross-protective immunity. Infect Immun. 2000;68:5610–8.

48. Horaud T, Le Bouguenec C, Pepper K. Molecular genetics of resistance to macrolides, lincosamides and streptogramin B (MLS) in *streptococci*. J Antimicrob Chemother. 1985;16:111–35.

49. Abdelkareem MZ, Sayed M, Hassuna NA, Mahmoud MS, Abdelwahab SF. Multi-drug-resistant *Enterococcus faecalis* among Egyptian patients with urinary tract infection. J Chemother. 2017;29:74–82.

50. McKenna JP, Cox C, Fairley DJ, Burke R, Shields MD, Watt A, et al. Loop-mediated isothermal amplification assay for rapid detection of *Streptococcus agalactiae* (group B *Streptococcus*) in vaginal swabs – a proof of concept study. J Med Microbiol. 2017;66:294–300.

51. WMJr D, Holland-Staley CA. Comparison of NNA agar culture and selective broth culture for detection of group B streptococcal colonization in women. J Clin Microbiol. 1998;36:2298–300.

9

Automated electrohysterographic detection of uterine contractions for monitoring of pregnancy: feasibility and prospects

C. Muszynski[1,2]* iD, T. Happillon[1], K. Azudin[1], J.-B. Tylcz[1], D. Istrate[1] and C. Marque[1]

Abstract

Background: Preterm birth is a major public health problem in developed countries. In this context, we have conducted research into outpatient monitoring of uterine electrical activity in women at risk of preterm delivery. The objective of this preliminary study was to perform automated detection of uterine contractions (without human intervention or tocographic signal, TOCO) by processing the EHG recorded on the abdomen of pregnant women. The feasibility and accuracy of uterine contraction detection based on EHG processing were tested and compared to expert decision using external tocodynamometry (TOCO) .

Methods: The study protocol was approved by local Ethics Committees under numbers ID-RCB 2016-A00663-48 for France and VSN 02-0006-V2 for Iceland.

Two populations of women were included (threatened preterm birth and labour) in order to test our system of recognition of the various types of uterine contractions.

EHG signal acquisition was performed according to a standardized protocol to ensure optimal reproducibility of EHG recordings. A system of 18 Ag/AgCl surface electrodes was used by placing 16 recording electrodes between the woman's pubis and umbilicus according to a 4×4 matrix. TOCO was recorded simultaneously with EHG recording. EHG signals were analysed in real-time by calculation of the nonlinear correlation coefficient H^2. A curve representing the number of correlated pairs of signals according to the value of H^2 calculated between bipolar signals was then plotted. High values of H^2 indicated the presence of an event that may correspond to a contraction.

Two tests were performed after detection of an event (fusion and elimination of certain events) in order to increase the contraction detection rate.

Results: The EHG database contained 51 recordings from pregnant women, with a total of 501 contractions previously labelled by analysis of the corresponding tocographic recording. The percentage recognitions obtained by application of the method based on coefficient H^2 was 100% with 782% of false alarms. Addition of fusion and elimination tests to the previously obtained detections allowed the false alarm rate to be divided by 8.5, while maintaining an excellent detection rate (96%).

Conclusion: These preliminary results appear to be encouraging for monitoring of uterine contractions by algorithm-based automated detection to process the electrohysterographic signal (EHG). This compact recording system, based on the use of surface electrodes attached to the skin, appears to be particularly suitable for outpatient monitoring of uterine contractions, possibly at home, allowing telemonitoring of pregnancies. One of the advantages of EHG processing is that useful information concerning contraction efficiency can be extracted from this signal, which is not possible with the TOCO signal.

Keywords: Electrohysterogram, Automated contraction detection, Uterine contraction, Premature delivery

* Correspondence: muszynski.charles@chu-amiens.fr
[1]Sorbonne Universités, Université de Technologie de Compiègne, CNRS, BMBI UMR 7338, 60200 Compiègne, France
[2]Département de gynécologie et obstétrique, CHU Amiens-Picardie, avenue Laënnec, 80480 Salouël, France

Background

The preterm delivery rate in Europe is between 5.5 and 11.1% and preterm delivery is the leading cause of perinatal morbidity and mortality [1]. Almost one in every two preterm deliveries is the result of spontaneous preterm labour [2]. Preterm delivery rates have remained stable for several years despite the routine use of monitoring tools in clinical practice [3].

In this context, with the support of the SAFE pregnancy@home research project (European Eurostars project), we have conducted research on an outpatient uterine electrical activity monitoring device that could be used for women at risk of preterm delivery. Uterine contraction is the direct result of the electrical activity of the myometrium. Recording of the electrical activity of the myometrium by surface electrodes (electrohysterography [EHG]), a noninvasive technique, can be used to identify changes of the electrical signal related to the type of uterine contraction, Braxton-Hicks contractions of normal pregnancy (inefficient) or labour contractions (efficient) [4–6].

The objective of this preliminary study was to perform automated detection of uterine contractions (without human intervention or TOCO signal using) based on EHG recording and analysis in pregnant women an. The feasibility and accuracy of electrohysterographic detection of contractions was compared to those of external tocodynamometry (TOCO).

Methods

Patient characteristics

Pregnant women, included in two university hospitals (France and Iceland, Icelandic database [7]) between 2015 and 2017, were classified into two categories. The first group, the Pregnancy group, consisted of women at 26 to 35 weeks of gestation (WG), during their normal pregnancy follow-up, or admitted for threatened preterm labour. Admissions for threatened preterm labour were defined by the presence of contractions experienced by the woman and/or present on tocography, associated with cervical changes, i.e. short cervical length on pelvic examination or vaginal ultrasound measurement (transvaginal cervical length < 25 mm). The second group, the Labour group, consisted of women in labour at term, defined by at least 4 cm of cervical dilatation associated with regular uterine contractions. Women in were recorded either at the first stage or second stage of labour but none of them were recorded during the pushing stage. These two populations of women were included in order to test our system of recognition of the various types of uterine contractions (Braxton-Hicks contractions and labour contractions). Women with pathological pregnancies (maternal or obstetric disease) other than threatened preterm labour were not included in this study. All women were over the age of 18 years,

with a BMI < 35, covered by national health insurance in the country concerned, and provided their written informed consent to participate in the study and to publish data and results in scientific journals. The study protocol was approved by local Ethics Committees under numbers ID-RCB 2016-A00663-48 for France and VSN 02-0006-V2 for Iceland.

Electrohysterography

In each centre, informed consent was obtained from each woman by the same person who also performed EHG recordings.

EHG signal acquisition was performed according to a standardized protocol to ensure optimal reproducibility of EHG recordings in the two maternity units [7]. Before applying the electrodes, the woman's skin was prepared by applying exfoliating cream to reduce inter-electrode impedance and to increase the signal-to-noise ratio of the recorded signals. A system of 18 Ag/AgCl surface electrodes was used by placing 16 recording electrodes between the woman's pubis and umbilicus according to a 4×4 matrix and two reference electrodes on each of the woman's hips. The 4×4 electrode matrix was shifted slightly to the right due to physiological dextrorotation of the uterus, as indicated in Fig. 1a. The sixteen 13-mm diameter electrodes were separated from each other by intervals of 17.5 mm (centre to centre). Electrical signals were recorded at a sampling frequency of 200 Hz and were then transferred by Wifi to a laptop computer for processing by TMSi PolyBench® software. All components of the EHG signal recording system are CE marked.

Signal preprocessing

The 16 unipolar signals distributed over the 4×4 matrix were subtracted two by two, according to the vertical axis, to obtain 12 bipolar signals, as indicated in Fig. 1b (Vbi, $i = 1$ to 12). Analysis of bipolar electrical signals has the advantage of increasing the signal-to-noise ratio and consequently increasing the signal quality. A bandpass filter was then applied to only select the 0.1-3 Hz frequency band, corresponding to the frequency spectrum of uterine contractions recorded by electrohysterography [8].

Characterization of series of uterine contractions

In this study, all EHG signals of uterine contractions were collected simultaneously with external tocodynamometry (TOCO) recordings. Although the accuracy of external TOCO has been reported to be poor, external TOCO was the only reference examination available in this study for experts to identify the presence of a contraction and to define the start and end times of EHG signals, while reviewing all signals. The start and end times of each contractile event, obtained by this peer

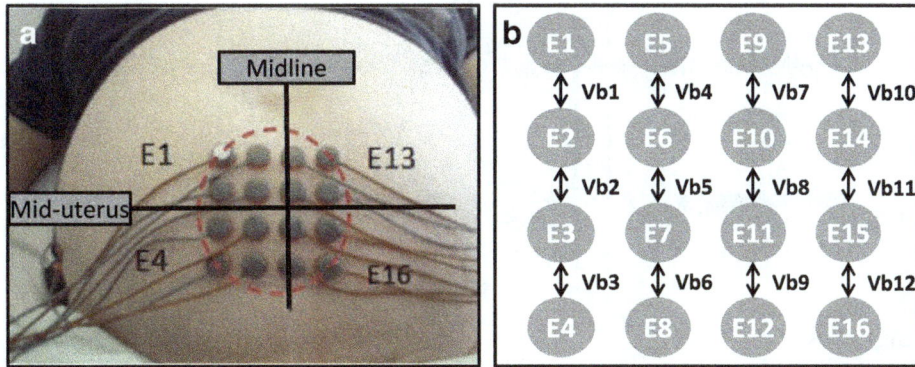

Fig. 1 a Positioning of the 16 electrodes (Ei, i ∈ [1–16]) according to a 4 × 4 matrix. This matrix is shifted slightly towards the right due to the physiological dextrorotation of the uterus. **b** Twelve bipolar signals are obtained (Vbi, i ∈ [1–12]) by vertical subtraction of 2 adjacent unipolar signals

review of TOCO and EHG signals, were used as the basis to test the feasibility and performance of algorithm-based automated EHG detection of uterine contractions.

Application of the nonlinear correlation coefficient H^2

EHG signals were analysed in real-time by calculation of the nonlinear correlation coefficient H^2. Each H^2 value was situated between 0 (non-correlated signals) and 1 (strongly correlated signals), as, in a previous study [9], we observed that EHG signals were correlated with high H^2 values during uterine contractions, while low H^2 values were observed for baseline signals between two contractions (Fig. 2). A sliding window, with a width equal to 800 acquisition points (i.e. 4 s), scanned the 12 bipolar EHG signals with a 400-point increment. At each position of this window, 36 H^2 values were calculated from the 36 laterally adjacent pairs of bipolar signals (for example between Vb1 and Vb4, between Vb4 and Vb7, between Vb2 and Vb5, etc.). A first cutoff for H^2, S1, was tested and defined to determine whether or not a pair of bipolar signals can be considered to be correlated. For each position of the sliding window, the number of H^2 values greater than S1 was then counted (corresponding to the number of correlated pairs among the 36 pairs tested for each window position), resulting in a curve representing the number of correlated pairs of signals for each position of the sliding window.

Detection of contractions with H^2

The values of the curve obtained in the previous step were compared according to a second cutoff, S2, corresponding to the limit of detection. H^2 values higher than S2 indicate the presence of an event (i.e. a sufficient number among the 36 pairs of signals are correlated over a given interval) (Fig. 3).

Fusion and elimination

Two tests were performed after the detection of events. The first test studied the interval between one event and the previous event. These two events were then fused when they were situated sufficiently close to each other (i.e. separated by a difference less than a tested and defined value, D1).

The second test studied the duration of the events detected. An event was eliminated when it did not exceed a minimal duration tested and defined in this study (D2).

Methodology of evaluation of the performance of automated detection of uterine contractions

All events detected for each recording were then compared to the reference labels of contractions previously identified by the experts. Three situations were observed: i) an event was detected in the absence of any identified contraction, and was therefore considered to be a "False alarm"; ii) an event was detected during a contraction and its start and end limits coincided with the reference labels (within an acceptable margin), and was therefore considered to be a "Full detection"; iii) when the limits of the event did not coincide with the reference labels, but covered only a part of the duration of the contraction or contained the baseline signal, it was therefore considered to be a "Partial detection" (Fig. 4).

Results

The EHG database contained 51 recordings from pregnant women, with a total of 501 contractions previously labelled by analysis of the corresponding tocographic recording. The percentages and number of recognitions obtained (full detections, partial detections and false alarms) by application of the first step of the method based on coefficient H^2 only are presented in Table 1.

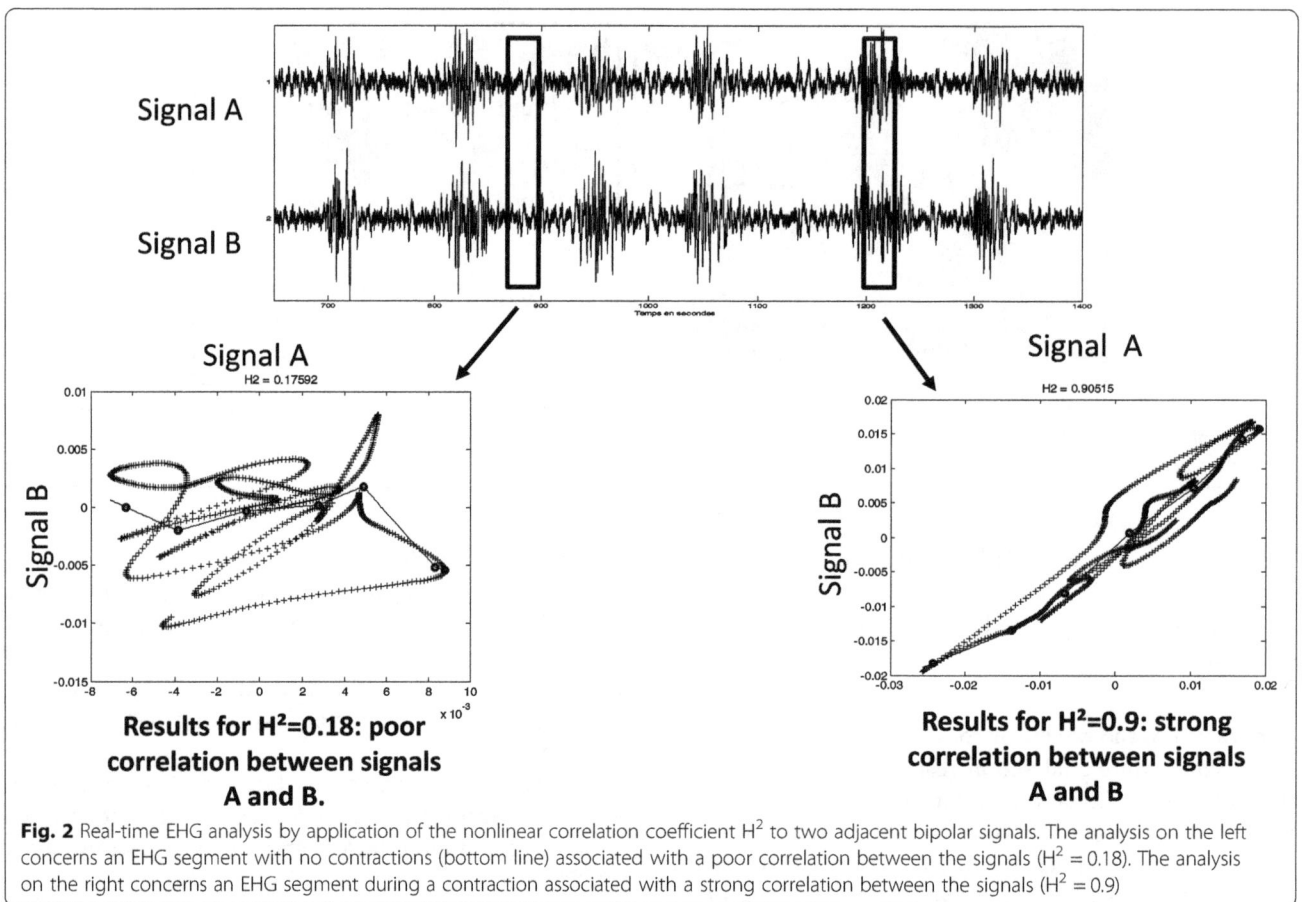

Fig. 2 Real-time EHG analysis by application of the nonlinear correlation coefficient H^2 to two adjacent bipolar signals. The analysis on the left concerns an EHG segment with no contractions (bottom line) associated with a poor correlation between the signals ($H^2 = 0.18$). The analysis on the right concerns an EHG segment during a contraction associated with a strong correlation between the signals ($H^2 = 0.9$)

The results obtained after adding fusion and elimination steps to the previously obtained detections are shown in Table 2.

The automated detection algorithm based on H^2 coefficients, followed by fusion and elimination steps, detected 96% of contractions (485 contractions out of a total of 501 contractions), with 62% of full detections. As explained previously (Fig. 4), a fully detected contraction is a contraction for which the segment detected by the algorithm corresponds (with a short time difference) to the limits indicated by the experts; a "partial detection" was noted when only part of the contraction or some noise was included in the detected segment. The number of false alarms (segments detected that did not correspond to a contraction identified by the experts) was 496 for 501 real contractions present on the EHG signals.

Discussion

Algorithm-based (automated) detection of uterine contractions is a major prerequisite to the use of EHG for the monitoring of at-risk pregnancies. The use of EHG has several advantages over tocography. Application of EHG electrodes adherent to the woman's skin avoids the problems of electrode displacement, in contrast with the

tocodynamometer, which must always be correctly maintained by a belt in order to detect uterine contractions. External tocography, can be used to evaluate intrauterine pressure by recording deformation of the uterine fundus across the maternal abdominal wall [10]. Displacement or poor positioning of the external pressure transducer can therefore modify the signals recorded during contraction. Internal tocography has therefore been developed to overcome the lack of precision of external tocography, mainly in terms of quantification of the amplitude of contraction [11]. However, internal tocography requires rupture of the amniotic membranes and is therefore an invasive procedure that can only be performed during labour. Electrohysterographic recording of uterine activity was therefore developed in this context. Electrohysterography is an appropriate tool to evaluate intrauterine pressure and consequently the mechanical effect of a contraction using surface electrodes [12]. It is therefore a noninvasive procedure that can be used to monitor contractions during pregnancy. The present study used a small signal recording system that can be attached to the woman's hip, facilitating outpatient monitoring, in contrast with external tocography, which usually requires immobilization of the patient

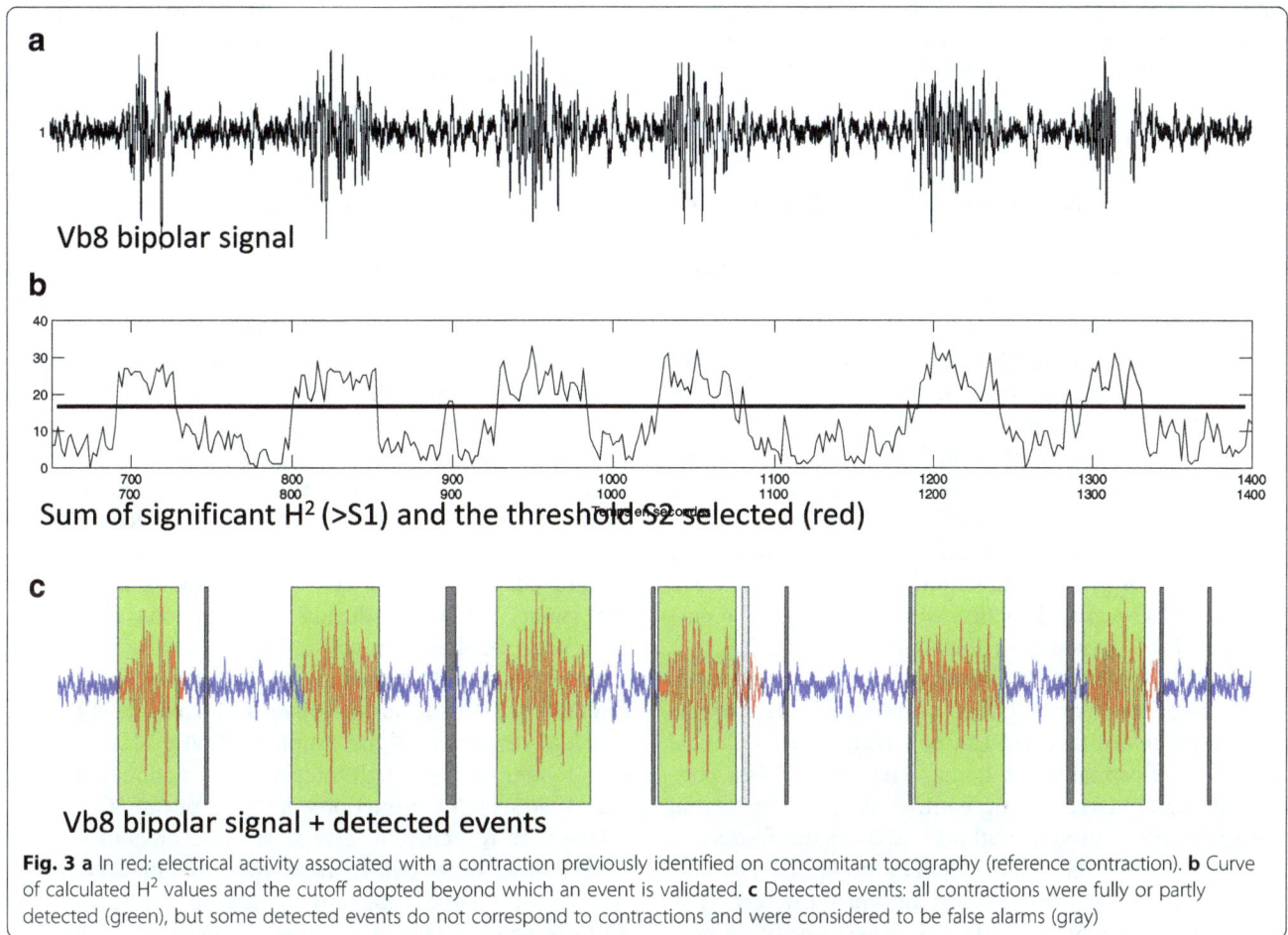

Fig. 3 a In red: electrical activity associated with a contraction previously identified on concomitant tocography (reference contraction). **b** Curve of calculated H^2 values and the cutoff adopted beyond which an event is validated. **c** Detected events: all contractions were fully or partly detected (green), but some detected events do not correspond to contractions and were considered to be false alarms (gray)

next to the apparatus. EHG allows mobilization during recording, making it a particularly attractive tool for outpatient monitoring, possibly at home. Another advantage of EHG is that, in the presence of contractions, it is able to discriminate between labour contractions and Braxton-Hicks contractions, and EHG analysis during pregnancy can be used to predict the risk of labour [13–18]. EHG could therefore be a potentially useful tool for the monitoring of patients with threatened preterm labour.

The automated detection of contraction based on EHG processing was compared to reference labels of contractions identified by experts using TOCO in order

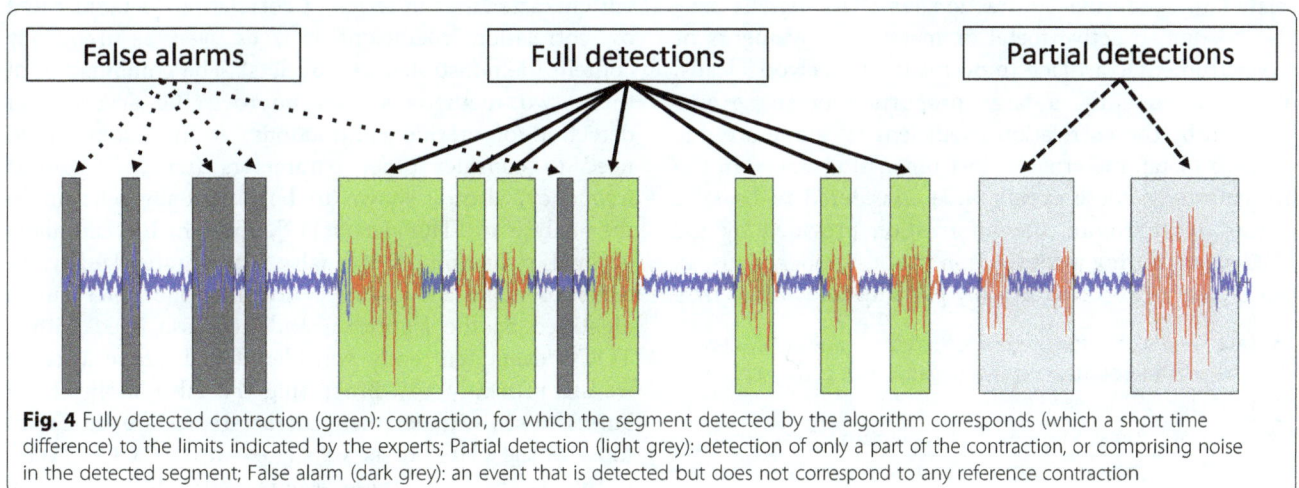

Fig. 4 Fully detected contraction (green): contraction, for which the segment detected by the algorithm corresponds (which a short time difference) to the limits indicated by the experts; Partial detection (light grey): detection of only a part of the contraction, or comprising noise in the detected segment; False alarm (dark grey): an event that is detected but does not correspond to any reference contraction

Table 1 Results of automated detection of uterine contractions by analysis based on the nonlinear correlation coefficient H^2 alone. The database used contains 501 labelled contractions

Full detections	Partial detections	Total detections	False alarms
62.5% (313/501)	37.5% (188/501)	100% (501/501)	782% (3918/501)

to evaluate the performance of detection of uterine contractions by EHG signals. Although the use of TOCO has not been able to decrease the premature delivery rate over recent years, it can be used to diagnose the number of contractions. However, TOCO does not provide any information on the type of contraction (physiological or pathological) in contrast with EHG analysis. Although intrauterine pressure determination appears to be slightly more accurate than EHG to detect uterine contraction, this device cannot be widely used during labour (risk of infections) and cannot be used during pregnancy with intact membranes [19]. To evaluate the accuracy of contraction detection in clinical practice, we compare EHG signal detection with the only device currently available in routine clinical practice, TOCO.

However, continuous automated detection of EHG spikes associated with uterine contractions must first be performed before this tool can be widely used in clinical practice in hospital or at home. The first studies concerning EHG detection of contractions, performed in the early 2000s, used a method based on the frequency content of the EHG signal [20]. The preliminary results of our study on algorithm-based automated detection of uterine contractions by EHG based exclusively on correlation coefficient H^2 showed a high level of accuracy of detection, but with a very high false alarm rate (3918 false alarms for 501 contractions), which can be explained by the fact that this method of detection is based on interpretation of the various correlations observed for the signals throughout signal acquisition. However, a strong correlation observed between signals recorded at a given point in time is not necessarily related to a uterine contraction, as these signals may also be due to active foetal or maternal movements or an instrumental artifact (movement of electrode leads, etc.). Consequently, a large proportion of the events detected by the correlation coefficient H^2 alone are due to these foetal, maternal or instrumental artifacts. In the present study, these events were considered to be false alarms. Furthermore, the information provided by the EHG signal during a contraction is not homogeneous, as some contractions may be only partially detected or may

be divided into several events (oversegmentation), resulting in detection of several events for a single uterine contraction. Inversely, the contraction detection rate (complete and partial detection) was 100%, which confirms that a strongly correlated electrical activity was responsible for the mechanical activity of the uterus. In this study, in order to decrease the number of false alarms, we have developed a technique of fusion and elimination of events according to their duration and the time intervals between events. Events closely related in time were fused, as they are considered to correspond to the same contraction, thereby decreasing oversegmentation (reduction of the number of events during the same contraction). Event fusion therefore increases the number of complete detections by decreasing the number of partial detections. Elimination of brief events decreased the number of events related to brief foetal or maternal movements, but also eliminated brief events detected within a contraction that were not fused during the previous step. This procedure resulted in a reduction of the false alarm rate (from 3918 to 496), as well as the short partial detection rate. Overall, this fusion-elimination technique allowed a ninefold reduction of the number of false alarms, while maintaining a very high uterine contraction detection rate of 96% (485 contractions detected out of 501).

However, the current false alarm rate obviously needs to be further decreased to allow effective clinical application of automated detection of uterine contractions by EHG. A study is currently underway in order to link this method of analysis based on correlation of EHG signals with a method based on EHG wavelet decomposition, taking frequency data into account. Linking of these two methods is designed to further decrease the false alarm rate, while also making detection of contractions more reliable, based on both their correlation and their frequency content. EHGs recorded during contractions, rest phases or in the presence of artifacts, present different characteristics in terms of correlation (demonstrated by correlation coefficient H^2), as well as frequency content (demonstrated by wavelets). The combination of these two methods should improve the accuracy of detection of uterine contractions. A final step would need to consider other parameters (temporal and/or frequency) already shown to be potentially relevant to the analysis of EHG signals [19], and which could allow optimal reduction of the false alarm rate. Finally, in order to make a decision concerning the EHG bursts identified by the algorithm and not associated with a TOCO event (currently considered to be false alarms), we are presently post-processing the false alarms EHG bursts to see whether their characteristics are similar to those of the EHG bursts associated with a TOCO event. If this is the case, these events will subsequently be

Table 2 Results of automated detection of uterine contractions after the addition of fusion and elimination steps. The database used contains 501 labelled contractions

Full detections	Partial detections	Total detections	False alarms
63% (316/501)	30.7% (154/501)	92.6% (464/501)	92.6% (464/501)

considered to be contractions, and will be used for clinical diagnosis. If their characteristics differ, they will remain classified as false alarms.

After ensuring reliable detection of uterine contractions, this EHG database, recorded at various terms of pregnancy and during labour, could then be used to determine whether EHG is able to discriminate between these various events. We would therefore be able to study EHG parameters specific to the type of contractions during pregnancy (physiological or pathological) and during labour, allowing real-time estimation of the intensity of each contraction detected and therefore the risk of preterm delivery. Apart from simple counting of uterine contractions, EHG monitoring of pregnant women would allow estimation of the efficiency of these contractions, thereby providing an estimation of the risk of subsequent labour over the days following the recording. This objective constitutes the subject of ongoing studies on available and further EHG databases.

Conclusions

These preliminary results appear to be encouraging for the diagnosis and algorithm-based automated monitoring of uterine contractions by electrohysterography (EHG). We are currently pursuing our research in order to reduce the number of false alarms, while maintaining, or even increasing, the good detection rates obtained in this study.

Finally, this compact recording system, comprising surface electrodes attached to the skin, appears to be particularly suitable for outpatient monitoring of uterine contractions, possibly at home, allowing telemonitoring of pregnancies.

Abbreviations
EHG: Electrohysterography; H^2: Nonlinear correlation coefficient; TOCO: External tocodynamometry; WG: Weeks of gestation

Acknowledgements
The authors are grateful to the midwives who contributed to data collection in the maternity unit and to the women who participated in the study.

Funding
The Safe.pregnancy@home project was funded by la Banque Publique d'Investissement (BPI) France with award number DOS0041193/00. The funding body had no role in the design of the study, collection, analysis, interpretation of data, and writing of the manuscript.

Authors' contributions
CMa and DI designed and conducted the research. CMu was responsible for data collection (EHG recording) and wrote the initial manuscript. CMu, TH, J-BT and KA analysed data. CMa and DI critically reviewed the manuscript. CMu had primary responsibility for final content. All authors read and approved the final manuscript.

Competing interests
The authors have no conflicts of interest to disclose. The authors have no financial relationships to disclose relevant to this article.

References
1. Zeitlin J, Szamotulska K, Drewniak N, Mohangoo AD, Chalmers J, Sakkeus L, et al. Preterm birth time trends in Europe: a study of 19 countries. BJOG Int J Obstet Gynaecol. 2013;120(11):1356–65.
2. Delorme P, Goffinet F, Ancel P-Y, Foix-L'Hélias L, Langer B, Lebeaux C, et al. Cause of preterm birth as a prognostic factor for mortality. Obstet Gynecol. 2016;127(1):40–8.
3. Beck S, Wojdyla D, Say L, Betran AP, Merialdi M, Requejo JH, Rubens C, Menon R, Van Look PF. The worldwide incidence of preterm birth: a systematic review of maternal mortality and morbidity. Bull World Health Organ. 2010;88(1):31–8.
4. Muszynski C, Terrien J, Dréan Y, Chkeir A, Hassan M, Marque C, et al. Evolution of electrohysterogram signals synchronization according to term of pregnancy: interest for preterm labor diagnosis. Gynecol Obstet Fertil. 2012;40(6):344–9.
5. Alamedine D, Khalil M, Marque C. Comparison of different EHG feature selection methods for the detection of preterm labor. Comput Math Methods Med. 2013;2013:485684.
6. Garfield RE, Maul H, Maner W, Fittkow C, Olson G, Shi L, et al. Uterine electromyography and light-induced fluorescence in the management of term and preterm labor. J Soc Gynecol Investig. 2002;9(5):265–75.
7. Alexandersson A, Steingrimsdottir T, Terrien J, Marque C, Karlsson B. The Icelandic 16-electrode electrohysterogram database. Sci Data. 2015 [cited 2015 Jun 19];2. Available from: http://www.ncbi.nlm.nih.gov/pmc/articles/PMC4431509/
8. Lange L, Vaeggemose A, Kidmose P, Mikkelsen E, Uldbjerg N, Johansen P. Velocity and directionality of the electrohysterographic signal propagation. PLoS One. 2014;9(1):e86775.
9. Happillon T., Muszynski C., Istrate D., Marque C. Automatic and real-time detection of contractions applying the non-linear correlation coefficient h2 on electrohysterograms. VII International Conf. Computational Bioengineering (ICCB 2017), Sept. 2017, Compiègne, France.
10. Eswaran H, Wilson JD, Murphy P, Siegel ER, Lowery CL. Comparing the performance of a new disposable pneumatic tocodynamometer with a standard tocodynamometer. Acta Obstet Gynecol Scand. 2016;95(3):319–28.
11. Miles AM, Monga M, Richeson KS. Correlation of external and internal monitoring of uterine activity in a cohort of term patients. Am J Perinatol. 2001;18(3):137–40.
12. Rabotti C, Mischi M, van Laar JOEH, Oei GS, Bergmans JWM. Estimation of internal uterine pressure by joint amplitude and frequency analysis of electrohysterographic signals. Physiol Meas. 2008;29(7):829–41.
13. de Lau H, Rabotti C, Bijloo R, Rooijakkers MJ, Mischi M, Oei SG. Automated conduction velocity analysis in the electrohysterogram for prediction of imminent delivery: a preliminary study. Comput Math Methods Med. 2013; 2013:627976.
14. Lucovnik M, Maner WL, Chambliss LR, Blumrick R, Balducci J, Novak-Antolic Z, et al. Noninvasive uterine electromyography for prediction of preterm delivery. Am J Obstet Gynecol. 2011;204(3):228. e1-10
15. Euliano TY, Marossero D, Nguyen MT, Euliano NR, Principe J, Edwards RK. Spatiotemporal electrohysterography patterns in normal and arrested labor. Am J Obstet Gynecol. 2009;200(1):54. e1-7
16. de Lau H, Rabotti C, Oosterbaan HP, Mischi M, Oei GS. Study protocol: PoPE-prediction of preterm delivery by Electrohysterography. 2014;14:192.
17. Leman H, Marque C, Gondry J. Use of the EHG signal for the characterization of contraction during pregnancy. IEEE Trans Biomed Eng. 1999;46(10):1222–9.
18. Marque C, Terrien J, Rihana S, Germain G. Preterm labour detection by use of a biophysical marker: the uterine electrical activity. BMC Pregnancy and Childbirth. 2007;7(Suppl 1):S5.
19. Hayes-Gill B., Hassan S., Mirza FG., Ommani S., Himsworth J., Solomon M., Brown R., Schifrin BS., Cohen WR. Accuracy and reliability of uterine contraction identification using abdominal surface electrodes, Clin Med Insights Womens Health 2012, v5 65–75.
20. Khalil M, Duchêne J, Marque C. An autoregressive-based technique for event extraction associated with multiscale classification in non stationary signals. Smart Engineering Systems Design. 2000;2:147–58.

10

Short term sequelae of preeclampsia: a single center cohort study

Michael Girsberger[1]* ⓘ, Catherine Muff[2], Irene Hösli[2] and Michael Jan Dickenmann[1]

Abstract

Background: Data on the prevalence of persistent symptoms in the first year after preeclampsia are limited. Furthermore, possible risk factors for these sequelae are poorly defined. We investigated kidney function, blood pressure, proteinuria and urine sediment in women with preeclampsia 6 months after delivery with secondary analysis for possible associated clinical characteristics.

Methods: From January 2007 to July 2014 all women with preeclampsia and 6-months follow up at the University Hospital Basel were analyzed. Preeclampsia was defined as new onset of hypertension (≥140/90 mmHg) and either proteinuria or signs of end-organ dysfunction. Hypertension was defined as a blood pressure ≥ 140/90 mmHg or the use of antihypertensive medication. Proteinuria was defined as a protein-to-creatinine ratio in a spot urine > 11 mg/mmol. Urine sediment was evaluated by a nephrologist. Secondary analyses were performed to investigate for possible parameters associated with persistent symptoms after preeclampsia.

Results: Two hundred two women were included into the analysis. At a mean time of follow up of 172 days (+/− 39.6) after delivery, mean blood pressure was 124/76 mmHg (+/− 14/11, range 116–182/63–110) and the mean serum-creatinine was 61.8 μmol/l (33–105 μmol/l) (normal < 110 μmol/l). Mean estimated glomerular filtration rate using CKD-EPI was 110.7 mml/min/1.73m^2 (range 59.7–142.4 mml/min/1.73m^2) (normal > 60 mml/min/1.73m^2). 20.3% (41/202) had a blood pressure of 140/90 mmHg or higher (mean 143/89 mmHg) or were receiving antihypertensive medication (5.5%, 11/202). Proteinuria was present in 33.1% (66/199) (mean 27.5 mg/mmol). Proteinuria and hypertension was present in 8% (16/199). No active urine sediment (e.g. signs of glomerulonephritis) was observed. Age and gestational diabetes were associated with persistent proteinuria and severe preeclampsia with eGFR decline of ≥ 10 ml/min/1.73m^2.

Conclusion: Hypertension and proteinuria are common after 6 months underlining the importance of close follow up to identify those women who need further care.

Keywords: Preeclampsia, Follow-up, Sequelae

Background

Preeclampsia is a pregnancy related disease defined as new onset of hypertension and either proteinuria or signs of other end-organ dysfunction (e.g. hepatic abnormality, pulmonary edema, thrombocytopenia). Preeclampsia occurs in approximately 5% of pregnancies [1], and is therefore a frequent disorder complicating gestation. Apart from the high morbidity with sometimes even life-threatening implications for mother and child during the acute phase of the disease, there are also concerns about

long-term sequelae. Studies in the past have shown an increased risk of kidney biopsy [2] indicating kidney disease or end-stage renal failure [3, 4]. There is also evidence of increased risk of chronic hypertension following an episode of preeclampsia [5–7].

To identify those with chronic hypertension or proteinuria after delivery, it is important to know the usual time of resolution of these symptoms. Guidelines state that blood pressure should normalize in the first 3 months [8] and referral is considered if hypertension or proteinuria persists after three to 6 months [9, 10]. However, there is data indicating that hypertension persists in almost 40% of patients after 3 months and still is

* Correspondence: mgirsberger@hotmail.com
[1]Clinic for Transplantation Immunology and Nephrology, University Hospital Basel, Petersgraben 4, 4031 Basel, Switzerland
Full list of author information is available at the end of the article

present in 18% after 2 years [11]. In one study almost 29% of patients were hypertensive after 5 years, although sample size was small [12]. Therefore, the time to define chronicity of symptoms remains unclear. In regard to the few existing studies, we hypothesized that a significant part of patients still show sequelae of preeclampsia 6 months after pregnancy. The aim of the study was to determine the frequency of hypertension, proteinuria and eGFR (estimated glomerular filtration rate) decline 6 months after preeclampsia and to search for possible parameters associated with these endpoints.

Methods

From January 2007 to July 2014 all women with pre-eclampsia at the University Hospital Basel referred to our nephrology clinic were included into the study. As by our hospital policy, all patients with preeclampsia are referred for nephrology follow-up after 6 months. Patients were closely followed by their family doctor or obstetrician and referred earlier if necessary. Preeclampsia was defined as new onset of hypertension (≥140/90 mmHg) after the 20th gestational week or worsening hypertension (defined as blood pressure values ≥20/10 mmHg higher than previously measured during pregnancy) in patients with pre-existing elevated blood pressure and either proteinuria or other signs of end-organ dysfunction. The gynaecology department of the University Hospital of Basel had been in the practice of defining preeclampsia without the proteinuria requirement, as was later confirmed by the ACOG 2013 guidelines [13]. Hypertension was defined as a blood pressure ≥ 140/90 mmHg or the use of antihypertensive medication. This definition was used for inclusion into the study as well as at follow up. The presence of severe hypertension (≥160/110 mmHg), acute renal failure or oliguria, eclamptic seizure, pulmonary lung oedema, signs of HELLP-Syndrome, hyperreflexia, severe headaches, visual disturbances or intra uterine growth retardation with or without pathological Doppler ultrasound resulted in a diagnosis of severe preeclampsia [14]. Acute kidney injury was defined as a rise in serum creatinine concentration of more than 50% from baseline during hospitalisation. The presence of pre-existing conditions like hypertension, diabetes mellitus or kidney disease was gathered from medical records. Proteinuria was defined as a protein-to-creatinine ratio in a spot urine > 11 mg/mmol [15]. Decline of kidney function was defined as a decrease in eGFR ≥10 ml/min/1.73m². Urine sediments were evaluated by a staff nephrologist. For secondary analyses, a multivariate logistic regression model was applied. Univariate analysis was conducted in all variables with at least 15 observations and variables with a p-value < 0.2 were added to the model. Wilcoxon Mann Whitney test was used to compare medians due to skewed distribution of the baseline characteristics in the subgroups; chi-

squared test was used to compare frequencies. Different denominators in the results section are due to missing data in a few patients.

Results

Of the 225 women referred to our nephrology clinic, 23 were lost to follow-up (10%). Two hundred two were included in the analysis. The mean time of the follow up visit was 172 days (+/– 39.6) after delivery. Mean age of the 202 women was 32 years (18–45 years). 58.2% (117/201) were pregnant for the first time (primigravida). In 22.2% (43/194) of the patient's preeclampsia occurred before 34 weeks of gestation. Severe preeclampsia was observed in 67% (132/197) and eclampsia as the most severe form was seen in 2% (4/198). 90.1% (181/201) had no pre-existing diseases before pregnancy (diabetes mellitus, chronic kidney disease or hypertension). Baseline characteristics are shown in Table 1.

Distribution of blood pressure and urinary protein excretion at follow-up are shown in Fig. 1a and b. The mean blood pressure at 6-months follow up was 124/76 mmHg (+/– 14/11, range 116–182/63–110) and the mean serum-creatinine was 61.8 μmol/l (33–105 μmol/l) (normal < 110 μmol/l). Mean estimated glomerular filtration rate (eGFR) using CKD-EPI (chronic kidney disease epidemiology collaboration) was 110.7 ml/min/1.73m² (59.7–142.4 ml/min/1.73m²) (normal > 60 mml/min/1.73m²). 20.3% (41/202) had a blood pressure of 140/90 mmHg or higher (mean 143/89 mmHg) or received antihypertensive medication (5.5%, 11/202). Proteinuria was present in 33.1% (66/199) (mean 27.5 mg/mmol, range 12–261 mg/mmol). Proteinuria and hypertension were present in 8% (16/199) (Fig. 2). 54.3% (108/199) had none of the investigated sequelae at follow up. No active urine sediment (e.g. glomerular

Table 1 Baseline characteristics

Age mean (±SD)	32 (± 5.9)
Onset of preeclampsia (gestational week) mean (±SD)	36 + 3 (± 3.9 weeks)
Early Onset (< 34 weeks of gestation) (43/195)	22.1%
Nulliparous (150/199)	75.4%
Multiple pregnancy (twins, triplets) (27/202)	13.4%
In vitro fertilisation (13/202)	6.4%
Diabetes before pregnancy (4/201)	1.99%
Gestational diabetes (19/202)	9.4%
Previous hypertension (16/202)	7.9%
HELLP (41/198)	20.7%
Eclampsia (4/198)	2.0%
Severe preeclampsia (132/197)	67%
Acute kidney injury (17/197)	8.6%
Chronic kidney disease (4/201)	1.99%

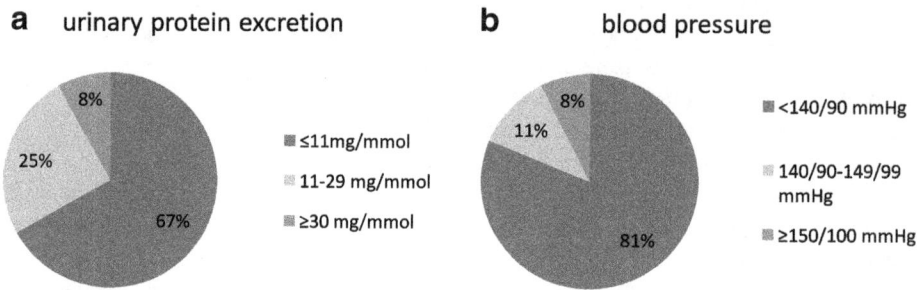

Fig. 1 a and **b** Distribution of urinary protein excretion and blood pressure at follow-up

microhematuria, casts, signs of glomerulonephritis) was observed.

Baseline characteristics in women with sequelae at follow-up are shown in Tables 2, 3 and 4. Multivariate logistic regression analyses showed an association of age and gestational diabetes with proteinuria > 11 mg/mmol and proteinuria ≥30 mg/mmol at follow-up, respectively. Additionally, severe preeclampsia was associated with an eGFR decline ≥10 ml/min/1.73m^2. None of the investigated parameters were associated with persistent hypertension (Table 5).

Discussion

Persistent proteinuria and hypertension after preeclampsia have been reported in several studies. Proteinuria in the first few months after preeclampsia is common [11, 16, 17], and can be detected up to several years. Hypertension can also persist for months and even for years [11, 12, 18]. Decreased kidney function is uncommon even after short term follow up in contrast to persistent hypertension and proteinuria [4, 12, 16, 19]. However, there is data indicating that the risk of chronic kidney disease after preeclampsia might be increased later

in life [2–4]. To our knowledge, our study is the largest on short term sequelae after preeclampsia. It shows that a significant part of patients with preeclampsia have ongoing sequelae 6 months after delivery. 20% remain hypertensive and one third have persistent proteinuria. 8% have combined hypertension and proteinuria. If hypertension or proteinuria persists 6 months after delivery, different guidelines state that referral for internal medicine or nephrology and further diagnostics should be considered [9, 10].

Berks et al. [11] reported proteinuria in 14% of patients after 3 months and 8% after 2 years. When applying, a proteinuria cut off of 0.3 g/d as done by this group, proteinuria was present in 8% in our study after 6 months, which is consistent with the 14% after 3 months in Berks' study. However, Berks et al. measured proteinuria by 24-h urine collection, whereas a creatinine-protein ratio to estimate proteinuria was used in this study, which makes a direct comparison of this low range proteinuria results more difficult. In a study by Chua et al. [20], proteinuria was absent after 3 months, but a relatively high cut off of 0.5 g/24 h was used. Again, proteinuria was measured with 24-h urine

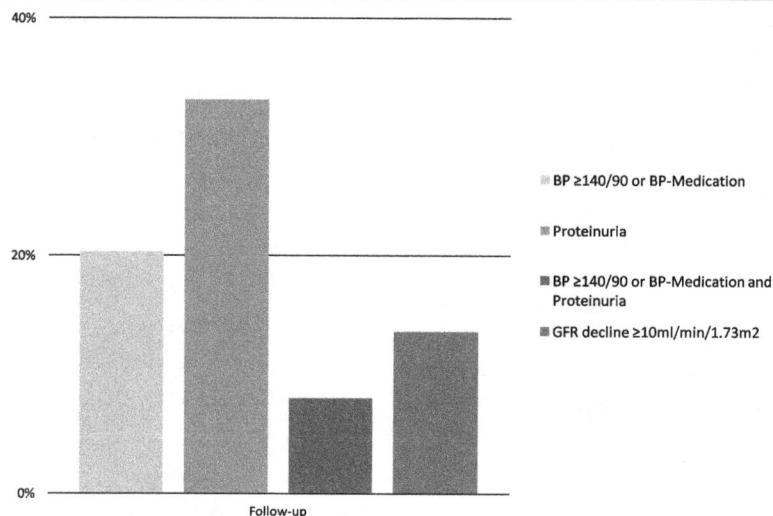

Fig. 2 Prevalence of hypertension, proteinuria and eGFR decline at mean follow-up of 172 days (± 39.6) after delivery

Table 2 Baseline characteristics (median (IQR)) of women with hypertension at follow-up

	No HT (n = 164)	BP ≥140/90 (n = 38)	p-value	No HT (n = 187)	BP ≥ 150/100 (n = 15)	p-value
Age	32 (28–36)	34 (30–37)	0.16	32 (28–36)	32 (29–40)	0.59
Onset (d)	260 (241–274)	250 (233–267)	0.08	259 (241–273)	250 (217–263)	0.12
Early onset	20.3% (32/158)	29.7% (11/37)	0.21	21.1% (38/180)	33.3% (5/15)	0.27
Nulliparous	75.6% (124/162)	68% (26/38)	0.30	75.1% (139/185)	73.3% (11/15)	0.88
Time to f/u (d)	180 (155–191)	182 (132–190)	0.33	180 (153–191)	176 (121–187)	0.18
MP	14.0% (23/164)	10.5% (4/38)	0.57	14.4% (27/187)	0% (0/15)	0.11
IVF	6.7% (11/164)	5.7% (2/38)	0.74	7.0% (13/187)	0% (0/15)	0.29
GD	7.9% (13/164)	15.8% (6/38)	0.13	9.1% (17/187)	13.3% (2/15)	0.56
HELLP	21.9% (35/160)	15.8% (6/38)	0.40	21.9% 40/183	6.7% (1/15)	0.16
Severe PE	67.3% (107/159)	64.1% (25/39)	0.86	67.0% (122/182)	66.7% (10/15)	0.97
AKI	9.7% (14/145)	5.3% (3/38)	0.86	7.7% (14/182)	20.0% 3/15	0.10

HT Hypertension, *BP* Blood pressure in mmHg, *PE* Preeclampsia, *AKI* Acute kidney injury, *GD* gestational diabetes; *f/u* follow-up, *d* days

collection. Another study reported persistent Microalbuminuria in up to 60% of patients 2–4 months after preeclampsia and in still 40% after 3–5 years using a considerably low cut off for microalbuminuria of 14 mg/24 h [19]. Overall, despite conflicting evidence proteinuria seems to be a relevant short-term sequela after preeclampsia. In our secondary analysis, older age at baseline was associated with proteinuria > 11 mg/mmol, but not with proteinuria > 30 mg/mmol. Gestational diabetes was associated with proteinuria > 30 mg/mmol. However, given the large confidence interval with the lower range close to 1, this finding might be significant by chance. Furthermore, as we know from diabetic kidney disease, it usually takes years of abnormal glucose metabolism to result in kidney damage with proteinuria, making this finding also clinically unlikely.

In our study, 20% of women were hypertensive after 6 months. In the study by Berks et al., 39% of women had hypertensive blood pressure values after 3 months and 18% were still hypertensive after 2 years [11]. These findings suggest that there is no further resolution of hypertension after 6 months in contrast to proteinuria which was only present in 2% after 2 years. Another explanation might be the difference in severe preeclampsia of 67% in our study to 89% in the study by Berks et al. and thereby a faster resolution of symptoms in our study. In another study from Japan [16] 17% (9/52) of women with preeclampsia still had hypertensive blood pressure values or received antihypertensive medication after 2 years. This value is close to the 18% of women with hypertension after 2 years in the study by Berks et al., although the percentage of patients with severe preeclampsia was not reported in the Japanese study. In a third study from Iran [12], 29% (10/35) were still hypertensive after a median follow up of 5.7 years. We could not identify any clinical parameters associated with persistent hypertension in our secondary analysis. In a subgroup analysis in 129 women with available data on peak hypertensive values at baseline, peak systolic blood pressure was significantly associated ($p = 0.04$) with

Table 3 Baseline characteristics (median (IQR)) of women with proteinuria at follow-up

	No UPE (n = 134)	UPE > 0.11 (n = 66)	p-value	No UPE (n = 184)	UPE ≥30 (n = 16)	p-value
Age	31 (28–35)	35 (28–38)	0.16	32 (29–36)	34 (25–38)	0.80
Onset (d)	260 (238–272)	258 (246–272)	0.61	259 (240–272)	266 (248–279)	0.29
Early onset	24.8% (32/129)	14.1% (9/64)	0.09	22.6% (40/177)	6.25% (1/16)	0.13
Nulliparous	75.2% (100/133)	73.9% (48/65)	0.84	73.6% (134/182)	87.5% (14/16)	0.22
Time to f/u (d)	183 (157–191)	172 (138–187)	0.06	180 (154–190)	160 (114–195)	0.42
MP	12.7% (17/134)	15.2% (10/66)	0.61	14.1% (26/184)	6.3% (1/16)	0.34
IVF	4.5% (6/134)	10.6% (7/66)	0.10	6.5%(12/184)	6.3% (1/16)	0.97
GD	7.5% (10/134)	16.7% (9/66)	0.16	8.2%(15/184)	25.0% (4/16)	0.02
HELLP	22.7% (30/132)	16.9% (11/65)	0.35	22.1% (40/181)	6.3% (1/16)	0.13
Severe	67.2% (88/131)	66.2%(43/65)	0.89	66.1% (119/180)	75% (12/16)	0.45
AKI	9.9% (13/131)	6.2%(4/65)	0.34	8.3% (15/180)	12.5% (2/16)	0.57

UPE urinary protein excretion, *HT* Hypertension, *BP* Blood pressure in mmHg, *PE* Preeclampsia, *AKI* Acute kidney injury, *GD* gestational diabetes; *f/u* follow-up; *d* days

Table 4 Baseline characteristics (median (IQR)) of women with decline in eGFR ≥10 ml/min/1.73 m2 at follow-up

	No eGFR decline (*n* = 170)	eGFR decline (*n* = 27)	*p*-value
Age	33 (28–37)	31 (27–35)	0.20
Onset (d)	258 (240–272)	261 (241–273)	0.64
Early onset	21.8% (36/165)	18.5% (5/27)	0.70
Nulliparous	75.7% (128/169)	66.7% (18/27)	0.32
Time to f/u (d)	180 (152–190)	179 (154–190)	0.93
MD	15.3% (26/170)	3.7% (1/27)	0.10
IVF	7.7% (13/170)	0% (0/27)	0.14
GD	8.8% (15/170)	14.8% (4/27)	0.33
HELLP	21.2% (36/170)	18.5% (5/27)	0.75
Severe PE	70% (119/170)	48.2% (13/27)	0.03
AKI	10.1% (17/169)	0% (0/27)	0.09

HT Hypertension, *BP* Blood pressure in mmHg, *PE* Preeclampsia, *AKI* Acute kidney injury, *GD* gestational diabetes, *f/u* follow-up; *d* days

Table 5 Multivariate logistic regression analysis for hypertension, proteinuria and eGFR at follow-up

	Odds ratio	p-value	95% conf. interval
BP ≥140/90 mmHg			
Age	1.05	0.18	0.98–1.12
Time to f/u (d)	0.99	0.08	0.98–1.00
Onset (d)	0.99	0.20	0.99–1.00
GD	2.16	0.16	0.74–6.34
		0.06	
BP ≥ 150/100 mmHg			
Time to f/u (d)	0.99	0.20	0.98–1.00
Onset (d)	0.99	0.12	0.98–1.00
HELLP	0.24	0.18	0.03–1.96
AKI	2.7	0.17	0.65–11.23
		0.08	
UPE > 11 mg/mmol			
Age	1.06	0.03	1.01–1.13
GD	1.71	0.21	0.70–4.81
Early onset	0.46	0.09	0.21–1.11
		0.02	
UPE ≥ 30 mg/mmol			
GD	3.67	0.049	1.01–13.37
HELLP	0.27	0.21	0.03–2.13
Early onset	0.35	0.45	0.02–5.46
Onset (d)	1.01	0.77	0.97–1.04
		0.08	
eGFR decline			
Severe PE	0.40	0.03	0.17–0.91

UPE urinary protein excretion, *BP* Blood pressure in mmHg, *PE* Preeclampsia, *AKI* Acute kidney injury, *GD* gestational diabetes *f/u* follow-up, *d* days

persistent hypertensive values ≥ 150/100 mmHg at follow-up, but not persistent proteinuria or eGFR decline.

Data on kidney function in the first months to years after preeclampsia are limited. In the study by Shahbazian et al. [12] the mean estimated glomerular filtration rate (eGFR) after a mean follow up of 5.7 years was 108 ml/min (+/− 14 ml/min). Bar et al. found a mean creatinine of 79.2 μmol/l and 70.4 μmol/l after 2 to 4 months and after 3 to 5 years, respectively [19]. Shammas and others described no difference in renal function 10 years after hypertensive disorder in pregnancy in comparison to healthy women [17]. In our study, the mean eGFR at 6-months follow up was 110.7 ml/min/1.73m^2. Only one woman had an eGFR below 60 ml/min/1.73m^2. Thus, a reduced eGFR early after preeclampsia is uncommon. Our results correspond well with an analysis from Vikse et al. that showed a 0.1% risk of ESRD after preeclampsia after 30 years [4]. The improbability of chronic structural kidney disease is underlined by the absence of pathologic urine sediment findings in our study.

We arbitrarily defined kidney decline as a decrease in kidney function by ≥10 ml/min/1.73m^2, which was present in 27 women. The clinical significance of this decline is difficult to interpret. Since physiologic glomerular hyperfiltration is still present at the end of pregnancy, the reported "decline" could really be a return to baseline before pregnancy. On the other hand, it was only present in a minority of patients and significantly associated with severe preeclampsia, both arguments against a physiological process. However, although a significant difference (*p* < 0.00) in medians in eGFR in women with a decline in eGFR (103 ml/min/1.73m^2) and women without (114 ml/min/1.73m^2) was present, both were within normal range. Furthermore, as mentioned above the risk of ESRD after preeclampsia is far lower than the 13% (27/197) of women with an eGFR delcine in our study, thus the clinical significance remains unclear.

Our study has several strengths. To the best of our knowledge, this is the largest study on short term sequelae of preeclampsia. Furthermore, information on urine sediments has not been reported in this setting before. Due to a standardized protocol for follow-up after preeclampsia at our clinic, a low number of patients were lost to follow-up. The collection of several baseline characteristics allowed for secondary analysis for risk factors.

There are also several limitations. Being designed as a cohort study, there is no control group as a reference. We did not have information on GFR during pregnancies, since there were no routine blood tests before preeclampsia symptoms occurred with mostly initiation of delivery short thereafter. An analysis on possible sociodemographic differences between the patients lost to follow-up and the patients included in our study would have been of interest, but was not possible due to unavailability of sociodemographic data. There seems to be a selection bias with a high incidence for severe preeclampsia (67%), most likely due to our hospital being a tertiary center with referral of more complicated deliveries. Additionally, even though all patients with preeclampsia in our center are supposed to be referred for nephrology follow-up after 6 months, we cannot exclude that some patients with mild forms of preeclampsia were not referred for follow-up leading to a higher incidence of severe preeclampsia.

Conclusion

Given the high frequency of sequelae 6 months after preeclampsia, this study underlies the importance of close follow-up. To identify those women at risk for persistent symptoms, knowing what features of preeclampsia are associated with these short-term sequelae would be important. We identified age and gestational diabetes as risk factors for proteinuria and severe preeclampsia for a decline in eGFR. However, further studies are need to define the clinical relevance of these findings.

Abbreviations
CKD-EPI: Chronic kidney disease epidemiology collaboration; eGFR: Estimated glomerular filtration rate; ESRD: End-Stage Renal Disease; HELLP: Hemolysis, Elevated Liver Enzymes, Low Platelet; SD: Standard Deviation

Authors' contributions
MG contributed to conception and design, collected, analyzed and interpreted the data and wrote the manuscript. IH was involved in critically revising the manuscript and gave approval to publish the manuscript. CM contributed to interpreting the data and gave approval to publish the manuscript. MD made major contributions to conception and design of the study and analyzing the data. He was a major contributor in writing the manuscript and gave approval of the manuscript to be published. All authors read and approved the final manuscript for publication.

Competing interests
The authors declare that they have no competing interests.

Author details
[1]Clinic for Transplantation Immunology and Nephrology, University Hospital Basel, Petersgraben 4, 4031 Basel, Switzerland. [2]Department of Gynaecology and Obstetrics, University Hospital Basel, Spitalstrasse 21, 4031 Basel, Switzerland.

References
1. Abalos E, Cuesta C, Grosso AL, Chou D, Say L. Global and regional estimates of preeclampsia and eclampsia: a systematic review. Eur J Obstet Gynecol Reprod Biol. 2013;170:1–7. https://doi.org/10.1016/j.ejogrb.2013.05.005.
2. Vikse BE, Irgens LM, Bostad L, Iversen BM. Adverse perinatal outcome and later kidney biopsy in the mother. J Am Soc Nephrol. 2006;17:837–45. https://doi.org/10.1681/ASN.2005050492.
3. Wang I-K, Muo C-H, Chang Y-C, Liang C-C, Chang C-T, Lin S-Y, et al. Association between hypertensive disorders during pregnancy and end-stage renal disease: a population-based study. CMAJ. 2013;185:207–13. https://doi.org/10.1503/cmaj.120230.
4. Vikse BE, Irgens LM, Leivestad T, Skjaerven R, Iversen BM. Preeclampsia and the risk of end-stage renal disease. N Engl J Med. 2008;359:800–9. https://doi.org/10.1056/NEJMoa0706790.
5. Chesley LC, Annitto JE, Cosgrove RA. American journal of obstetrics and gynecology, volume 124, 1976: the remote prognosis of eclamptic women. Sixth periodic report. Am J Obstet Gynecol. 2000;182 1 Pt 1:247. discussion 248. http://www.ncbi.nlm.nih.gov/pubmed/10649186. Accessed 14 Oct 2016
6. Sibai BM, el-Nazer A, Gonzalez-Ruiz A. Severe preeclampsia-eclampsia in young primigravid women: subsequent pregnancy outcome and remote prognosis. Am J Obstet Gynecol. 1986;155:1011–6. http://www.ncbi.nlm.nih.gov/pubmed/3777042. Accessed 14 Oct 2016
7. Fisher KA, Luger A, Spargo BH, Lindheimer MD. Hypertension in pregnancy: clinical-pathological correlations and remote prognosis. Medicine (Baltimore). 1981;60:267–76. http://www.ncbi.nlm.nih.gov/pubmed/7242320. Accessed 14 Oct 2016
8. Report of the National High Blood Pressure Education Program Working Group on high blood pressure in pregnancy. Am J Obstet Gynecol. 2000; 183:S1–22. http://www.ncbi.nlm.nih.gov/pubmed/10920346. Accessed 14 Oct 2016
9. Magee LA, Pels A, Helewa M, Rey E, von Dadelszen P. SOGC hypertension guideline committee. Diagnosis, evaluation, and management of the hypertensive disorders of pregnancy: executive summary. J Obstet Gynaecol Canada. 2014;36:575–6. http://www.ncbi.nlm.nih.gov/pubmed/25184972. Accessed 14 Oct 2016
10. Federführende Leitlinien der deutschen Gesellschaft für Gynäkologie und Geburtshilfe; Diagnostik und Therapie hypertensiver Schwangerschaftserkrankungen. 2013.
11. Berks D, Steegers EAP, Molas M, Visser W. Resolution of hypertension and proteinuria after preeclampsia. Obstet Gynecol. 2009;114:1307–14. https://doi.org/10.1097/AOG.0b013e3181c14e3e.
12. Shahbazian N, Shahbazian H, Ehsanpour A, Aref A, Gharibzadeh S. Hypertension and microalbuminuria 5 years after pregnancies complicated by pre-eclampsia. Iran J Kidney Dis. 2011;5:324–7. http://www.ncbi.nlm.nih.gov/pubmed/21876309. Accessed 14 Oct 2016
13. American College of Obstetricians and Gynecologists, Task Force on Hypertension in Pregnancy. Hypertension in pregnancy. Obstet Gynecol. 2013;122:1122–31. https://doi.org/10.1097/01.AOG.0000437382.03963.88.
14. Severe Pre-eclampsia/Eclampsia, Management (Guideline No. 10A). R Coll Obstet Gynecol.
15. Fulks M, Stout RL, Dolan VF. Urine protein/creatinine ratio as a mortality risk predictor in non-diabetics with normal renal function. J Insur Med. 2012;43:76–83. http://www.ncbi.nlm.nih.gov/pubmed/22876411. Accessed 11 Oct 2017
16. Suzuki H, Watanabe Y, Arima H, Kobayashi K, Ohno Y, Kanno Y. Short- and long-term prognosis of blood pressure and kidney disease in women with a past history of preeclampsia. Clin Exp Nephrol. 2008;12:102–9. https://doi.org/10.1007/s10157-007-0018-1.
17. Shammas AG, Maayah JF. Hypertension and its relation to renal function 10

years after pregnancy complicated by pre-eclampsia and pregnancy induced hypertension. Saudi Med J. 2000;21:190–2. http://www.ncbi.nlm.nih.gov/pubmed/11533780. Accessed 21 Oct 2016

18. Nisell H, Lintu H, Lunell NO, Möllerström G, Pettersson E. Blood pressure and renal function seven years after pregnancy complicated by hypertension. Br J Obstet Gynaecol. 1995;102:876–81. http://www.ncbi.nlm.nih.gov/pubmed/8534622. Accessed 14 Oct 2016

19. Bar J, Kaplan B, Wittenberg C, Erman A, Boner G, Ben-Rafael Z, et al. Microalbuminuria after pregnancy complicated by pre-eclampsia. Nephrol Dial Transplant. 1999;14:1129–32. http://www.ncbi.nlm.nih.gov/pubmed/10344350. Accessed 14 Oct 2016

20. Chua S, Redman CW. Prognosis for pre-eclampsia complicated by 5 g or more of proteinuria in 24 hours. Eur J Obstet Gynecol Reprod Biol. 1992;43:9–12. http://www.ncbi.nlm.nih.gov/pubmed/1737613. Accessed 21 Oct 2016

11

Common carotid artery intima-media thickness increases throughout the pregnancy cycle

Nancy Anderson Niemczyk[1,2]*(iD), Marianne Bertolet[1], Janet M. Catov[1,3,4], Mansi Desai[1], Candace K. McClure[1], James M. Roberts[1,3,4,5], Akira Sekikawa[1], Ping Guo Tepper[1] and Emma J. Barinas-Mitchell[1]

Abstract

Background: High parity is associated with greater cardiovascular disease (CVD) among mid-life and older women. Prospective studies of arterial change throughout pregnancy are needed to provide insight into potential mechanisms. This study assessed vascular adaptation across pregnancy in healthy first-time pregnant women.

Methods: The Maternal Vascular Adaptation to Healthy Pregnancy Study (Pittsburgh, PA, 2010–2015) assessed 37 primigravid women each trimester, 6–8 weeks after delivery and 1–5 years postpartum, with B-mode ultrasound imaging of common carotid artery (CCA) intima-media thickness (IMT) and inter-adventitial diameter (IAD) to assess associations with physical and cardiometabolic measures.

Results: Thirty-seven women (age 28.2 ± 4.5 years, pre-pregnant BMI 24.4 ± 3.2 kg/m^2) experienced uncomplicated pregnancies. After adjustment for age and pre-pregnancy BMI, mean (SE) IAD (mm) increased each trimester, from 6.38 (0.08) in the 1st trimester to 6.92 (0.09) in the 3rd trimester, and then returned to 1st trimester levels postpartum (6.35 [0.07], $P < 0.001$). In contrast, mean (SE) CCA IMT (mm) increased from the 2nd trimester (i.e., 0.546 [0.01]) onward, and remained higher at an average of 2.7 years postpartum (0.581 [0.02], $P = 0.03$). Weight partially explained changes in IAD.

Conclusions: In uncomplicated first pregnancies, IAD increased and returned to 1st trimester levels postpartum. In contrast, CCA IMT remained increased 2 years postpartum. Maternal weight explained vascular changes better than did metabolic changes. Increased postpartum CCA IMT may persist and contribute to long-term CVD risk.

Keywords: Common carotid artery intima-media thickness, Inter-adventitial diameter, Pregnancy, Cardiovascular disease, Vascular remodeling

Background

High parity is associated with greater cardiovascular disease (CVD) risk in women [1]. Although some of this risk may be due to socio-economic status and lifestyle factors associated with greater parity, acute physiologic changes during pregnancy also may contribute to CVD

risk [1–4]. For example, either weight gain or the atherogenic metabolic changes of pregnancy may instigate persistent unhealthy vascular changes [5, 6]. However, studies that could illuminate these relationships have been limited by 1) sample sizes inadequate to detect significant differences in vessel measures [7, 8], 2) failure to collect serial arterial measures [6], 3) use of non-standard techniques to assess the vasculature [5, 9], 4) short follow-up [7, 8], and 5) lack of biomarker collection across the pregnancy cycle [5–10].

Structural arterial changes during pregnancy can be assessed using B-mode ultrasonography of the carotid

* Correspondence: nan37@pitt.edu
[1]Department of Epidemiology, Graduate School of Public Health, University of Pittsburgh, 130 De Soto Street, Pittsburgh, PA 15261, USA
[2]Department of Health Promotion and Development, School of Nursing, University of Pittsburgh, 3500 Victoria Street, 440 Victoria Building, Pittsburgh, PA 15261, USA
Full list of author information is available at the end of the article

artery, a well-established, non-invasive, reproducible technique [11]. Abnormal values of two measures of arterial structure—greater intima-media thickness (IMT) and inter-adventitial diameter (IAD) of the common carotid artery (CCA)—are associated with greater CVD risk factor burden [12–14], arterial aging [15], and higher incidence of CVD [13, 16, 17]. The normal changes that occur in the CCA IMT and IAD during and after a healthy pregnancy have not been well established.

The primary objective of our *Maternal Vascular Adaptation to Healthy Pregnancy* (MVP) study was to assess vascular changes in normal first pregnancies, using an adequate sample size, serial measures, a standardized technique to assess vasculature, and including collection of biomarkers. We hypothesized that the vasculature would transiently adapt to the increased blood volume and metabolic requirements of healthy pregnancy, and that these adaptations would be associated with pregnancy weight gain and changes in levels of cardiometabolic factors.

Methods
Study design and population
The MVP study prospectively assessed common carotid artery measures in a cohort of healthy primigravid women. Eligible participants recruited from the community were healthy, non-smoking primigravid women, aged ≤40 years, at less than 38 weeks of gestational age. Exclusion criteria were the following: 1) vasoactive medication use; 2) infertility history—defined as either experiencing a period of at least 12 months marked by the inability to achieve pregnancy or using fertility medications to achieve pregnancy; 3) family history of premature coronary artery disease; 4) previous abortion; 5) multiple gestation.

Study visits were scheduled at 12–14, 24–26, and 36–38 weeks of pregnancy, and 6–8 weeks postpartum; all visits were conducted between in 2010 to 2013. After telephone screening for eligibility, women began the study at any one of the pregnancy visits. Each visit involved physical measures (e.g., height and weight) and ultrasound measures of the carotid artery. We calculated that 31 women were needed as participants to generate 80% power to detect a 0.5 SD difference for change in CCA IMT and IAD given an assumed 0.5 correlation among the repeated observations. Because we estimated that 1) 10–20% of women develop a pregnancy complication and 2) our study would experience 25% attrition, we targeted recruitment of 46. The study enrolled 44 women, of whom 43 had multiple visits, and six developed pregnancy complications (one preeclampsia; 3 gestational hypertension; 2 preterm births, one of which had a placental abruption), which left 37 participants with uncomplicated pregnancies and full term births of

normal weight newborns in the analytic sample for our analysis.

These participants were invited to return for a follow-up visit 1–5 years after their first postpartum visit. Fourteen had moved out of the region and were unable to participate. Participants (i.e., five women) were excluded if they were pregnant or if they had given birth within the previous 4 months, which generated seventeen potential participants. Of these seventeen, fourteen experienced uncomplicated first pregnancies and were, therefore, included in our analysis. These follow-up visits occurred between 2014 and 2015. Participants signed an informed consent document approved by the University of Pittsburgh, Human Research Protection Office.

Carotid artery measures
Carotid ultrasounds were performed by a trained research vascular sonographer from the University of Pittsburgh, Ultrasound Research Laboratory (URL). Participants were placed supine, with a right hip wedge for comfort if necessary, and the common carotid artery was scanned bilaterally with high-resolution B-mode ultrasound (ACUSON Cypress System, Malvern, PA.) Digitized images of the common carotid artery were obtained at end diastole, 1 cm proximal to the carotid bulb, and IMT was measured as the distance from the media-adventitial interface to the intima-lumen interface of both the near and far wall of the artery. Approximately 140 measurements of thickness were made for each 1-cm segment, and the mean of each segment was calculated. IMT reported represents the mean value for near and far wall bilaterally. IAD was measured as distance from the adventitial-medial interface of the near arterial wall to the media-adventitial interface of the arterial wall using the same CCA segment. Images were read by one reader, using a computerized, semi-automated reading program system [18]. Reproducibility of carotid measures at the URL was excellent during the time period of the study, with an intraclass correlation coefficient within reader of over 0.91 for CCA IMT and over 0.99 for IAD.

Demographic, pregnancy history, physical, and laboratory measures
At the initial visit, participants completed a self-administered demographic form. Research staff 1) measured the height of participants using a stadiometer and 2) weighed the participants on a standard balance scale. The mean value of two readings for each measure was recorded. Pre-pregnancy weight was identified preferentially as the pre-pregnancy weight documented in the prenatal record or, if not available, as a documented weight in the medical record in the 3 months prior to the last menstrual period. Pre-pregnancy BMI was

calculated as pre-pregnancy weight in kilograms divided by height in meters, squared. Weight change was calculated as the difference between current and pre-pregnancy weight.

Pulse and blood pressure were measured, according to a standardized protocol. Three measurements of each were taken, and the mean of the last two measurements was recorded and used for our analysis. Data resulting from both demographic and physical measures and records reviews were collected and managed using REDCap electronic data capture tools hosted at the University of Pittsburgh [19].

Laboratory assays of fasting serum samples collected at each visit were performed at the Heinz Nutrition Laboratory at the University of Pittsburgh, Graduate School of Public Health, and the following parameters were determined using standard laboratory procedures: total cholesterol, high density lipoprotein (HDL-c), low density lipoprotein (LDL-c) [20], triglycerides [21], and glucose [22]. Insulin was measured using a standard radio-immune assay (Linco Research, St. Charles, MO). HOMA-IR, a measure of insulin resistance, was calculated as (glucose (mg/dl) x insulin (µU/ml))/405 [23]. High-sensitivity C-reactive protein (hsCRP) was measured with an enzyme-linked immunoassay (Alpha Diagnostics International Inc., San Antonio, TX).

Prenatal and birth records were reviewed after the first postpartum study visit to exclude women with complications, which included gestational hypertension, preeclampsia, and preterm birth. Participants completed an interval reproductive and health history form at the second postpartum visit.

Statistical analysis

Measures with normal distributions were evaluated as means ± standard deviations. Measures with non-normal distributions (i.e., hsCRP and HOMA-IR) were analyzed as medians with interquartile range and log-transformed for our analysis. Categorical variables (e.g., employment) were presented as percentages. Linear mixed models featuring random intercepts and Toeplitz variance and covariance structure were used to estimate means for CCA IMT and IAD.

Baseline maternal age and pre-pregnancy BMI were included a priori in all models. Separate models were constructed for systolic blood pressure, weight, and weight change. For CCA IMT, models were also constructed including IAD, since over time increases in IAD can cause increases in CCA IMT. Predictors with a significance level of $P \leq 0.2$ were then placed into models together, and predictors with a significance level of $P \leq 0.1$ were retained. Next, biomarkers were tested individually in the final models identified for each outcome. Biomarkers with a significance level of $P \leq 0.1$ were then

placed into the best models together, and significant predictors were retained. A sensitivity analysis was performed to eliminate three extreme outlier values for hsCRP (i.e. ≥ 60 mg/L). P values of 0.05 or less were considered statistically significant for the analysis. As a sensitivity analysis, the analysis was repeated using only data from women who completed all four initial visits. Associations between physical and carotid measures were not assessed for the second postpartum visit because 1) associations may differ during pregnancy as a result of dramatic hematologic and hormonal changes and 2) the sample size was smaller (i.e., 14) for this visit. Statistical analyses were performed using SAS statistical software releases 9.3 and 9.4 (SAS Institute, Cary, NC).

Results

The mean number of initial study visits was 3.3 (range 2–4), and 15 participants (41%) completed all 4 visits. The average participant age was 28.4 ± 4.6 years, and the average participant pre-pregnancy BMI was 24.3 ± 3.3. Participants were predominantly white (91.9%), married or living as married (89.2%), well-educated (89.1% college graduate or greater), and employed (64.9% full-time; 24.3% part-time). Mean birth weight was 3427.2 ± 224.5 g and mean gestational age at birth was 39.7 ± 1.3 weeks. Route of birth was vaginal for 91.2% of women, and no newborns had apgar scores less than 7 at 1 or 5 min of life. At the 6–8-week postpartum visit, 88% of participants were breastfeeding their infants exclusively. Fourteen participants completed the second postpartum visit 1–5 years (mean 2.7 years) after their first birth, and seven of these participants had experienced subsequent pregnancies (i.e., five participants reported having one additional birth, one participant reported having two additional births, and one participant having a spontaneous abortion).

Among the participants, IAD increased throughout pregnancy from a mean (SE) of 6.47 (.12) mm in the 1st trimester to 6.89 (.10) mm in the 3rd trimester (all $P < 0.05$). IAD then returned to early pregnancy values (i.e., 6.36 [.07] mm, $P = 0.76$) by the first postpartum visit, and we observed no further decrease at the second postpartum visit (6.42 [0.11] mm) (Table 1). Adjustment for maternal age and pre-pregnancy BMI minimally affected these estimates (Fig. 1). CCA IMT remained stable between the 1st and 2nd trimesters and then increased in the 3rd trimester and through the postpartum period (i.e., 1st trimester mean [SE] 0.547 [.02] mm, first postpartum 0.565 [.01] mm, second postpartum 0.581 [0.02] mm) (Table 1). These values changed minimally when adjusted for maternal age and pre-pregnancy BMI (Fig. 2).

Changes in weight, blood pressure, heart rate, lipid, glucose, and hsCRP concentrations followed expected

Table 1 Unadjusted values for vascular measures and biomarkers by trimester and postpartum

Measure	1st trimester $n = 17$	2nd trimester $n = 32$	3rd trimester $n = 37$	1st postpartum $n = 35$	2nd postpartum $n = 14$	Overall P-value
Inter-adventitial diameter (mm)	6.47 (0.12)	6.79 (0.08)	6.89 (0.10)	6.36 (0.07)	6.42 (0.11)	< 0.0001
CCA intima-media thickness (mm)	0.547 (0.02)	0.546 (0.01)	0.553 (0.01)	0.565 (0.01)	0.581 (0.02)	0.03
Weight (kg)	68.7 (2.2)	73.1 (1.6)	79.5 (1.8)	69.2 (1.5)	70.2 (1.9)	< 0.0001
Weight change (kg)	0.55 (0.46)	7.27 (0.62)	14.4 (0.91)	4.3 (0.75)	3.7 (1.1)	< 0.0001
Systolic blood pressure (mm Hg)	103.7 (2.1)	106.0 (1.7)	110.4 (1.4)	106.2 (1.7)	102.9 (2.5)	< 0.0001
Heart rate (bpm)	78.0 (2.4)	79.8 (1.6)	82.0 (1.5)	68.1 (1.5)	63.6 (2.5)	< 0.0001
Total cholesterol (mg/dl)	201.7 (8.9)	257.3 (7.0)	273.1 (7.2)	191.4 (5.5)	194.8 (8.4)	< 0.0001
LDL-c (mg/dl)	111.2 (7.0)	148.0 (6.3)	155.5 (6.6)	114.7 (4.8)	121.9 (7.0)	< 0.0001
Triglycerides (mg/dl)	108.3 (10.5)	176.5 (10.2)	250.7 (13.6)	77.3 (7.0)	87.1 (9.6)	< 0.0001
HDL-c (mg/dl)	68.8 (2.2)	74.0 (3.1)	66.8 (2.3)	61.2 (1.8)	55.6 (2.9)	< 0.0001
Glucose (mg/dl)	79.3 (1.5)	77.2 (1.1)	77.0 (1.2)	82.6 (1.2)	88.5 (1.9)	< 0.0001
Insulin (μU/ml)	8.84 (0.78)	11.25 (0.98)	11.95 (0.81)	8.59 (0.50)	10.76 (0.82)	0.0008
HOMA-IR	1.64 [1.32, 2.09]	2.16 [1.56, 2.56]	2.28 [1.67, 2.51]	1.72 [1.34, 2.13]	2.20 [1.76, 2.87]	0.03
hsCRP (mg/L)	3.58 [2.16, 5.57]	3.36 [2.31, 5.49]	3.29 [2.24, 7.01]	1.20 [.77, 2.44]	0.96 [0.37, 1.50]	< 0.0001

Normally distributed values presented as mean (SE) and P value from mixed models. Skewed values presented as median [IQR] and P-value from Wilcoxon rank-sum test. CCA is common carotid artery. Weight change is change from pre-pregnancy weight

patterns for healthy pregnancies [24] (Table 1). Greater weight was associated marginally with greater IAD, and attenuated the increase in IAD that occurred throughout pregnancy (Table 2, Model 3). When metabolic factors were considered, higher triglyceride concentrations were associated ($P < 0.0001$) with lower IAD, but higher hsCRP was associated ($P = 0.0002$) with greater IAD (Table 2, Model 5, and Table 3).

Higher SBP was associated with greater CCA IMT; nonetheless, accounting for SBP did not attenuate the postpartum increase in CCA IMT (Table 4, Model 2). Greater weight gain was marginally associated with thinner CCA IMT (Table 4, Models 5, 6, 7), and greater IAD was associated with thicker CCA IMT (Table 4, Model 6). In addition, when metabolic factors were considered, greater HOMA-IR was associated with lower CCA IMT

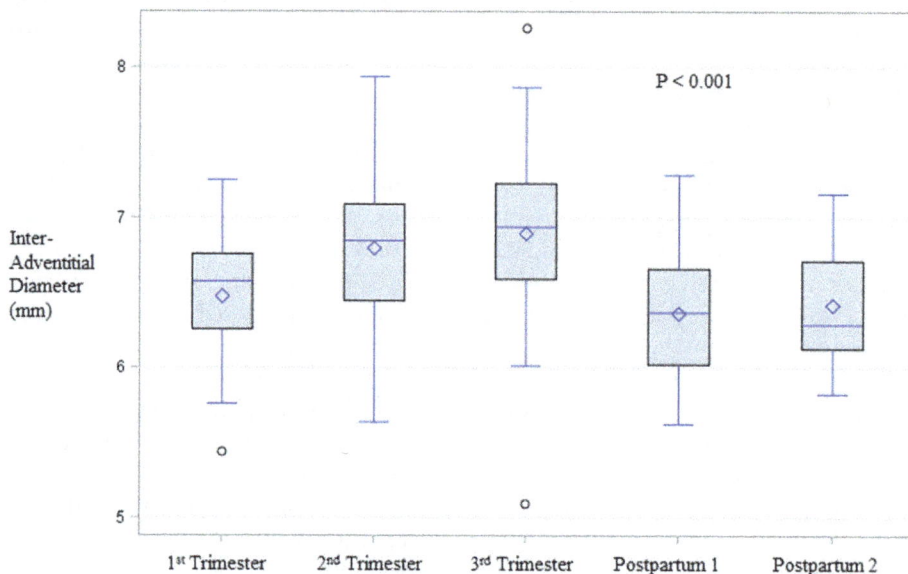

Fig. 1 Changes in inter-adventitial diameter across pregnancy, adjusted for maternal age and pre-pregnancy BMI. All pairwise comparisons significant at $P < .0001$ except: 1st Trimester vs. 1st Postpartum $P = .99$, 1st Trimester vs. 2nd Postpartum $P = 0.80$, 2nd Trimester vs. 3rd Trimester $P = .03$, 1st postpartum vs. 2nd postpartum $P = 0.73$. Adjusted for age and pre-pregnancy body mass index. The diamond represents the mean and the horizontal line represents the median

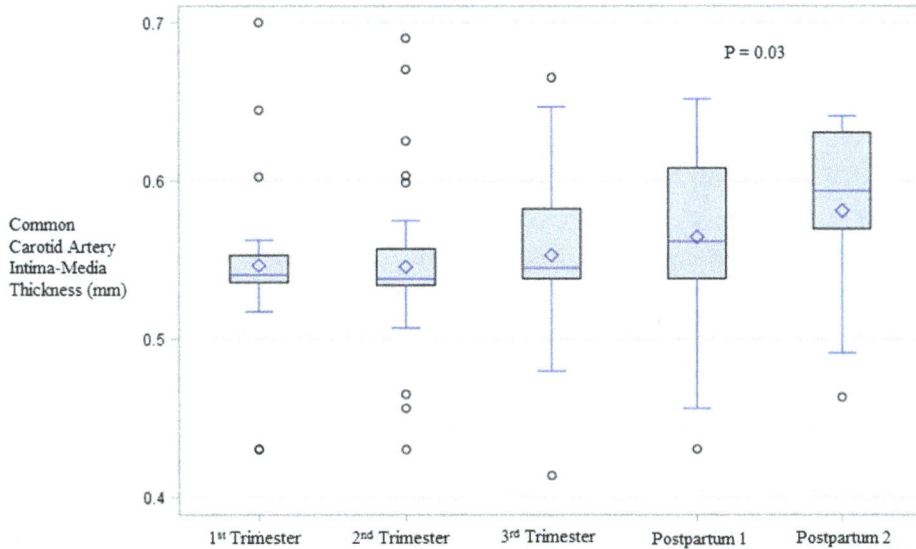

Fig. 2 Changes in CCA IMT across pregnancy, adjusted for maternal age and pre-pregnancy BMI. Statistically significant differences are as follows: 1st Trimester vs. 1st Postpartum $P = 0.03$, 1st Trimester vs. 2nd Postpartum $P = 0.01$, 2nd Trimester vs. 1st Postpartum $P = 0.01$, 2nd Trimester vs. 2nd Postpartum $P = 0.01$. The diamond represents the mean and the horizontal line represents the median

Table 2 Associations[a] between inter-adventitial diameter, physical predictors, and significant metabolic predictors

Predictor	Unadjusted		Model 1[b]		Model 2[b]	
	ß (SE)	P-value	ß (SE)	P-value	ß (SE)	P-value
Trimester 1	Ref		Ref		Ref	
Trimester 2	0.361 (.07)[c]	0.0001	0.361 (.07)[c]	< 0.0001	0.389 (.07)[c]	< 0.001
Trimester 3	0.498 (.07)[cd]	0.0001	0.499 (.07)[cd]	< 0.0001	0.511 (.07)[c]	< 0.001
Postpartum	−0.015 (.05)	0.74	−0.014 (.05)	0.76	0.010 (.04)	0.81
Age (years)			−0.004 (.02)	0.81	−0.003 (.02)	0.83
Pre-pregnancy BMI (kg/m²)			0.046 (.02)	0.06	0.042 (.02)	0.09
SBP (mmHG)					0.004 (.00)	0.29
Predictor	Model 3[b]		Model 4[b]		Model 5[b]	
	ß (SE)	P-value	ß (SE)	P-value	ß (SE)	P-value
Trimester 1	Ref		Ref	0.84	Ref	
Trimester 2	0.294 (.09)[c]	0.001	0.321 (.09)[c]	< 0.001	0.456 (.07)[c]	< 0.0001
Trimester 3	0.338 (.13)[c]	0.009	0.392 (.14)[c]	0.008	0.683 (.12)[cd]	< 0.0001
Postpartum	−0.032 (.05)	0.49	−0.020 (.05)	0.69	− 0.029 (.04)	0.44
Age (years)	0.004 (.02)	0.82	− 0.001 (.02)	0.93	−0.006 (.02)	0.73
Pre-pregnancy BMI (kg/m²)	0.013 (.03)	0.67	0.047 (.02)	0.06	0.006 (.03)	0.85
Weight (kg)	0.015 (.01)	0.08			0.011 (.01)	0.12
Weight change (kg)			0.010 (.01)	0.29		
Triglycerides (mg/dl)					−0.002 (.00)	< 0.0001
Log hsCRP (mg/L)					0.070 (.02)	0.0002

[a]Linear mixed models
[b]Model 1: Adjusted for age & pre-pregnancy BMI. Model 2: Model 1 plus SBP. Model 3: Model 1 plus weight. Model 4: Model 1 plus weight change. Model 5: Model 3 plus triglycerides and Log hsCRP
[c]Different from postpartum at $p < .01$. [d]Different from second trimester at $p < .05$
Weight change is from pre-pregnancy weight. β represents change in millimeters

Table 3 Associations[a] of individual biomarkers with inter-adventitial diameter and common carotid artery intima-media thickness

Biomarker	Inter-adventitial Diameter[b]		Common Carotid Artery Intima-Media Thickness[b]	
	β (SE)	P-value	β (SE)	P-value
Total Cholesterol (mg/dl)	−0.001 (0.1)	0.18	−0.000 (.00)	0.95
HDL-c (mg/dl)	0.002 (.00)	0.52	−0.000 (.00)	0.39
Triglycerides (mg/dl)	−0.001 (.00)	0.01	0.000 (.00)	0.45
LDL-c (mg/dl)	−0.001 (.00)	0.38	−0.000 (.00)	0.80
hsCRP (mg/L)	0.004 (.00)	0.03	0.000 (.00)	0.54
Fasting insulin (µU/ml)	0.004 (.01)	0.55	−0.002 (.00)	0.13
Fasting glucose (mg/dl)	−0.005 (.00)	0.13	−0.001 (.00)	0.09
Log HOMA-IR	−0.013 (.07)	0.86	−0.029 (.01)	0.02

[a]Linear mixed models
[b]Models include time point in pregnancy cycle (trimester or postpartum), age, pre-pregnancy BMI, systolic blood pressure, and weight change from pre-pregnancy baseline
β represents change in millimeters

values (Table 4, Model 7). Accounting for HOMA-IR did not affect the increased CCA IMT observed postpartum (Table 4, Model 7).

Results of sensitivity analyses limited to women who completed all four initial visits and that excluded hsCRP outliers, were consistent with those from the primary analyses (Additional file 1: Table S1 and Additional file 2: Table S2). Moreover, for the second postpartum visit, no reproductive factors (e.g., number of interval pregnancies or breastfeeding status) were

Table 4 Associations[a] between common carotid artery intima-media thickness, physical predictors, and significant metabolic predictors

Predictor	Unadjusted		Model 1[b]		Model 2[b]		Model 3[b]	
	ß (SE)	P-value	ß (SE)	P-value	ß (SE)	P-value	ß (SE)	P-value
Trimester 1	Ref		Ref		Ref		Ref	
Trimester 2	0.001 (.01)	0.89	0.001 (.01)	0.89	0.002 (.01)	0.85	0.007 (.01)	0.56
Trimester 3	0.013 (.01)	0.24	0.013 (.01)	0.24	0.009 (.01)	0.43	0.022 (.02)	0.22
Postpartum	0.027 (.01)[c]	0.02	0.027 (.01) [c]	0.02	0.026 (.01)[cd]	0.03	0.031 (.01)[c]	0.01
Age (yr)			0.004 (.00)	0.03	0.004 (.00)	0.02	0.003 (.00)	0.08
Pre-pregnancy BMI (kg/m²)			−0.001 (.00)	0.78	−0.002 (.00)	0.45	0.000 (.00)	0.93
SBP (mm Hg)					0.001 (.00)	0.08		
Weight (kg)							−0.000 (.00)	0.66

Predictor	Model 4[b]		Model 5 [b]		Model 6[b]		Model 7[b]	
	ß (SE)	P-value	ß (SE)	P-value	ß (SE)	P-value	ß (SE)	P-value
Trimester 1	Ref		Ref		Ref		Ref	
Trimester 2	0.016 (.01)	0.19	0.018 (.01)	0.17	0.007 (.01)	0.59	0.009 (.01)	0.51
Trimester 3	0.042 (.02)[c]	0.04	0.041 (.02)[c]	0.046	0.027 (.02)	0.19	0.033 (.02)[c]	0.13
Postpartum	0.036 (.01)[d]	0.003	0.035 (.01)[d]	0.005	0.034 (.01)[c]	0.006	0.027 (.01)[d]	0.03
Age (years)	0.002 (.00)	0.11	0.003 (.00)	0.07	0.003 (.002)	0.05	0.003 (.00)	0.12
Pre-pregnancy BMI (kg/m²)	−0.001 (.00)	0.70	−0.002 (.00)	0.35	−0.004 (.00)	0.15	−0.002 (.00)	0.55
Weight change (kg)	−0.002 (.00)	0.13	−0.002 (.00)	0.07	−0.002 (.00)	0.06	−0.002 (.00)	0.08
SBP (mmHg)			0.001 (.00)	0.04	0.001 (.00)	0.04	0.001 (.00)	0.03
Inter-adventitial diameter					0.026 (.01)	0.02	0.017 (.01)	0.17
Log HOMA-IR							−0.028 (.01)	0.03

[a]Linear mixed models
[b]Model 1: Adjusted for age & pre-pregnancy BMI. Model 2: Model 1 plus SBP. Model 3: Model 1 plus weight. Model 4: Model 1 plus weight change. Model 5: Model 1 plus SBP and weight change. Model 6: Model 5 plus inter-adventitial diameter. Model 7: Model 6 plus HOMA-IR
[c]Different from second trimester at $p < .05$. [d]Different from third trimester at $p < .05$
BMI is body mass index. SBP is systolic blood pressure. Weight change is from pre-pregnancy weight. β represents change in millimeters

statistically significantly associated with either carotid measure (data not shown).

Discussion

Among our participants with normal first pregnancies, CCA IMT thickened late in pregnancy and remained thickened at 2.7 years postpartum; IAD, however, increased throughout pregnancy and returned to early pregnancy levels, postpartum. Although our results mirror those described in two classic studies [7, 8], our study is the first to follow women for more than 1 year postpartum. With more participants (i.e., 43) than those studies [7, 8] combined, our study establishes statistically significant changes in CCA IMT and IAD. While a recent study did not demonstrate that CCA IMT was increased in the 3rd trimester, it assessed women earlier in the trimester than we did [10]. Our results demonstrate that unhealthy change in CCA IMT is partially explained by changes in IAD and weight—not atherogenic metabolic changes.

An increase in CCA IMT beginning late in pregnancy and persisting postpartum beyond 2 years, in addition to lifestyle changes involved with parenthood and socio-economic profile of women with large families, could help explain the greater CVD risk that occurs for women of high parity [1, 3]. Greater IMT is a risk factor for CVD because thickened arteries are 1) less capable of responding to changes in blood pressure [25] and 2) more prone to atherosclerosis [26]. Although studies have identified greater CCA IMT in women of higher parity [6, 27–29], the cause remains unknown. However, we observed thicker CCA IMT among our participants more than 2 years after childbirth, which suggests that the acute negative effect of pregnancy on CCA IMT may persist and could serve as a risk factor for CVD.

The observed changes in CCA IMT and IAD are consistent with the literature concerning hemodynamic changes in pregnancy and the effect of hemodynamic changes on arteries [30–34]. Importantly, we provide serial measures in pregnancy to characterize this vascular remodeling and evaluate concomitant metabolic markers. Vascular remodeling is largely due to hemodynamic factors. Arterial walls adapt to maintain homeostasis between the two main stresses of blood flow: shear and tensile stress. First, shear stress is the frictional force of blood flowing along the arterial wall. Increased shear stress causes blood vessels to increase in diameter [30–32]. Cardiac output increases early in the 1st trimester of pregnancy [33] and peaks at 30–60% above the non-pregnant level in the late 2nd or early 3rd trimester [33]. Increased cardiac output should increase IAD resulting from increased shear stress, as our results demonstrate. Second, tensile stress is the force of blood perpendicular to the arterial wall, and this force

increases as arterial diameter increases, which causes arterial walls to thicken [30, 34]. CCA IMT would thicken during pregnancy as IAD increases, to normalize arterial wall stresses, as our results confirm [25].

In contrast to the effects of body weight and change in IAD, the metabolic changes during pregnancy that may be considered atherogenic in non-pregnant adults (i.e., increased total cholesterol, LDL-c, triglycerides, HOMA-IR, and hsCRP) do not explain the increased IAD and CCA IMT that we observed. As expected, we observed an association between higher hsCRP and greater IAD. Without pregnancy, higher hsCRP concentrations are associated with greater carotid IMT [35–37], which is associated with greater IAD. However, in our study, hsCRP concentrations did not explain the observed changes in IAD. Our finding that higher triglyceride concentrations were associated with smaller IAD [12] was unexpected, because this relationship differs from that observed in non-pregnant adult women.

Triglyceride concentrations increase dramatically during healthy pregnancy to support fetal growth, and no accepted threshold value exists for what constitutes high triglyceride concentrations in pregnancy [24]. However, triglyceride concentrations can be excessive in pregnancy, as triglyceride concentrations in the upper percentiles have been associated with preeclampsia and preterm birth [38–40]. Both high triglyceride concentrations and smaller IAD indeed could be associated with less healthy pregnancies. Our results suggest that paradigms of CVD prediction may not be applicable to the wellness state of pregnancy.

Our study benefited from the use of a highly valid and reproducible measure of carotid structure (i.e., B-mode ultrasonography), and high participant retention (i.e., 98%) in the initial study. We also collected serial vascular and biomarker measures during and after pregnancy, which strengthens this study, but the lack of pre-pregnancy measures poses a limitation. Limitations of the study are largely due to the rapidly changing hormonal and hemodynamic milieus of pregnancy and the postpartum period. Because the hemodynamic changes of pregnancy begin as early as 5 weeks of gestation [33], our 1st trimester values may not represent a true pre-pregnancy baseline. For example, thinning of the CCA IMT may have occurred before we could assess it. Similarly, because most participants (94%) were breastfeeding at the first postpartum visit, their hormonal and cardiovascular status had not attained new postpartum "normal" status. CCA IMT may regress after weaning. Our results also might not reflect those for women who formula-feed. Additionally, at the second postpartum visit, participants exhibited a varying number of subsequent pregnancies, which makes interpretation difficult. However, our results are consistent with those of the Cardiovascular Risk in Young Finns study, which found that young women who gave birth over a 6-year period had greater progression of CCA IMT than those who had not [6], and with epidemiologic studies showing greater CCA IMT in midlife women of higher parity [27–29]. Moreover, although our largely white, well-educated participants do not represent all first-time pregnant women in the United States, our study provides valuable baseline data against which arterial remodeling in other demographic groups can be assessed.

Future work should follow a life course approach, and seek to enroll women during the preconception period to obtain a true baseline and then follow them through at least a several month period after weaning. Retention for the postpartum visits is critical. Additional studies should explore vascular adaptation to pregnancy in women in subsequent pregnancies, from different racial and ethnic groups, and with higher BMI. Collection of serum folate levels might provide valuable insights into the role folate deficiency during pregnancy plays in differences in vascular adaptation.

Conclusions

We found that IAD increased throughout a healthy first pregnancy and decreased by 8 weeks postpartum. In contrast, postpartum CCA IMT thickening persisted for more than 2 years. These adaptations can be explained—partially—by pregnancy-related changes in weight and IAD; moreover, they are not substantially explained by changes in metabolic measures. Therefore, our results suggest that pregnancy represents a unique setting of rapid physiologic changes that maintain homeostasis during a period of acute stress.

Understanding normal vascular adaptation to pregnancy can not only engender an improved understanding of the physiology of pregnancy complications, but also better identify women at risk for complications early in pregnancy. If it persists, the greater CCA IMT detected postpartum may help explain the higher CVD risk in women of higher parity.

Additional files

Additional file 1: Table S1 Associations between inter-adventitial diameter, physical predictors, and significant metabolic predictors for the 15 women who completed all 4 study visits. These are data about carotid measures, physical predictors, and significant metabolic predictors for the 15 women who completed all 4 initial study visits.

Additional file 2: Table S2 Associations between common carotid artery intima-media thickness, physical predictors, and significant metabolic predictors for the 15 women who completed all 4 study visits. These are data about carotid measures, physical predictors, and significant metabolic predictors for the 15 women who completed all 4 initial study visits.

Abbreviations

BMI: Body mass index; CCA IMT : Common carotid artery intima-media thickness; CVD : Cardiovascular disease; HDL-c : High density lipoprotein concentration; hsCRP : High-sensitivity C-reactive protein; IAD : Inter-adventitial diameter; LDL-c : Low density lipoprotein concentration; MVP : Maternal Vascular Adaptations to Healthy Pregnancy; SBP : Systolic blood pressure; SE : Standard error; URL : Ultrasound Research Laboratory

Acknowledgments

The authors gratefully acknowledge William B. Greene, EdD, Scientific Editor and Writer at the University of Pittsburgh, School of Nursing, for his assistance with the preparation of this manuscript, and Alyssa Oakes, SN, for her assistance with development of the tables.

Funding

NAN was supported by NICHD grant T32HD0055162–04 and NHBLI grant T32HL083825 to the University of Pittsburgh. The project described was supported by the National Institutes of Health through Grant Numbers UL1 RR024153 and UL1TR000005. The funding bodies had no role in design of the study; collection, analysis, and interpretation of data; or in writing the manuscript.

Authors' contributions

NAN performed the original study visits; analyzed the data; and wrote the first, second, and third drafts of the manuscript. MB provided statistical support, contributed to interpretation of results, and read and approved the final manuscript. JC contributed to interpretation of results, and read and approved the final manuscript. MD designed the follow up study, performed study visits, and read and approved the final manuscript. CKM designed the original study, contributed to interpretation of results, and read and approved the final manuscript. JMR contributed to interpretation of results, and read and approved the final manuscript. AS contributed to interpretation of results and read and approved the final manuscript. PGT provided statistical support, contributed to interpretation of results, and read and approved the final manuscript. EBM contributed to interpretation of results, and read and approved the final manuscript.

Competing interests

The authors declare that they have no competing interests.

Author details

[1]Department of Epidemiology, Graduate School of Public Health, University of Pittsburgh, 130 De Soto Street, Pittsburgh, PA 15261, USA. [2]Department of Health Promotion and Development, School of Nursing, University of Pittsburgh, 3500 Victoria Street, 440 Victoria Building, Pittsburgh, PA 15261, USA. [3]Department of Obstetrics and Gynecology, School of Medicine, University of Pittsburgh, 3550 Terrace Street, Pittsburgh, PA 15213, USA. [4]Department of Clinical and Translational Research, School of Medicine, University of Pittsburgh, 3550 Terrace Street, Pittsburgh, PA 15213, USA. [5]Magee-Womens Research Institute, Magee-Womens Hospital of University of Pittsburgh Medical Center (UPMC), 204 Craft Avenue, Pittsburgh, PA 15213, USA.

References

1.   Parikh NI, Cnattingius S, Dickman PW, Mittleman MA, Ludvigsson JF, Ingelsson E. Parity and risk of later-life maternal cardiovascular disease. Am Heart J. 2010;159(2):215–21. e216

2. Bertuccio P, Tavani A, Gallus S, Negri E, La Vecchia C. Menstrual and reproductive factors and risk of non-fatal acute myocardial infarction in Italy. Eur J Obstet Gynecol Reprod Biol. 2007;134(1):67–72.

3. Ness RB, Harris T, Cobb J, Flegal KM, Kelsey JL, Balanger A, Stunkard AJ, D'Agostino RB. Number of pregnancies and the subsequent risk of cardiovascular disease. NEnglJMed. 1993;328(21):1528–33.

4. Ness RB, Schotland HM, Flegal KM, Shofer FS. Reproductive history and coronary heart disease risk in women. EpidemiolRev. 1994;16(2):298–314.

5. Akhter T, Larsson A, Larsson M, Wikstrom AK, Naessen T. Artery wall layer dimensions during normal pregnancy: a longitudinal study using noninvasive high-frequency ultrasound. Am J Physiol Heart Circ Physiol. 2013;304(2):H229–34.

6. Skilton MR, Bonnet F, Begg LM, Juonala M, Kahonen M, Lehtimaki T, Viikari JS, Raitakari OT. Childbearing, child-rearing, cardiovascular risk factors, and progression of carotid intima-media thickness: the cardiovascular risk in young Finns study. Stroke. 2010;41(7):1332–7.

7. Mersich B, Rigo J Jr, Besenyei Z, Lenard Z, Studinger P, Kollai M. Opposite changes in carotid versus aortic stiffness during healthy human pregnancy. ClinSci(Lond). 2005;109(1):103–7.

8. Visontai Z, Lenard Z, Studinger P, Rigo J Jr, Kollai M. Impaired baroreflex function during pregnancy is associated with stiffening of the carotid artery. Ultrasound ObstetGynecol. 2002;20(4):364–9.

9. Sator MO, Joura EA, Gruber DM, Obruca A, Zeisler H, Egarter C, Huber JC. Non-invasive detection of alterations of the carotid artery in pregnant women with high-frequency ultrasound. Ultrasound ObstetGynecol. 1999;13(4):260–2.

10. Iacobaeus C, Andolf E, Thorsell M, Bremme K, Jorneskog G, Ostlund E, Kahan T. Longitudinal study of vascular structure and function during normal pregnancy. Ultrasound Obstet Gynecol. 2017;49(1):46–53.

11. Stein JH, Korcarz CE, Hurst RT, Lonn E, Kendall CB, Mohler ER, Najjar SS, Rembold CM, Post WS. Use of carotid ultrasound to identify subclinical vascular disease and evaluate cardiovascular disease risk: a consensus statement from the American Society of Echocardiography carotid intima-media thickness task force. Endorsed by the Society for Vascular Medicine. J Am Soc Echocardiogr. 2008;21(2):93–111. quiz 189-190

12. Bonithon-Kopp C, Touboul PJ, Berr C, Magne C, Ducimetiere P. Factors of carotid arterial enlargement in a population aged 59 to 71 years: the EVA study. Stroke. 1996;27(4):654–60.

13. Polak JF, Wong Q, Johnson WC, Bluemke DA, Harrington A, O'Leary DH, Yanez ND. Associations of cardiovascular risk factors, carotid intima-media thickness and left ventricular mass with inter-adventitial diameters of the common carotid artery: the multi-ethnic study of atherosclerosis (MESA). Atherosclerosis. 2011;

14. Joensuu T, Salonen R, Winblad I, Korpela H, Salonen JT. Determinants of femoral and carotid artery atherosclerosis. J Intern Med. 1994;236(1):79–84.

15. Lakatta EG, Levy D. Arterial and cardiac aging: major shareholders in cardiovascular disease enterprises: part I: aging arteries: a "set up" for vascular disease. Circulation. 2003;107(1):139–46.

16. Eigenbrodt ML, Sukhija R, Rose KM, Tracy RE, Couper DJ, Evans GW, Bursac Z, Mehta JL. Common carotid artery wall thickness and external diameter as predictors of prevalent and incident cardiac events in a large population study. CardiovascUltrasound. 2007;5:11.

17. Kozakova M, Morizzo C, La Carrubba S, Fabiani I, Della Latta D, Jamagidze J, Chiappino D, Di Bello V, Palombo C. Associations between common carotid artery diameter, Framingham risk score and cardiovascular events. Nutr Metab Cardiovasc Dis. 2017; 27(4):329–34.

18. Wendelhag I, Gustavsson T, Suurkula M, Berglund G, Wikstrand J. Ultrasound measurement of wall thickness in the carotid artery: fundamental principles and description of a computerized analysing system. Clin Physiol. 1991;11(6):565–77.

19. Harris PA, Taylor R, Thielke R, Payne J, Gonzalez N, Conde JG. Research electronic data capture (REDCap)–a metadata-driven methodology and workflow process for providing translational research informatics support. J Biomed Inform. 2009;42(2):377–81.

20. Friedewald W, Levy R, Fredrickson D. Estimation of the concentration of low-density lipoprotein cholesterol in plasma, without use of the preparative ultracentrifuge. Clin Chem. 1972;18(6):499–502.

21. Bucolo G, David H. Quantitative determination of serum triglycerides by the use of enzymes. Clin Chem. 1973;19(5):476–82.

22. Bondar RJ, Mead DC. Evaluation of glucose-6-phosphate dehydrogenase from Leuconostoc mesenteroides in the hexokinase method for determining glucose in serum. Clin Chem. 1974;20(5):586–90.

23. Matthews D, Hosker J, Rudenski A, Naylor B, Treacher D, Turner R. Homeostasis model assessment: insulin resistance and beta-cell function from fasting plasma glucose and insulin concentrations in man. Diabetologia. 1985;28(7):412–9.

24. Liu LX, Arany Z. Maternal cardiac metabolism in pregnancy. Cardiovasc Res. 2014;101(4):545–53.

25. Carallo C, Irace C, Pujia A, De Franceschi MS, Crescenzo A, Motti C, Cortese C, Mattioli PL, Gnasso A. Evaluation of common carotid hemodynamic forces. Relations with wall thickening. Hypertension. 1999;34(2):217–21.

26. Lakatta EG. Arterial and cardiac aging: major shareholders in cardiovascular disease enterprises: part III: cellular and molecular clues to heart and arterial aging. Circulation. 2003;107(3):490–7.

27. Humphries KH, Westendorp IC, Bots ML, Spinelli JJ, Carere RG, Hofman A, Witteman JC. Parity and carotid artery atherosclerosis in elderly women: the Rotterdam study. Stroke. 2001;32(10):2259–64.

28. Wolff B, Volzke H, Robinson D, Schwahn C, Ludemann J, Kessler C, John U, Felix SB. Relation of parity with common carotid intima-media thickness among women of the study of health in Pomerania. Stroke. 2005;36(5):938–43.

29. Skilton MR, Serusclat A, Begg LM, Moulin P, Bonnet F. Parity and carotid atherosclerosis in men and women: insights into the roles of childbearing and child-rearing. Stroke. 2009;40(4):1152–7.

30. Pries AR, Reglin B, Secomb TW. Remodeling of blood vessels: responses of diameter and wall thickness to hemodynamic and metabolic stimuli. Hypertension. 2005;46(4):725–31.

31. Herity NA, Ward MR, Lo S, Yeung AC. Review: clinical aspects of vascular remodeling. J Cardiovasc Electrophysiol. 1999;10(7):1016–24.

32. Kiechl S, Willeit J. The natural course of atherosclerosis. Part II: vascular remodeling. Bruneck Study Group. Arterioscler Thromb Vasc Biol. 1999; 19(6):1491–8.

33. Abbas AE, Lester SJ, Connolly H. Pregnancy and the cardiovascular system. IntJCardiol. 2005;98(2):179–89.

34. Bokov P, Chironi G, Orobinskaia L, Flaud P, Simon A. Carotid circumferential wall stress homeostasis in early remodeling: theoretical approach and clinical application. J Clin Ultrasound. 2012;40(8):486–94.

35. Toprak A, Kandavar R, Toprak D, Chen W, Srinivasan S, Xu JH, Anwar A, Berenson GS. C-reactive protein is an independent predictor for carotid artery intima-media thickness progression in asymptomatic younger adults (from the Bogalusa heart study). BMC Cardiovasc Disord. 2011;11:78.

36. Ciccone MM, Scicchitano P, Zito A, Cortese F, Boninfante B, Falcone VA, Quaranta VN, Ventura VA, Zucano A, Di Serio F, et al. Correlation between inflammatory markers of atherosclerosis and carotid intima-media thickness in obstructive sleep apnea. Molecules. 2014;19(2):1651–62.

37. Ock SY, Cho KI, Kim HJ, Lee NY, Kim EJ, Kim NK, Lee WH, Yeo GE, Heo JJ, Han YJ, et al. The impacts of C-reactive protein and atrial fibrillation on carotid atherosclerosis and ischemic stroke in patients with suspected ischemic cerebrovascular disease: a single-center retrospective observational cohort study. Korean Circ J. 2013;43(12):796–803.

38. Gallos ID, Sivakumar K, Kilby MD, Coomarasamy A, Thangaratinam S, Vatish M. Pre-eclampsia is associated with, and preceded by, hypertriglyceridaemia: a meta-analysis. BJOG. 2013;120(11):1321–32.

39. Mudd LM, Holzman CB, Catov JM, Senagore PK, Evans RW. Maternal lipids at mid-pregnancy and the risk of preterm delivery. Acta Obstet Gynecol Scand. 2012;91(6):726–35.

40. Catov JM, Bodnar LM, Kip KE, Hubel C, Ness RB, Harger G, Roberts JM. Early pregnancy lipid concentrations and spontaneous preterm birth. Am J Obstet Gynecol. 2007;197(6):610 e611–7.

12

Population-based trends and risk factors of early- and late-onset preeclampsia in Taiwan 2001–2014

Shu-Han You[1], Po-Jen Cheng[1], Ting-Ting Chung[2], Chang-Fu Kuo[3], Hsien-Ming Wu[1*] and Pao-Hsien Chu[4*]

Abstract

Background: Preeclampsia, a multisystem disorder in pregnancies complicates with maternal and fetal morbidity. Early- and late-onset preeclampsia, defined as preeclampsia developed before and after 34 weeks of gestation, respectively. The early-onset disease was less prevalent but associated with poorer outcomes. Moreover, the risk factors between early -and late- onset preeclampsia could be differed owing to the varied pathophysiology. In the study, we evaluated the incidences, trends, and risk factors of early- and late- onset preeclampsia in Taiwan.

Methods: This retrospective population-based cohort study included all ≧20 weeks singleton pregnancies resulting in live-born babies or stillbirths in Taiwan between January 1, 2001 and December 31, 2014 ($n = 2,884,347$). The data was collected electronically in Taiwanese Birth Register and National Health Insurance Research Database. The incidences and trends of early- and late-onset preeclampsia were assessed through Joinpoint analysis. Multivariate logistic regression was used to analyze the risk factors of both diseases.

Results: The age-adjusted overall preeclampsia rate was slightly increased from 1.1%(95%confidence interval [CI], 1.1–1.2) in 2001 to 1.3% (95%CI, 1.2–1.3) in 2012 with average annual percentage change (AAPC) 0.1%/year (95%CI, 0–0.2%). However, the incidence was remarkably increased from 1.3% (95%CI, 1.3–1.4) in 2012 to 1.7% (95%CI, 1.6–1.8) in 2014 with AAPC 1.3%/year (95%CI,0.3–2.5). Over the study period, the incidence trend in late-onset preeclampsia was steadily increasing from 0.7% (95%CI, 0.6–0.7) in 2001 to 0.9% (95%CI, 0.8–0.9) in 2014 with AAPC 0.2%/year (95%CI, 0.2–0.3) but in early-onset preeclampsia was predominantly increase from 0.5% (95%CI, 0.4–0.5) in 2012 to 0.8% (95%CI, 0.8–0.9) in 2014 with AAPC 2.3%/year (95%CI, 0.8–4.0). Advanced maternal age, primiparity, stroke, diabetes mellitus, chronic hypertension, and hyperthyroidism were risk factors of preeclampsia. Comparing early- and late-onset diseases, chronic hypertension (ratio of relative risk [RRR], 1.71; 95%CI, 1.55–1.88) and older age (RRR, 1.41; 95%CI 1.29–1.54) were more strongly associated with early-onset disease, whereas primiparity (RRR 0.71, 95%CI, 0.68–0.75) had stronger association with late-onset preeclampsia.

Conclusions: The incidences of overall, and early- and late-onset preeclampsia were increasing in Taiwan from 2001 to 2014, predominantly for early-onset disease. Pregnant women with older age and chronic hypertension had significantly higher risk of early-onset preeclampsia.

Keywords: Preeclampsia, Incidence, Risk factors, Early onset, Late onset, Hypertension

* Correspondence: danielwu@cgmh.org.tw; taipei.chu@gmail.com
[1]Department of Obstetrics and Gynecology, Chang Gung Memorial Hospital, Linkou, Taiwan
[4]Department of Cardiology, Chang Gung Memorial Hospital, Linkou, Taiwan
Full list of author information is available at the end of the article

Background

Worldwide 2.0 to 8.0% pregnancies were complicated by preeclampsia [1–5] with variation across regions [2]. Preeclampsia, the progressive disorder during pregnancy is strongly associated with maternal and fetal complications including eclampsia, acute renal failure, coagulopathy, placenta abruption, postpartum hemorrhage, intrauterine growth restriction, medically indicated preterm birth, and maternal and fetal death [1, 6, 7]. In a systemic analysis from World Health Organization (WHO), hypertensive disorders including preeclampsia accounted for 14.0% maternal death between 2003 and 2009 [8]. Moreover, the risk of severe obstetric morbidities in women with eclampsia or severe preeclampsia was increasing [9]. Although most of the maternal dysfunctions resolved gradually in postpartum, these women were at higher risk of developing chronic hypertension, recurrent preeclampsia in the next pregnancy, and later-life cardiovascular diseases [10].

Preeclampsia is recognized as a heterogenous syndrome with different pathophysiology and be divided in two subtypes according to the disease onset [7, 11, 12]. Early-onset preeclampsia, diagnosed less than 34 gestational weeks was less prevalent than late-onset preeclampsia, occurring at 34 or more weeks of gestation [13]. The incidences of early- and late-onset preeclampsia were 0.3 and 2.7%, respectively [14, 15]; nevertheless, the early-onset disease contributed to more unfavorable maternal and fetal outcomes [14, 16, 17]. Around ten-fold increased risk of perinatal death and maternal death in women with early-onset preeclampsia and two-fold higher risk of perinatal death and threefold increased risks of maternal death in women with late-onset disease were observed, comparing with normal pregnancy [14, 15]. In addition, some studies showed biological variations and different spectrums of pathophysiology between early- and late-onset preeclampsia [18–20].

Clinical factors associated with risk of preeclampsia included primiparity, advanced maternal age, previous preeclampsia, family history of preeclampsia, multiple gestation, obesity, African-American race, diabetes mellitus, chronic hypertension, chronic renal disease, and presence of antiphospholipid antibodies were identified [21, 22]. Besides, there were evidences that stroke and hyperthyroidism increased the risk of preeclampsia [23, 24]. Further studies comparing predisposing factors of early- versus late-onset preeclampsia demonstrated similar risk factors but the strengths of association were differed among the factors. There were only two population-based studies, to our knowledge to evaluate each risk factor between early- and late-onset preeclampsia [14, 16]. One study, carried out by Lisonkova et al. revealed African-American race, chronic hypertension, and older age were more strongly associated with

early-onset disease, whereas women with nulliparity and diabetes mellitus had higher risk to develop late-onset disease [14]. The other study conducted by Iacobelli et al. showed older age and higher prevalence of chronic hypertension in the group of early-onset disease [16].

The incidence of preeclampsia in Taiwan was significantly increased from 0.87 to 1.21% between 1998 and 2010 [25]. However, there was limited data of early- and late-onset preeclampsia rate and the associated factors in Taiwan has not been determined yet. The aim of the study was to investigate the population-based trends of early- and late-onset preeclampsia and examine the maternal risk factors in Taiwanese population.

Methods

Study design and data source

The population-based cohort study retrospectively included all ≥20 weeks singleton deliveries, comprising live births and stillbirths in Taiwan from January 1, 2001 to December 31, 2014. Two databases were used to obtain data electronically in this study. One was Taiwanese birth registration system in Health Promotion Administration, Ministry of Health and Welfare (https://www.hpa.gov.tw/EngPages/Index.aspx), which included information of birth date, gestational age, and fetal weights of all neonates and stillbirths with gestational age ≥20 weeks. Another was National Health Insurance Database (NHIRD, https://nhird.nhri.org.tw/en/index.html), which could be linked from Taiwanese birth registration system for details of maternal general data and diagnosis. Both databases have been encrypted to generate the unique identification to anonymous identification.

In Taiwan, birth certificates of all neonates and stillbirths with gestational age ≥20 weeks or gestational age < 20 weeks but fetal birth weights ≥500 g are issued at the hospital or medical institution and registered in the Ministry of Health and Welfare. The birth register can be linked to NHIRD, which was a database contained information of insured people, including demographic data, dates of hospitalization and clinical visits, and diagnostic codes as International Classification of Diseases, the 9th version (ICD-9) during the study period.

Participants

There were 2,973,989 registered deliveries in Taiwan from January 1, 2001 to December 31, 2014. Women who were younger than 15-year-old or older than 55-year-old, with multiple gestation including twins, triplets, or quadruplets, and with gestational age at delivery less than 20 weeks were excluded. To identify the incidences of early- and late-onset preeclampsia, all the included delivers were categorized to ongoing pregnancy at 20 weeks of gestation and 34 weeks of gestation according to the gestational age at delivery, and each of which were the denominators of early- and late-onset preeclampsia rate, respectively [14, 15, 26].

The diagnostic criteria of preeclampsia was two occasions of hypertension at least 140/90 mmHg after 20 weeks of gestation accompanied by proteinuria > 300 mg/day or ≧1+ on dipstick based on International Society for the Study of Hypertension in Pregnancy (ISSHP) by 2014 [10, 26, 27]. All included delivers associated with diagnosis of preeclampsia were identified from NHIRD ICD-9 diagnostic codes 642.4, 6424.5, 6424.6, and 6424.7 [14, 15]. To obtain the gestational week of onset of preeclampsia for determing early- and late-onset preeclampsia, which were occurring less than and later than 34 weeks of gestation, the date of diagnosis was subtracted from the date at delivery, and calculated the gestational age according to the information of gestational weeks at birth in birth registers. A flow chart illustrating patient inclusion is showed in Fig. 1. The study was approved by Institutional Review Board of the Chang Gung Memorial Hospital (IRB No.201600657B0).

Definition of variables

Maternal characteristics including maternal age (15–24, 25–34, and 35–55 years old), parity (number of prior≧20 weeks births, 0 vs. ≧1), place of residence (urban, suburban, rural), income (quintiles 1 to 5), and clinical factors associated with risk of preeclampsia were examined for potential variables [14, 16, 22–24, 28, 29]. The clinical factors were identified in NHIRD, including acute coronary syndrome (ICD-9 codes, 410, 412 and 413), chronic ischemic heart disease (ICD-9 codes, 4140, 4148 and 4149), stroke (ICD-9 codes, 43,301, 43,311, 43,321, 43,331, 43,381, 43,391, 43,401, 43,411, 43,491, 435, 436, 4371, 4379 and 438), diabetes mellitus (ICD-9, 250), chronic hypertension (ICD-9 codes, 401–405) and hyperthyroidism (ICD-9 codes, 242).

Statistical analysis

The standardized preeclampsia incidence was adjusted based on the age distribution in 2014 and 95% confidence intervals (CI) were derived from the Poisson distribution. The linear trends in proportion were assessed using Joinpoint Regression Program version 4.2.0.2 (National Cancer Institute, Bethesda, MD, USA) to estimate temporal trends in standardized incidence of preeclampsia. Bayesian information criterion was used to generate 'joinpoints' over time according to the changes of trend and average annual percentage change (AAPC) and 95%CI for each segment were calculated.

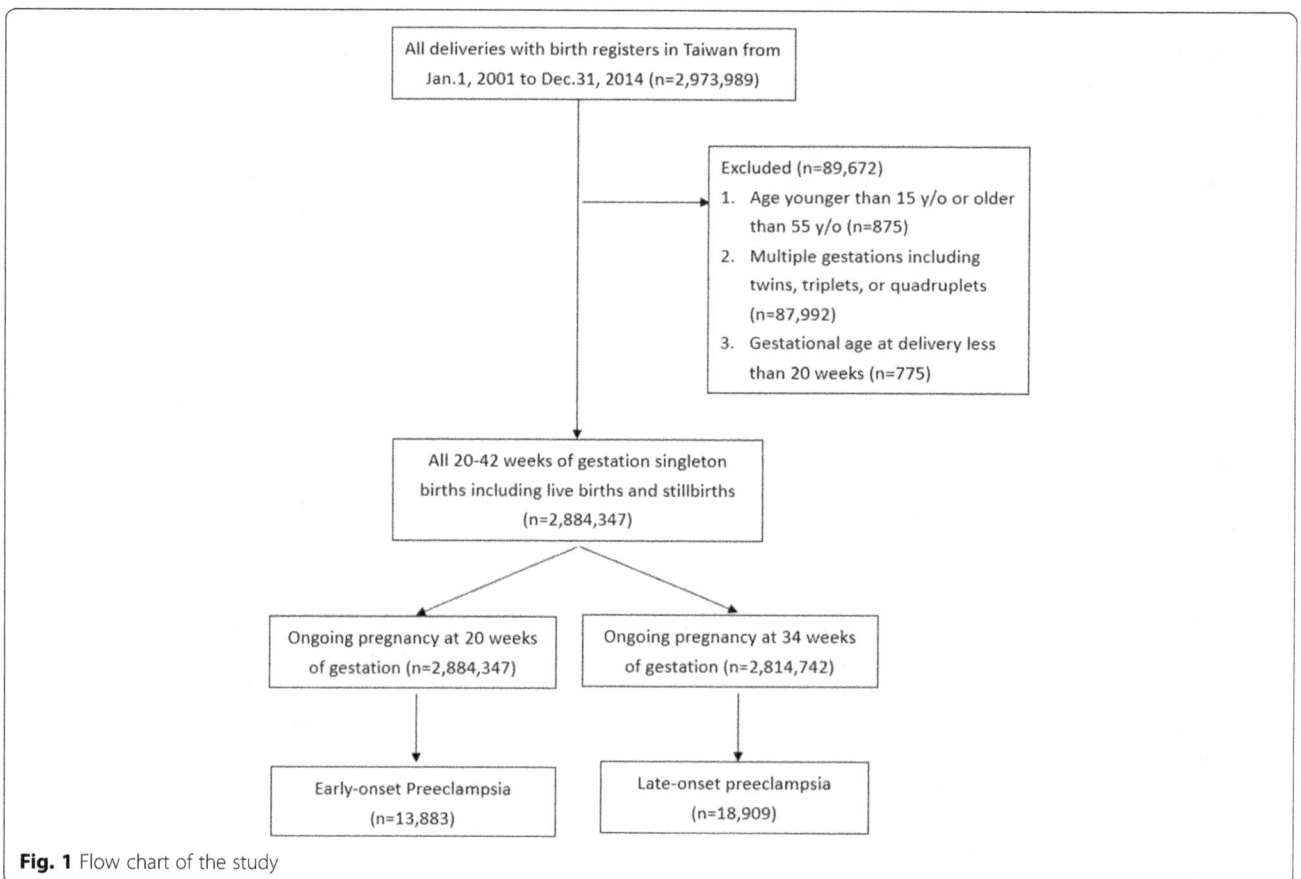

Fig. 1 Flow chart of the study

Multivariate logistic regression was used to obtain adjusted relative risks (ARR) and 95% CIs adjusted for the variables including maternal characteristics and clinical factors to examine the association with preeclampsia. The association between the clinical risk factors and early- or late-onset preeclampsia was further compared through the ratio of relative risks (RRR). Analyses were carried out using SAS, version 9.4 (SAS Institute, Cary, NC, USA). A 2-tailed $P < 0.05$ was considered significant. All tests of statistical hypothesis were done on the 2-sided 5% level of significance.

Results

Among 2,973,989 delivers over the 14 years period, 2,884,347 delivers were included and 32,742 preeclampsia events were identified. The subgroups of early- and late- onset preeclampsia were 13,833 (42.3%) and 18,909 (57.6%) deliveries, respectively (Fig. 1).

The overall preeclampsia incidence increased from 1.1% (95%CI, 1.1–1.2) in 2001 to 1.7% (95%CI, 1.6–1.8) in 2014. Table 1 reveals crude and age-adjusted overall preeclampsia rates each year in the study period. The analysis of the overall, early-onset, and late-onset incidence trends through average annual percentage change is presented in Table 2. The overall preeclampsia rate was slightly increased from 1.1% (95%CI, 1.1–1.2) in 2001 to 1.3% (95%CI, 1.2–1.3) in 2012 with average annual percentage change (AAPC) 0.1%/year (95%CI, 0–0.2%). However, the incidence was remarkably increased from 1.3% (95%CI, 1.3–1.4) in 2012 to 1.7% (95%CI, 1.6–1.8) in 2014 with AAPC 1.3%/year (95%CI,0.3–2.5).

Over the 14 years study period, the incidence trends in late-onset preeclampsia was steadily increasing from 0.7% (95%CI, 0.6–0.7) in 2001 to 0.9% (95%CI, 0.8–0.9) in 2014 with AAPC 0.2%/year (95%CI, 0.2–0.3). However, in early-onset preeclampsia, similar to the trend of overall preeclampsia, the incidence was relatively steady around 0.5% (95%CI, 0.4–0.5) in 2001 and 0.5% (95%CI, 0.5–0.6) in 2012 but predominantly increase from 0.5% (95%CI, 0.4–0.5) in 2012 to 0.8% (95%CI, 0.8–0.9) in 2014 with AAPC 2.3%/year (95%CI, 0.8–4.0). Figure 2 illustrates the trends in overall preeclampsia, early-onset, and late-onset disease.

Maternal characteristics (age, parity, place of residence, and income) and clinical factors (acute coronary syndrome, chronic ischemic heart disease, stroke, diabetes mellitus, chronic hypertension, and hyperthyroidism) are described in Table 3. In multivariate logistic regression, all maternal characteristics and clinical factors listed in Table 3 were adjusted as possible confounders. Women with older age, nulliparity, chronic hypertension, diabetes mellitus, stroke, and hyperthyroidism were more likely to develop preeclampsia (all p values< 0.01), while acute coronary syndrome and

chronic ischemic heart disease were not significantly associated with preeclampsia. The ARR of each clinical factor of overall preeclampsia are displayed in Table 4. Of note, women with chronic hypertension had much higher risk of preeclampsia (ARR, 12.1; 95%CI, 11.5–12.8).

For subgroup analysis of early- and late-onset preeclampsia, the clinical factors associated with early- or late-onset diseases were identical to overall preeclampsia, detailed in Table 5. To compare the strength of the association among the risk factors between early- and late-onset preeclampsia, RRR of each clinical factor was calculated according to the ARR of early- and late preeclampsia. Advanced maternal age (> 35 years) (RRR, 1.4; 95%CI, 1.3–1.5, $p < 0.01$) and chronic hypertension (RRR, 1.7; 95%CI, 1.6–1.9, p < 0.01) had higher risk to develop early-onset preeclampsia. In the contrary, primiparity (RRR, 0.7; 95%CI, 0.7–0.8, p < 0.01) was more strongly associated with late-onset disease. Other risk factors of preeclampsia including diabetes mellitus, stroke, and hyperthyroidism revealed no statistical difference in the association of early- and late-onset preeclampsia (Table 5).

Discussion

The incidences of overall, and early- and late-onset preeclampsia were increasing in Taiwan between 2001 and 2014, predominantly for early-onset disease. Pregnant women with advanced maternal age, primiparity, chronic hypertension, stroke, diabetes mellitus, and hyperthyroidism had significantly higher risk of developing preeclampsia. Among the factors, older age and hypertension were more strongly associated with early-onset disease.

Our study has certain limitations. First, overall preeclampsia was identified by diagnostic codes; thus, the artificial coding error and misclassification bias could not be avoided. Second, NHIRD included 99% of Taiwanese residents, which led to around 1.2% deliveries in birth registration not be linked to hospital records. The missing data could be susceptible to underascertainment, resulting in slightly underestimation of the incidence. Third, if a patient had neither antenatal exam nor delivered in hospitals, or developed postpartum preeclampsia without hospitalization, the diagnostic code could not be obtained from the hospital record. The such undetermined were few and less severe but may cause underestimation as well. Fourth, we did not classify the severity of preeclampsia or determine the subgroup using aspirin for prevention, both of which may give more information to interpret the trends of preeclampsia. In addition, we failed to assess certain risk factors including BMI, preeclampsia history in prior pregnancy, and family history of preeclampsia, as well as

Table 1 Preeclampsia incidence between January 1, 2001 and December 31, 2014 (n = 2,884,347)

	Total				Early onset				Late onset			
Year	Total Delivery (n)	No of event	Crude IR, per 1000 births (95% CI)	Standardised IR, per 1000 births (95%CI)	Ongoing pregnancies at 20 weeks (n)	No of event	Crude IR, per 1000 births (95% CI)	Standardised IR, per 1000 births (95%CI)	Ongoing pregnancies at 34 weeks (n)	No of event	Crude IR, per 1000 births (95% CI)	Standardised IR, per 1000 births (95%CI)
2001	243,357	2150	8.83 (8.46–9.21)	11.1 (10.5–11.6)	243,357	838	3.44 (3.21–3.68)	4.68 (4.31–5.05)	237,933	1312	5.51 (5.22–5.81)	6.56 (6.13–6.98)
2002	237,134	2186	9.22 (8.83–9.60)	11.6 (11.0–12.1)	237,134	950	4.01 (3.75–4.26)	5.37 (4.97–5.76)	231,862	1236	5.33 (5.03–5.63)	6.36 (5.93–6.78)
2003	221,232	2077	9.39 (8.98–9.79)	11.9 (11.3–12.5)	221,232	843	3.81 (3.55–4.07)	5.16 (4.76–5.56)	216,470	1234	5.70 (5.38–6.02)	6.88 (6.43–7.33)
2004	213,433	2014	9.44 (9.02–9.85)	11.7 (11.2–12.3)	213,433	839	3.93 (3.66–4.20)	5.10 (4.71–5.49)	208,461	1175	5.64 (5.31–5.96)	6.82 (6.37–7.27)
2005	203,137	1950	9.60 (9.17–10.0)	11.7 (11.1–12.3)	203,137	765	3.77 (3.50–4.03)	4.89 (4.51–5.27)	198,580	1185	5.97 (5.63–6.31)	6.98 (6.54–7.43)
2006	201,335	2306	11.5 (11.0–11.9)	13.3 (12.7–13.9)	201,335	968	4.81 (4.51–5.11)	5.76 (5.36–6.16)	196,617	1338	6.81 (6.44–7.17)	7.76 (7.30–8.23)
2007	199,389	2278	11.4 (11.0–11.9)	12.7 (12.1–13.3)	199,389	961	4.82 (4.51–5.12)	5.61 (5.22–5.99)	194,687	1317	6.76 (6.40–7.13)	7.27 (6.85–7.70)
2008	192,819	2086	10.8 (10.4–11.3)	11.9 (11.4–12.4)	192,819	891	4.62 (4.32–4.92)	5.22 (4.85–5.58)	188,125	1195	6.35 (5.99–6.71)	6.86 (6.45–7.28)
2009	188,735	2192	11.6 (11.1–12.1)	12.7 (12.2–13.3)	188,735	943	5.00 (4.68–5.32)	5.58 (5.21–5.95)	184,184	1249	6.78 (6.41–7.16)	7.32 (6.90–7.75)
2010	162,932	1927	11.8 (11.3–12.4)	12.4 (11.8–13.0)	162,932	801	4.92 (4.58–5.26)	5.23 (4.86–5.60)	158,724	1126	7.09 (6.68–7.51)	7.38 (6.94–7.82)
2011	194,095	2460	12.7 (12.2–13.2)	13.3 (12.7–13.8)	194,095	969	4.99 (4.68–5.31)	5.31 (4.97–5.65)	189,049	1491	7.89 (7.49–8.29)	8.18 (7.76–8.60)
2012	228,774	2885	12.6 (12.2–13.1)	13.0 (12.5–13.5)	228,774	1204	5.26 (4.97–5.56)	5.48 (5.17–5.79)	223,249	1681	7.53 (7.17–7.89)	7.73 (7.36–8.10)
2013	191,022	2775	14.5 (14.0–15.1)	14.6 (14.1–15.2)	191,022	1185	6.20 (5.85–6.56)	6.26 (5.91–6.62)	185,916	1590	8.55 (8.13–8.97)	8.59 (8.17–9.02)
2014	206,953	3506	16.9 (16.4–17.5)	16.9 (16.4–17.5)	206,953	1726	8.34 (7.95–8.73)	8.34 (7.95–8.73)	200,885	1780	8.86 (8.45–9.27)	8.86 (8.45–9.27)

Abbreviation: IR incidence rate

Table 2 Joinpoint analysis of trend of preeclampsia incidence in Taiwan between 2001 and 2014

	Standardised IR, per 1000 births		AAPC		Trend 1		Trend 2	
	2001	2014			Year	AAPC (95%CI)	Year	AAPC (95%CI)
Trend of entire cohort	11.1 (10.5–11.6)	16.9 (16.4–17.5)	3.01	(1.50 to 4.54)*	2001–2012	1.25 (0.36 to 2.14)*	2012–2014	13.3 (2.55 to 25.1) *
by onset weeks								
< 34 weeks	4.68 (4.31–5.05)	8.34 (7.95–8.73)	3.67	(1.67 to 5.72)*	2001–2012	0.58 (− 0.63 to 1.80)	2012–2014	22.5 (7.50 to 39.6) *
≥ 34 weeks	6.56 (6.13–6.98)	8.86 (8.45–9.27)	2.21	(1.51 to 2.91)*				

AAPC average annual percent change
*P < 0.05

the maternal and neonatal outcomes due to limited information.

The overall preeclampsia rate in Taiwan was relatively lower than the worldwide studies though, 42.3% preeclampsia events identified as early-onset disease was remarkable. The incidence of preeclampsia was 1.1 to 1.7% in Taiwan compared with 2 to 8% incidence of preeclampsia worldwide with regional variations [2]. The lower incidence could be owing to the majority of Asian race in the population, which had lower risk of developing preeclampsia, 2.0–3.0%according to previous studies [26, 30]. We did not collect data of races in this study but over 95% of the population is Han Chinese, who are regarded as East Asian ethnic group based on the data in Ministry of Interior. Besides, there could possibly be slight underestimation because of missing data in NHIRD or the artificial bias of disease coding. Nevertheless, NHIRD was one of the powerful tools in assessment of the epidemiology in Taiwan because of the high coverage of National Health Insurance program, financing around 99% Taiwanese residents [31]. In the current study, the unidentified anonymous identification between birth register system and NHIRD was around 1.2%. In addition, compared with the study by Chan et al., who revealed the increased incidence of preeclampsia in Taiwan was notable from 0.87 to 1.21% between 1998 and 2010 [25]. Therefore, the interpretation of exact preeclampsia rate could be somewhat underestimated owing to the unavoidable bias but the persisted increasing

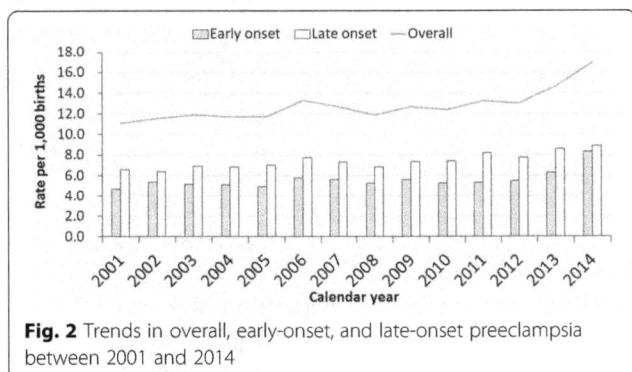

Fig. 2 Trends in overall, early-onset, and late-onset preeclampsia between 2001 and 2014

incidence of preeclampsia in the population-based study was thoroughly informative.

Our data suggested that the trend of preeclampsia was increasing between 2001 and 2014 after age ajustment, especially in early-onset disease from 2012 to 2014. We analyzed the subgroup trends of preeclampsia depend on maternal age and women with or without hypertension, respectively [Additional file 1 and Additional file 2]. Additional file 1 shows increased trend in all three age groups (age 15–25, 25–35, and 35–55). However, Additional file 2 reveals no significant incidence change in women with our without hypertension during the study period. The subgroup analysis indicated that the increasing trend of preeclampsia occurred in all age groups and possibly the growing number of women with hypertension. Interestingly, the rise rate of preeclampsia was not universally consistent, for instance, studies for the entire USA from 1999 to 2004 showed plateaued rate [32] and in Western New York from 1999 to 2003 [33] and European countries during the past ten years [34] reported slight declines in preeclampsia. However, the increase in preeclampsia in our population could partially affected by the revision of diagnostic criteria. American College of Obstetrician and Gynecologist (ACOG) in2013 and ISSHP in 2014 have excluded proteinuria as an necessary condition to establish diagnosis of preeclampsia in women presence of organ dysfunction of uteroplacental dysfunction [35, 36]. Therefore, the observation of significant rise in early-onset preeclampsia from 2012 to 2014 in this study was a conservative indication of increasing trend but the true percentage change should be followed since overall revision of the criteria in Taiwan.

The proportion of early-onset preeclampsia was significantly higher (42.3% in early-onset and 57.6% in late onset disease) than previous studies conducted other than Taiwan [14–16], about twofold to nine-fold of late-onset disease than early-onset preeclampsia. The difference could attributed to increasing prevalence of chronic hypertension as a result of a surge of risk rates of prehypertension, obesity and metabolic syndrome in Taiwan [37]. Genetic variation or epigenetic regulation such as DNA methylation or microRNA expression associated with preeclampsia in the population

Table 3 Maternal characteristics and clinical factors associated with early- and late-onset preeclampsia

Characteristics	Ongoing pregnancies at 20 weeks n = 2,884,347	Early-onset preeclampsia n = 13,883	Rate per 1000 (95% CI)	Ongoing pregnancies at 34 weeks n = 2,814,742	Late-onset preeclampsia n = 18,909	Rate per 1000 (95% CI)
Age at delivery						
15–24	525,457	1305	2.48 (2.35–2.62)	513,581	2447	4.76 (4.58–4.95)
25–34	1,956,147	8688	4.44 (4.35–4.53)	1,914,210	12,155	6.35 (6.24–6.46)
35–55	402,743	3890	9.66 (9.36–9.96)	386,951	4307	11.13 (10.8–11.5)
Number of prior ≧20 weeks births (parity)						
0	1,938,341	9559	4.93 (4.83–5.03)	1,893,197	14,611	7.72 (7.59–7.84)
≥ 1	946,006	4324	4.57 (4.43–4.71)	921,545	4298	4.66 (4.52–4.80)
Place of residence						
Urban	1681,534	7988	4.75 (4.65–4.85)	1,641,570	11,169	6.8 (6.68–6.93)
Suburban	826,656	4368	5.28 (5.13–5.44)	806,062	5645	7 (6.82–7.19)
Rural	192,141	1027	5.35 (5.02–5.67)	186,732	1403	7.51 (7.12–7.91)
Unknown	184,016	500	2.72 (2.48–2.96)	180,378	692	3.84 (3.55–4.12)
Income levels						
Quintile 1	558,314	2689	4.82 (4.63–5.00)	542,450	3825	7.05 (6.83–7.27)
Quintile 2	516,131	2560	4.96 (4.77–5.15)	503,177	3441	6.84 (6.61–7.07)
Quintile 3	566,360	3097	5.47 (5.28–5.66)	553,016	4140	7.49 (7.26–7.71)
Quintile 4	527,626	2508	4.75 (4.57–4.94)	516,050	3499	6.78 (6.56–7.01)
Quintile 5	540,007	2554	4.73 (4.55–4.91)	527,737	3351	6.35 (6.13–6.56)
Unknown	175,909	475	2.7 (2.46–2.94)	172,312	653	3.79 (3.50–4.08)
Acute Coronary syndrome						
No	2,878,429	13,809	4.8 (4.72–4.88)	2,809,040	18,854	6.71 (6.62–6.81)
Yes	5918	74	12.5 (9.66–15.4)	5702	55	9.65 (7.10–12.2)
Chronic ischemic heart disease						
No	2,877,398	13,767	4.78 (4.70–4.86)	2,808,117	18,801	6.7 (6.60–6.79)
Yes	6949	116	16.69 (13.7–19.7)	6625	108	16.3 (13.2–19.4)
Stroke						
No	2,877,911	13,792	4.79 (4.71–4.87)	2,808,569	18,824	6.7 (6.61–6.80)
Yes	6436	91	14.14 (11.2–17.0)	6173	85	13.77 (10.8–16.7)
Diabetes mellitus						
No	2,856,198	13,164	4.61 (4.53–4.69)	2,788,463	18,256	6.55 (6.45–6.64)
Yes	28,149	719	25.54 (23.7–27.4)	26,279	653	24.85 (22.9–26.8)
Chronic hypertension						
No	2,862,222	11,671	4.08 (4.00–4.15)	2,796,074	17,471	6.25 (6.16–6.34)
Yes	22,125	2212	99.98 (95.8–104)	18,668	1438	77.03 (73.0–81.0)
Hyperthyroidism						
No	2,813,030	13,316	4.73 (4.65–4.81)	2,745,618	18,231	6.64 (6.54–6.74)
Yes	71,317	567	7.95 (7.30–8.60)	69,124	678	9.81 (9.07–10.5)

[18, 38–40], and the theory of developmental origins of health and disease (DOHaD) that the early life environment impacting the risk of chronic disease from childhood to adulthood [41] could possibly cause the population vulnerable to early- or late-onset preeclampsia. However, none of the hypotheses has been verified. Therefore, higher proportion, almost half of early-onset preeclampsia women in the population warranted further investigation to provide addition insights into the variation of early- and late-onset preeclampsia incidences.

Table 4 Maternal characteristics and clinical risk factors associated with preeclampsia

	Incidence rate per 1000 births (95%CI)		Crude Relative risk (95%CI)		P Value	Adjusted Relative risk (95%CI)[a]		P Value
Age at delivery								
15–24	7.19	(6.96–7.42)	Reference			Reference		
25–34	10.77	(10.6–10.9)	1.48	(1.43–1.54)	< 0.01*	1.49	(1.44-1.55)	< 0.01*
35–55	20.78	(20.3–21.2)	2.78	(2.67–2.89)	< 0.01*	2.62	(2.51-2.73)	< 0.01*
Number of prior ≧20 weeks births (parity)								
0	12.63	(12.5–12.8)	1.35	(1.32–1.38)	< 0.01*	1.71	(1.67-1.76)	< 0.01*
≧ 1	9.2	(9.00-9.39)	Reference			Reference		
Acute Coronary syndrome[b]								
No	11.48	(11.4–11.6)	Reference			Reference		
Yes	22.28	(18.4–26.1)	1.93	(1.60–2.31)	< 0.01*	0.9	(0.74-1.10)	0.32
Chronic ischemic heart disease								
No	11.45	(11.3–11.6)	Reference			Reference		
Yes	33.31	(28.9–37.7)	2.83	(2.46–3.27)	< 0.01*	0.9	(0.77-1.06)	0.21
Stroke								
No	11.46	(11.3–11.6)	Reference			Reference		
Yes	28.12	(24.0–32.3)	2.44	(2.09–2.85)	< 0.01*	1.33	(1.13-1.58)	< 0.01*
Diabetes mellitus								
No	11.12	(11.0–11.2)	Reference			Reference		
Yes	51.24	(48.5–53.9)	4.28	(4.02–4.55)	< 0.01*	2.01	(1.86-2.16)	< 0.01*
Chronic hypertension								
No	10.29	(10.2–10.4)	Reference			Reference		
Yes	197.56	(191–204)	15.5	(14.8–16.2)	< 0.01*	12.14	(11.5-12.8)	< 0.01*
Hyperthyroidism								
No	11.34	(11.2–11.5)	Reference			Reference		
Yes	17.77	(16.8–18.8)	1.56	(1.46–1.65)	< 0.01*	1.21	(1.14-1.29)	< 0.01*

[a]Adjusted Relative risk: adjusted with age at delivery, income, urbanization, parity, acute coronary syndrome, chronic ischemic heart disease, stroke, diabetes mellitus, chronic hypertension and hyperthyroidism
[b]Acute Coronary syndrome included myocardial infarction and unstable angina
*$P < 0.05$

In the population between 2001 and 2014, our findings of the risk factors including advanced maternal age, primiparity, stroke, diabetes mellitus, chronic hypertension, or hyperthyroidism were consistent with commonly quoted clinical factors of preeclampsia [14, 16, 21, 22]. The subgroups of women with early- and late-onset preeclampsia were similar in terms of maternal risk factors but different association in age, parity, and chronic hypertension. Among the risk factors, advanced maternal age and chronic hypertension revealed stronger association with early-onset disease, while primiparity had higher risk of late-onset preeclampsia. The findings were similar to previous studies [14, 16]. To assess the possible interaction of old age and hypertension. We divided women according to different age groups (age 15–25. age 25–35, age 35–55)and women with or without hypertension, respectively [Additional file 3]. In Additional file 3: Table S6 reveals that chronic hypertension had highest ARR in all age groups and demonstrates old age was an independent risk factor either in women with or without hypertension. The different strength of association among the specific risk factors between early- and late-onset preeclampsia could be associated with the different pathophysiologic mechanisms including histology, hemodynamic change, or vascular adaption between early- and late-onset preeclampsia. Several evidences supported more typical histological change of defective trophoblast invasion and higher percentage of altered uterine artery Doppler in early-onset disease [18–20]. Cheng et al. revealed maternal serum markers associated with cardiovascular inflammatory response such as high-sensitive C-reactive protein and homocysteine were significantly higher in early-onset preeclampsia, which could be related to direct injury to vascular endothelial cells or increased oxidative stress and resulting in the sequence of placenta dysfunction and poorer outcomes [42]. Despite those

Table 5 Maternal characteristics and clinical risk factors associated with early- and late-onset preeclampsia

	Early onset preeclampsia				Late onset preeclampsia				Ratio of Relative risk (95%CI)	P Value
	Crude Relative risk (95%CI)	P Value	Adjusted Relative risk (95%CI)[a]	P Value	Crude Relative risk (95%CI)	P Value	Adjusted Relative risk (95%CI)[a]	P Value		
Age at delivery										
15–24	Reference		Reference		Reference		Reference		Reference	
25–34	1.79 (1.69–1.90)	< 0.01*	1.73 (1.63-1.84)	< 0.01*	1.33 (1.27-1.39)	< 0.01*	1.36 (1.30-1.43)	< 0.01*	1.27 (1.78-1.37)	< 0.01*
35–55	3.84 (3.60–4.10)	< 0.01*	3.21 (2.99-3.44)	< 0.01*	2.31 (2.19-2.42)	< 0.01*	2.28 (2.16-2.40)	< 0.01*	1.41 (1.29-1.54)	< 0.01*
Number of prior ≧20 weeks births (parity)										
0	1.06 (1.02–1.09)	< 0.01*	1.39 (1.34-1.44)	< 0.01*	1.65 (1.59-1.70)	< 0.01*	1.95 (1.89-2.02)	< 0.01*	0.71 (0.68-0.75)	< 0.01*
≥ 1	Reference		Reference		Reference		Reference		Reference	
Acute Coronary syndrome[b]										
No	Reference		Reference		Reference		Reference		Reference	
Yes	2.59 (2.04–3.28)	< 0.01*	1 (0.78-1.30)	0.98	1.45 (1.11–1.90)	< 0.01*	0.77 (0.58-1.02)	0.07	1.3 (0.89–1.90)	0.09
Chronic ischemic heart disease										
No	Reference		Reference		Reference		Reference		Reference	
Yes	3.44 (2.83–4.17)	< 0.01*	0.84 (0.68-1.04)	0.11	2.45 (2.02–2.98)	< 0.01*	0.92 (0.74-1.14)	0.45	0.91 (0.67–1.24)	0.28
Stroke										
No	Reference		Reference		Reference		Reference		Reference	
Yes	2.96 (2.37–3.68)	< 0.01*	1.33 (1.05-1.68)	0.02*	2.07 (1.67-2.58)	< 0.01*	1.28 (1.02-1.61)	0.03*	1.04 (0.75-1.44)	0.4
Diabetes mellitus										
No	Reference		Reference		Reference		Reference		Reference	
Yes	5.34 (4.91–5.81)	< 0.01*	1.9 (1.71-2.10)	< 0.01*	3.76 (3.46-4.08)	< 0.01*	2.03 (1.85-2.23)	< 0.01*	0.94 (0.82-1.08)	0.19
Chronic hypertension										
No	Reference		Reference		Reference		Reference		Reference	
Yes	22.73 (21.5–24.0)	< 0.01*	16.8 (15.7-18.0)	< 0.01*	12.21 (11.5-13.0)	< 0.01*	9.85 (9.19-10.6)	< 0.01*	1.71 (1.55-1.88)	< 0.01*
Hyperthyroidism										
No	Reference		Reference		Reference		Reference		Reference	
Yes	1.68 (1.53–1.83)	< 0.01*	1.18 (1.07-1.29)	< 0.01*	1.48 (1.36-1.60)	< 0.01*	1.21 (1.12-1.32)	< 0.01*	0.98 (0.86-1.10)	0.34

[a]Adjusted Relative risk: adjusted for with age at delivery, income, urbanization, parity, acute coronary syndrome, chronic ischemic heart disease, stroke, diabetes mellitus, chronic hypertension and hyperthyroidism
[b]Acute Coronary syndrome included myocardial infarction and unstable angina
*$P < 0.05$

evidences, there was yet no definite pathophysiology and mechanism to explain the development towards early- or late-onset preeclampsia. Thus, more investigations are needed to identify the specific correlation between old age or chronic hypertension and early-onset preeclampsia, and clinicians should be aware of preeclampsia prediction in women with clinical risk factors, particularly chronic hypertension, which had highest risk (ARR, 16.8, 95%CI, 15.7–18.0) of early-onset preeclampsia in the current study. Furthermore, early intervention such as aspirin prophylaxis may be considered in patients with evidence of higher risk, according to the ASPRE trial [43] to prevent severe maternal morbidities and poorer birth outcomes of early-onset preeclampsia [14, 16, 17]. On the other hand, Valensise et al. have found late-onset preeclampsia

appeared to be more frequent in patients with high body mass index (BMI) compared with early-onset disease [19]. However, we had no data of maternal BMI to assess and the mechanism between preeclampsia and obesity was yet completely understood. In general, maternal risk factors between early- and late- onset preeclampsia were similar but old age and chronic hypertension appeared stronger association to early-onset disease and primiparity had higher risk of late-onset preeclampsia.

This study was the first documented the increasing trend of preeclampsia in Taiwan between 2001 and 2014, predominantly in early-onset disease. The strength of the study includes a large cohort sample from a specific geographic area which is very representative of the regional population and the large study size provided reliability in statistics.

Conclusions

In conclusion, the population-base study showed a rise in the incidence of preeclampsia, particularly in early-onset disease in Taiwan from 2001 to 2014, suggesting the clinical early prediction, identification, and management of the diseases will increasingly challenge obstetricians. As increasing number of advanced maternal age and chronic hypertension in delivering population in Taiwan, preconceptional counseling and surveillance is warranted in pregnant women with higher risk of early-onset preeclampsia. Further study of the predominance of early-onset preeclampsia in the population and the stronger association with old age and hypertension and early-onset preeclampsia is required.

Additional files

Additional file 1 Trends of preeclampsia incidence according to different ages between 2001 and 2014 (blue: 15–25-year-old; red: 25–35-year-old; green:35–55-year-old).

Additional file 2 Trends of preeclampsia incidence according to women with or without hypertension (orange: women with hypertension; blue: women without hypertension). (TIF 1131 kb)

Additional file 3 Table S6 Maternal characteristics and clinical risk factors associated with preeclampsia by age group. **Table S7** Maternal characteristics and clinical risk factors associated with preeclampsia by hypertension.

Abbreviations

AAPC: average annual percentage change; ACOG: American College of Obstetrician and Gynecologist; ARR: adjusted relative risk; BMI: body mass index; CI: confidence interval; DOHaD: developmental origins of health and disease; ICD-9: International Classification of Diseases, the 9th version; ISSHP: International Society for the Study of Hypertension in Pregnancy; NHIRD: National Health Insurance Database; RRR: ratio of relative risk; WHO: World Health Organization

Funding

This work was funded by the National Science Council of Taiwan (project 104-2314-B-182A-047) and Chang Gung Memorial Hospital (project CMRPG3E1961) and was supported by the University of Nottingham in methodology and infrastructure.
Role of the sponsors: The sponsors of the study, the Chang Gung Memorial Hospital, the National Science Council, the University of Nottingham and the Arthritis Research UK had no role in design and conduct of the study; collection, management, analysis, and interpretation of the data; and preparation, review, or approval of the manuscript and decision to submit the manuscript for publication.

Authors' contributions

PHC initiated the concept and designed the study. TTC and CFK collected the data and analyzed the data. SHY wrote the initial manuscript. HMW, PJC, and PHC gave critical comments to the study design, interpretation, and revised the draft. All authors read and approved the final manuscript.

Competing interests

The authors declare that they have no competing interests.

Author details

[1]Department of Obstetrics and Gynecology, Chang Gung Memorial Hospital, Linkou, Taiwan. [2]Big data research office, Chang Gung Memorial Hospital, Linkou, Taiwan. [3]Division of Rheumatology, Allergy and Immunology, Chang Gung Memorial Hospital, Linkou, Taiwan. [4]Department of Cardiology, Chang Gung Memorial Hospital, Linkou, Taiwan.

References

1. Khan KS, Wojdyla D, Say L, Gulmezoglu AM, Van Look PF. WHO analysis of causes of maternal death: a systematic review. Lancet. 2006;367(9516):1066–74.
2. Abalos E, Cuesta C, Grosso AL, Chou D, Say L. Global and regional estimates of preeclampsia and eclampsia: a systematic review. Eur J Obstet Gynecol Reprod Biol. 2013;170(1):1–7.
3. Duley L. The global impact of pre-eclampsia and eclampsia. Semin Perinatol. 2009;33(3):130–7.
4. Abalos E, Cuesta C, Carroli G, Qureshi Z, Widmer M, Vogel JP, Souza JP, W.H.O.M.S.o. Maternal, and N. Newborn Health Research. Pre-eclampsia, eclampsia and adverse maternal and perinatal outcomes: a secondary analysis of the World Health Organization Multicountry Survey on Maternal and Newborn Health. BJOG. 2014;121(Suppl 1):14–24.
5. Roberts CL, Algert CS, Morris JM, Ford JB, Henderson-Smart DJ. Hypertensive disorders in pregnancy: a population-based study. Med J Aust. 2005;182(7):332–5.
6. Paruk F, Moodley J. Maternal and neonatal outcome in early- and late-onset pre-eclampsia. Semin Neonatol. 2000;5(3):197–207.
7. Sibai B, Dekker G, Kupferminc M. Pre-eclampsia. Lancet. 2005;365(9461):785–99.
8. Say L, Chou D, Gemmill A, Tuncalp O, Moller AB, Daniels J, Gulmezoglu AM, Temmerman M, Alkema L. Global causes of maternal death: a WHO systematic analysis. Lancet Glob Health. 2014;2(6):e323–33.
9. Kuklina EV, Ayala C, Callaghan WM. Hypertensive disorders and severe obstetric morbidity in the United States. Obstet Gynecol. 2009;113(6):1299–306.
10. English FA, Kenny LC, McCarthy FP. Risk factors and effective management of preeclampsia. Integr Blood Press Control. 2015;8:7–12.
11. Dekker G, Sibai B. Primary, secondary, and tertiary prevention of pre-eclampsia. Lancet. 2001;357(9251):209–15.
12. Ness RB, Roberts JM. Heterogeneous causes constituting the single syndrome of preeclampsia: a hypothesis and its implications. Am J Obstet Gynecol. 1996;175(5):1365–70.
13. von Dadelszen P, Magee LA, Roberts JM. Subclassification of preeclampsia. Hypertens Pregnancy. 2003;22(2):143–8.
14. Lisonkova S, Joseph KS. Incidence of preeclampsia: risk factors and outcomes associated with early- versus late-onset disease. Am J Obstet Gynecol. 2013;209(6):544 e1–544 e12.
15. Lisonkova S, Sabr Y, Mayer C, Young C, Skoll A, Joseph KS. Maternal morbidity associated with early-onset and late-onset preeclampsia. Obstet Gynecol. 2014;124(4):771–81.
16. Iacobelli S, Bonsante F, Robillard PY. Comparison of risk factors and perinatal outcomes in early onset and late onset preeclampsia: a cohort based study in Reunion Island. J Reprod Immunol. 2017;123:12–6.
17. Madazli R, Yuksel MA, Imamoglu M, Tuten A, Oncul M, Aydin B, Demirayak G. Comparison of clinical and perinatal outcomes in early- and late-onset preeclampsia. Arch Gynecol Obstet. 2014;290(1):53–7.
18. Mifsud W, Sebire NJ. Placental pathology in early-onset and late-onset fetal growth restriction. Fetal Diagn Ther. 2014;36(2):117–28.
19. Valensise H, Vasapollo B, Gagliardi G, Novelli GP. Early and late preeclampsia: two different maternal hemodynamic states in the latent phase of the disease. Hypertension. 2008;52(5):873–80.
20. Stergiotou I, Crispi F, Valenzuela-Alcaraz B, Bijnens B, Gratacos E. Patterns of maternal vascular remodeling and responsiveness in early- versus late-onset preeclampsia. Am J Obstet Gynecol. 2013;209(6):558 e1–558 e14.
21. Duckitt K, Harrington D. Risk factors for pre-eclampsia at antenatal booking: systematic review of controlled studies. BMJ. 2005;330(7491):565.
22. Bartsch E, Medcalf KE, Park AL, Ray JG, G. High Risk of Pre-eclampsia Identification. Clinical risk factors for pre-eclampsia determined in early

pregnancy: systematic review and meta-analysis of large cohort studies. BMJ. 2016;353:i1753.

23. Bushnell C, Chireau M. Preeclampsia and stroke: risks during and after pregnancy. Stroke Res Treat. 2011;2011:858134.

24. Aggarawal N, Suri V, Singla R, Chopra S, Sikka P, Shah VN, Bhansali A. Pregnancy outcome in hyperthyroidism: a case control study. Gynecol Obstet Investig. 2014;77(2):94–9.

25. Chan TF, Tung YC, Wang SH, Lee CH, Lin CL, Lu PY. Trends in the incidence of pre-eclampsia and eclampsia in Taiwan between 1998 and 2010. Taiwan J Obstet Gynecol. 2015;54(3):270–4.

26. Purde MT, Baumann M, Wiedemann U, Nydegger UE, Risch L, Surbek D, Risch M. Incidence of preeclampsia in pregnant Swiss women. Swiss Med Wkly. 2015;145:w14175.

27. Mol BWJ, Roberts CT, Thangaratinam S, Magee LA, de Groot CJM, Hofmeyr GJ. Pre-eclampsia. Lancet. 2016;387(10022):999–1011.

28. Tang CH, Wu CS, Lee TH, Hung ST, Yang CY, Lee CH, Chu PH. Preeclampsia-eclampsia and the risk of stroke among peripartum in Taiwan. Stroke. 2009; 40(4):1162–8.

29. Lin YS, Tang CH, Yang CY, Wu LS, Hung ST, Hwa HL, Chu PH. Effect of pre-eclampsia-eclampsia on major cardiovascular events among peripartum women in Taiwan. Am J Cardiol. 2011;107(2):325–30.

30. Lee CJ, Hsieh TT, Chiu TH, Chen KC, Lo LM, Hung TH. Risk factors for pre-eclampsia in an Asian population. Int J Gynaecol Obstet. 2000;70(3):327–33.

31. Wang YP, Liu CJ, Hu YW, Chen TJ, Lin YT, Fung CP. Risk of cancer among patients with herpes zoster infection: a population-based study. CMAJ. 2012; 184(15):E804–9.

32. Wallis AB, Saftlas AF, Hsia J, Atrash HK. Secular trends in the rates of preeclampsia, eclampsia, and gestational hypertension, United States, 1987-2004. Am J Hypertens. 2008;21(5):521–6.

33. Lawler J, Osman M, Shelton JA, Yeh J. Population-based analysis of hypertensive disorders in pregnancy. Hypertens Pregnancy. 2007;26(1):67–76.

34. Roberts CL, Ford JB, Algert CS, Antonsen S, Chalmers J, Cnattingius S, Gokhale M, Kotelchuck M, Melve KK, Langridge A, Morris C, Morris JM, Nassar N, Norman JE, Norrie J, Sorensen HT, Walker R, Weir CJ. Population-based trends in pregnancy hypertension and pre-eclampsia: an international comparative study. BMJ Open. 2011;1(1):e000101.

35. Tranquilli AL, Dekker G, Magee L, Roberts J, Sibai BM, Steyn W, Zeeman GG, Brown MA. The classification, diagnosis and management of the hypertensive disorders of pregnancy: a revised statement from the ISSHP. Pregnancy Hypertens. 2014;4(2):97–104.

36. American College of, O., Gynecologists, and P. Task Force on Hypertension in, Hypertension in pregnancy. Report of the American College of Obstetricians and Gynecologists' task force on hypertension in pregnancy. Obstet Gynecol. 2013;122(5):1122–31.

37. Chien KL, Hsu HC, Sung FC, Su TC, Chen MF, Lee YT. Incidence of hypertension and risk of cardiovascular events among ethnic Chinese: report from a community-based cohort study in Taiwan. J Hypertens. 2007; 25(7):1355–61.

38. Sheikh AM, Small HY, Currie G, Delles C. Systematic review of micro-RNA expression in pre-eclampsia identifies a number of common pathways associated with the disease. PLoS One. 2016;11(8):e0160808.

39. von Krogh AS, Kremer Hovinga JA, Romundstad PR, Roten LT, Lammle B, Waage A, Quist-Paulsen P. ADAMTS13 gene variants and function in women with preeclampsia: a population- based nested case- control study from the HUNT study. Thromb Res. 2015;136(2):282–8.

40. Mohammadpour-Gharehbagh A, Teimoori B, Narooei-Nejad M, Mehrabani M, Saravani R, Salimi S. The association of the placental MTHFR 3'-UTR polymorphisms, promoter methylation and MTHFR expression with preeclampsia. J Cell Biochem. 2018;119(2):346–1354.

41. Bianco-Miotto T, Craig JM, Gasser YP, van Dijk SJ, Ozanne SE. Epigenetics and DOHaD: from basics to birth and beyond. J Dev Orig Health Dis. 2017;8(5):513–9.

42. Cheng PJ, Huang SY, Su SY, Hsiao CH, Peng HH, Duan T. Prognostic value of cardiovascular disease risk factors measured in the first-trimester on the severity of preeclampsia. Medicine (Baltimore). 2016;95(5):e2653.

43. Rolnik DL, Wright D, Poon LC, O'Gorman N, Syngelaki A, de Paco Matallana C, Akolekar R, Cicero S, Janga D, Singh M, Molina FS, Persico N, Jani JC, Plasencia W, Papaioannou G, Tenenbaum-Gavish K, Meiri H, Gizurarson S, Maclagan K, Nicolaides KH. Aspirin versus placebo in pregnancies at high risk for preterm preeclampsia. N Engl J Med. 2017;377(7):613–22.

13

Assessment of quality of obstetric care in Zimbabwe using the standard primipara

Bothwell Takaingofa Guzha[1]*[iD], Thulani Lesley Magwali[1], Bismark Mateveke[1], Maxwell Chirehwa[2], George Nyandoro[3] and Stephen Peter Munjanja[1]

Abstract

Background: To improve maternity services in any country, there is need to monitor the quality of obstetric care. There is usually disparity of obstetric care and outcomes in most countries among women giving birth in different obstetric units. However, comparing the quality of obstetric care is difficult because of heterogeneous population characteristics and the difference in prevalence of complications. The concept of the standard primipara was introduced as a tool to control for these various confounding factors. This concept was used to compare the quality of obstetric care among districts in different geographical locations in Zimbabwe.

Methods: This was a substudy of the Zimbabwe Maternal and Perinatal Mortality Study. In the main study, cluster sampling was done with the provinces as clusters and 11 districts were randomly selected with one from each of the nine provinces and two from the largest province. This database was used to identify the standard primipara defined as; a woman in her first pregnancy without any known complications who has spontaneous onset of labour at term. Obstetric process and outcome indicators of the standard primipara were then used to compare the quality of care between rural and urban, across rural and across urban districts of Zimbabwe.

Results: A total of 45,240 births were recruited in the main study and 10,947 women met the definition of standard primipara. The maternal mortality ratio (MMR) and the perinatal mortality rate (PNMR) for the standard primiparae were 92/100000 live births and 15.4/1000 total births respectively. Compared to urban districts, the PNMR was higher in the rural districts (11/1000 total births vs 19/1000 total births, $p < 0.001$). In the urban to urban and rural to rural districts comparison, there were significant differences in most of the process indicators, but not in the PNMR.

Conclusions: The study has shown that the standard primipara can be used as a tool to measure and compare the quality of obstetric care in districts in different geographical areas. There is need to explore further how the quality of obstetric care can be improved in rural districts of Zimbabwe.

Keywords: Standard primipara, Quality of care, Obstetric process indicators, Obstetric outcome indicators, the perinatal mortality rate

Background

The previous millennium development goal (MDG) number 5 targeted to reduce maternal deaths by 75% by the year 2015. This unrealistic target was not achieved because there is still a great need for unrestricted access to high-quality emergency obstetric care to reduce the high risk of dying in pregnancy which is still prevalent in the low-resource countries [1]. Thus reducing this great risk of dying during pregnancy in low-resource countries is the new target in the developed sustainable development goal (SDG) number 3, targeting to reduce the global maternal mortality ratio to less than 70 per 100,000 live births by 2030.

The lifetime risk of dying due to pregnancy-related complications in Sub-Saharan Africa is 1 in 39 compared to 1 in 4600 in the United Kingdom and 1 in 3800 in high-income countries in general [2].

To improve maternity services, there is need to monitor and improve the quality of care women receive in different obstetric units. One limitation though is that

* Correspondence: bothwellguzha@gmail.com
[1]Department of Obstetrics and Gynaecology, University of Zimbabwe, College of Health Sciences, P.O. Box A178, Avondale, Harare, Zimbabwe

there is no universally agreed definition of quality of care (QoC). This explains the variation in obstetric outcomes like caesarean section, instrumental delivery and induction of labour rates among different health institutions within the same setting [3]. In most countries, there is a disparity of care and outcomes among different obstetric units [4]. For this to be corrected there is need to come up with a tool that can be used to compare the quality of care between the different institutions. The tool should be able to control for confounding factors like difference in patient characteristics and disease patterns.

In Zimbabwe, like in most countries, the difference in the quality of care among the different geographical areas is difficult to determine because of heterogeneous population characteristics and the difference in prevalence of complications in those areas. The concept of the standard primipara was introduced as a basis of inter-unit comparison in evaluating the quality of obstetric services to minimise the risks of bias [4]. Alfirevic et al. used this concept in comparing the impact of delivery suite guidelines on intrapartum care among different health institutions [5]. Some maternal and perinatal process and outcome indicators were then used as tools to compare the quality of obstetric care among the different geographical districts in Zimbabwe [6, 7].

The availability of comprehensive obstetric care in various settings depends on local conditions and the resources available. There is no available data looking at the quality of obstetric care among the different districts in the different Provinces of Zimbabwe. This study was done to identify the districts with poor quality of obstetric care. This data is important to improve maternity services in poorly performing districts to match those of areas that had better performance.

Methods

Zimbabwe is divided into 10 administrative Provinces, which are divided into 59 Districts. Harare, the biggest Province has urban districts only unlike all the other Provinces which are comprised of urban and rural districts. The Zimbabwe Maternal and Perinatal Mortality Study (ZMPMS) was a population-based descriptive and cross-sectional study of deaths of women in pregnancy and perinatal deaths in Zimbabwe. The study was done to estimate the maternal mortality ratio (MMR) and the perinatal mortality rate (PNMR) in Zimbabwe [8]. Data were collected from the 1st of May 2007 to the 30th April 2008. Cluster sampling was done with the 10 provinces as clusters and 11 districts were randomly selected with one from each of the 9 provinces and 2 from Harare which is the biggest province in Zimbabwe. In these 11 districts, pregnancy outcomes were collected prospectively on all women delivering after 22 weeks gestation for 11 months [8]. Data were collected from all

healthcare facilities and also from homes and villages. A data entry template was designed in Microsoft Access and used for data capture. Alfirevic et al. defined the standard primipara as a woman in her first pregnancy, with a singleton fetus in cephalic presentation, with spontaneous onset of labour between 37 + 0 weeks and 42 + 0 weeks, with no antenatal complications or previous hospital admission lasting more than 24 h [5]. This was the definition of the standard primipara used in this study. Data from all the districts in the main study were used to extract records for women who met the definition of the standard primipara; and subsequent data analyses were performed in Stata Version 9.0 (StataCorp LP, College Station, TX). The standard primiparae were then used to compare maternal and perinatal process and outcome indicators between rural and urban, across urban and across rural districts. Pearson chi-squared test was used to determine the association between the categorical variables. The quality of obstetric care was assessed using the following indicators:

a) Obstetric process indicators:Booking status (at least one antenatal visit), gestational age at booking, antenatal human immunodeficiency virus (HIV) screening rate, and initial place of onset of labour, utilisation of maternity waiting shelters in the rural districts, institutional delivery rate, intrapartum complication detection rate, and referral in labour rate, operative vaginal delivery rate, caesarean section rate and the postpartum referral rate.

b) Obstetric outcome indicators:PNMR.

Results

In the main study, a total of 45,240 births were recruited from the 11 districts and 10,947 women met the definition of standard primipara.

As shown in Table 1 below, the median (Q1; Q3) age of the women was 20 (18; 22) years.

As shown in Table 2 below, the vast majority of the standard primiparas booked their pregnancies (94.1%) and the median (Q1; Q3) gestation at booking was 24 (20; 28) weeks. Less than half of them (42.4%) were screened for HIV in the antenatal period. The institutional delivery rate was high at 87.8, and 8.8% of them were referred to higher levels of care for intrapartum complications. The caesarean section and vacuum delivery rates were low at 4.1 and 1.4% respectively. Compared to the rest of the women in the 11 districts, the standard primiparas had lower maternal mortality ratios (92/100000 live births vs 698/100000 live births, $p < 0.001$). The perinatal mortality rates were also lower in the standard primiparas (15.4/ 1000 total births vs 31.9/ 1000 total births, $p < 0.001$).

As shown in the Table 3 below, in the urban to rural districts comparison, there were significant differences

Table 1 Demographic characteristics of the standard primiparae, stratified by district

District/ Area	Sample size	Median age (years) (Q1; Q3)
Rural		
Bindura	837	19 (18;21)
Chivi	1394	20 (18;22)
Matobo	617	19 (17;20)
Mutoko	778	19 (18;21)
Tsholotsho	648	18 (17;20)
Zvimba	1005	20 (18;22)
Urban		
South Eastern district of Harare	444	23 (20;25)
Western district of Harare	1463	21 (19;23)
Kwekwe	1398	20 (18;23)
Nkulumane	1159	21.(19;23
Mutare	1204	20 (19;23)
Area		
Rural	6026	19 (18;21)
Urban	4921	21 (19;23)
Total	10,947	20 (18; 22)

Table 2 Obstetric indicators for the standard primiparae

Process Indicators	Standard primipara N = 10,947
Booking status (%)	94.1
Mean gestation at booking (weeks)	23.6
Antenatal HIV screening (%)	42.4
Initial place of onset of labour-institutional (%)	19.4
Institutional deliveries (%)	87.8
Intra partum complications detected (%)	12.3
Referrals in labour (%)	8.8
Caesarean section rate (%)	4.1
Vacuum delivery rate (%)	1.4
Post-partum referrals (%)	5.5
Outcome Indicators	
PNMR (N/1000 births)	15.4

Abbreviations: HIV human immunodeficiency virus, PNMR perinatal mortality rate

Table 3 Comparison between rural and urban districts

Process Indicators	Rural N = 6026	Urban N = 4921	*p-value
Booking status (%)	94.9	94.5	0.394
Mean gestation at booking (weeks)	22.4	25.3	< 0.001
Antenatal HIV screening (%)	37.8	60.1	< 0.001
Initial place of onset labour-institutional (%)	30.6	5.6	< 0.001
Institutional deliveries (%)	80.2	97.1	< 0.001
Intrapartum complications detected (%)	7.4	18.3	< 0.001
Referrals in labour (%)	3.1	15.8	< 0.001
Caesarean section rate (%)	2.2	6.5	< 0.001
Vacuum delivery rate (%)	0.5	2.5	< 0.001
Post-partum referrals (%)	0.4	1.2	< 0.001
Outcome Indicators			
PNMR (N/1000 births)	19	11	0.001

Abbreviations: HIV human immunodeficiency virus, PNMR perinatal mortality rate
*= Analysis of process and outcome indicators between districts

in the following process indicators: mean gestation at booking, antenatal HIV screening rate, initial place of onset of labour, institutional delivery rate, intrapartum complication detection rate, and referral in labour rate, caesarean section rate, vacuum delivery rate and post-partum referral rate. The urban districts had a significantly lower PNMR.

As shown in Table 4 below, across the urban districts, there were significant differences in the following process indicators: booking status, antenatal HIV screening rate, and initial place of onset of labour, institutional delivery rate, intrapartum complications detection rate, referral in labour rate, caesarean section rate, vacuum delivery rate and post-partum referral rate. There was no significant difference in the PNMR.

As shown in Table 5 below, across the rural districts, there were significant differences in the following process indicators: booking status, mean gestation at booking, antenatal HIV screening rate, initial place of onset of labour, institutional delivery rate, intrapartum complications detection rate, referral in labour rate and vacuum delivery rate. There was no significant difference in the PNMR.

As shown in Table 6 below, the standard primiparas had significantly better obstetric and process outcome indicators than the general obstetric population.

Discussion

Compared to the total ZMPMS population, the standard primiparas had a lower maternal mortality ratio and perinatal mortality rate (see Table 6). This confirms that this was a low-risk group and the differences in outcomes were probably due to variation in quality of service provision than patient-related factors.

Across urban and across rural districts (see Tables 4 and 5), there were significant differences in most of the obstetric process indicators. Some of the differences across the rural or urban districts were inexplicable considering that they get similar resources from the central Government. There is need to investigate why this is

Table 4 Comparison across urban districts

Process Indicators	South Eastern district of Harare	Western district of Harare	Kwekwe	Mutare	Nkulumane	*p-value
Booking status (%)	95.7	90.7	96.8	96.5	95.4	< 0.001
Mean gestation at booking (weeks)	23.8	26.0	23.7	24.7	26.6	0.122
Antenatal HIV screening (%)	31.0	52.5	49.5	61.6	86.6	< 0.001
Initial place of onset of labour-institutional (%)	2.7	5.6	2.2	15.2	1.3	< 0.001
Institutional deliveries (%)	98.0	96.6	97.4	98.3	96.3	0.033
Intrapartum complications detected (%)	28.4	19.5	19.6	12.5	17.0	< 0.001
Referrals in labour (%)	9.5	16.7	14.1	23.4	12.1	< 0.001
Caesarean section rate (%)	8.4	5.0	9.8	5.7	5.9	< 0.001
Vacuum delivery rate (%)	15.9	2.0	0.5	0.1	1.5	< 0.001
Post-partum referrals (%)	1.6	1.6	0.7	0.1	2.3	0.001
Outcome Indicators						
PNMR (N/1000 births)	7	12	14	11	9.5	0.777

Abbreviations: *HIV* human immunodeficiency virus, *PNMR* perinatal mortality rate
*= Analysis of process and outcome indicators between districts

happening and offer remedial action to enable standardised maternity care in Zimbabwe. Surprisingly these differences did not have an impact on the PNMR. The study was not powered to detect a difference in the MMR among the individual districts.

In the rural to urban districts comparison (see Table 3), the only obstetric process indicator that did not show a significant difference was the antenatal booking status. The provision of free antenatal care in the Government rural clinics could explain why booking rates are high in both the rural and urban districts of Zimbabwe [9]. Despite these high booking rates, antenatal HIV screening rates remain low in both urban and rural districts (60.1% vs 37.8%, $p < 0.001$). This probably explains why a quarter of maternal deaths in Zimbabwe are still due to HIV/AIDS

[8]. Zimbabwe has adopted the World Health Organisation (WHO) HIV guidelines which recommended that all HIV-infected pregnant women be put on anti-retroviral treatment regardless of their CD4+ or viral load count [10]. Therefore, there is need to put mechanisms in place to make sure that all pregnant women are screened for HIV and those infected are put on treatment to reduce the MMR and parents to child transmission rates of HIV.

More standard primiparae in the urban districts had access to skilled birth attendants (SBA) (97.1% vs 80.2%, $p < 0.001$) (see Table 3). The low rate of delivery by skilled birth attendants in the rural districts fell below the target of 90% set by the WHO [11]. Due to unavailability of transport, almost 20% of women ended up delivering outside institutions.

Table 5 Comparison across rural districts

Outcome Indicators	Bindura	Chivi	Kwekwe	Matobo	Mutare	Mutoko	Zvimba	Tsholotsho	*p-value
Booking status (%)	95.3	97.3	97.6	98.0	96.1	96.8	98.1	84.0	< 0.001
Mean gestation at booking (weeks)	21.6	19.3	25.0	25.7	23.4	23.3	23.9	23.0	< 0.001
Antenatal HIV screening (%)	34.7	10.4	14.9	43.6	69.0	40.2	70.6	55.0	< 0.001
Initial place of onset of labour (%)	1.1	48.0	3.5	58.0	18.3	26.6	0.1	55.7	< 0.001
Institutional deliveries (%)	71.1	90.7	67.1	85.6	87.8	75.4	81.1	77.7	< 0.001
Intra partum complications detected (%)	4.1	4.4	6.9	10.3	2.7	16.2	3.9	9.3	< 0.001
Referrals in labour (%)	4.6	4.4	3.3	1.3	3.1	0.8	1.1	4.4	< 0.001
Caesarean section rate (%)	2.3	1.9	2.3	1.8	1.0	2.4	3.0	2.1	0.645
Vacuum delivery rate (%)	0.5	0.4	0.0	2.3	0.0	0.1	0.0	0.5	< 0.001
Post-partum referrals (%)	0.4	0.2	0.0	0.9	0.0	0.4	0.3	1.0	0.066
Outcome Indicators									
PNMR (N/1000 births)	24	22	18	20	31	14	22	10	0.234

Abbreviations: *HIV* human immunodeficiency virus, *PNMR* perinatal mortality rate and
*= Analysis of process and outcome indicators between districts

Table 6 Comparison between the standard primipara and the general obstetric population

Process Indicators	Standard primipara N = 10,947	Non-Standard primipara N = 34,293	*p-value
Booking status (%)	94.1	76.7	< 0.001
Mean gestation at booking (weeks)	23.6	24.5	< 0.001
Antenatal HIV screening (%)	42.4	31.2	< 0.001
Initial place of onset of labour-institutional (%)	19.4	10.9	< 0.001
Institutional deliveries (%)	87.8	62.4	< 0.001
Intra partum complications detected (%)	12.3	11.7	0.091
Referrals in labour (%)	8.8	5.1	< 0.001
Caesarean section rate (%)	4.1	3.8	0.157
Vacuum delivery rate (%)	1.4	0.7	< 0.001
Post-partum referrals (%)	5.5	1.0	< 0.001
Outcome Indicators			
PNMR (N/1000 births)	15.4	31.9	< 0.001

Abbreviations: HIV human immunodeficiency virus, *PNMR* perinatal mortality rate
*= Analysis of process and outcome indicators between districts

In the urban districts, the number of standard primiparas delivering in comprehensive emergency obstetric units and caesarean section rates meet the minimum targets set by the WHO of 15 and 5%, respectively [1, 12]. In the rural districts, the caesarean section rate of 2.2% is way below the WHO recommendation. Coupled with this, the operative vaginal delivery rate of 0.5% is way below the 2.5% in the urban districts. The low caesarean and operative delivery rates in the rural districts could be as a result of lack of personnel who are trained to do the procedures and a reluctance to attempt vacuum deliveries in remote areas, and this could explain the higher PNMR. Although the Central Government through the Ministry of Health and Child Care (MOHCC) has started to enforce the policy of deploying recently qualified doctors to the rural districts, this might not have an impact in the long term unless maternity waiting shelters are fully utilised to improve the institutional delivery rates in these areas.

Conclusions

The study has shown that the standard primipara is a useful tool to measure the quality of obstetric care in different districts in Zimbabwe. Therefore every district should measure process and outcome indicators of the standard primipara. The MOHCC can use this tool to monitor improvement in obstetric care and to find out the specific reasons for the discrepancy in the different obstetric process indicators and how this variation in service provision can be corrected at local and national level.

To the best of our knowledge, no study has been done in Africa utilising this tool to measure the quality of obstetric care between institutions in one country. A pilot study can also be done to assess its feasibility in comparing the quality of obstetric care among different countries in Africa.

Abbreviations
AIDS: Acquired Immunodeficiency Syndrome; HIV: Human Immunodeficiency Virus; MDG: Millennium Development Goal; MMR: Maternal Mortality Ratio; MOHCC: Ministry of Health and Child Care; PNMR: Perinatal Mortality Rate; QoC: Quality of Care; SBA: Skilled Birth Attendant; SDG: Sustainable Development Goal; WHO: World Health Organization; ZMPMS: Zimbabwe Maternal and Perinatal Mortality Study

Acknowledgements
This was a substudy of the Zimbabwe Maternal and Perinatal Mortality Study (ZMPMS).

Funding
The main study, the Zimbabwe Maternal and Perinatal Mortality Study (ZMPMS) was funded by the United Kingdom (UK), Department for International Development (DfID). This sub-study was done utilising data from the main study. The funders of the main study had no role in the design, collection, analysis, and interpretation of data and in writing the manuscript.

Authors' contributions
BTG, TLM, BM, SPM, MC and GN designed the study; MC and GN did the data analysis; BTG and SPM wrote the manuscript with SPM being the senior author. All the authors read and approved the manuscript.

Competing interests
The authors declare that they have no competing interests.

Author details
[1]Department of Obstetrics and Gynaecology, University of Zimbabwe, College of Health Sciences, P.O. Box A178, Avondale, Harare, Zimbabwe. [2]Department of Medicine, Division of Clinical Pharmacology, University of Cape Town, K45 Old Main Building, Groote Schuur Hospital, Observatory, Cape Town 7925, South Africa. [3]Biomedical Research and Training Institute, 10 Seagrave Avenue, Avondale, Harare, Zimbabwe.

References
1. Paxton A, Maine D, Freedman L, Fry D, Lobis S. The evidence for emergency obstetric care. Int J Gynaecol Obstet. 2005;88(2):181–93. PubMed Abstract | Publisher Full Text
2. How many women and girls die in childbirth? http://www.maternityworldwide. org/the-issues. Accessed 26 Sept 2014
3. Faisel H, Pittrof R, El-Hosini M, Habib M, Azzam E. Using standard primipara method to compare quality of care in Cairo and London. J Obstet Gynaecol. 2009;29(4):284–7.
4. Cleary R, Beard RW, Chapple J, Colles J, Griffin M, Joffe M, Welch A. The standard primipara as a basis of inter-unit comparisons of maternity care. Br J Obstet Gynaecol. 1996;103(3):223–9.
5. Alfirevic Z, Edwards G, Platt MJ. The impact of delivery suite guidelines on

intrapartum care in standard primigravida. Eur J Obstet Gynecol Reprod Biol. 2004;115(1):28–31.

6.   AMDD. Program note: using UN process indicators to assess needs in emergency obstetric services: Morocco, Nicaragua and Sri Lanka. Int J Gynaecol Obstet. 2003;80(2):222–30. PubMed Abstract | Publisher Full Text

7.   Gottlieb P, Lindmark G. WHO indicators for evaluation of maternal health care services, applicability in least developed countries: a case study from Eritrea. Afr J Reprod Health. 2002;6(2):13–22.

8.   Munjanja SP, Nystrom L, Nyandoro M, Magwali T. Maternal and Perinatal Mortality Study. 2007. http://www.unicef.org/zimbabwe/ZMPMS_report.pdf.

9.   Raatikainen K, Heiskanen N, Heinonen S. Under-attending free antenatal care is associated with adverse pregnancy outcomes. BMC Public Health. 2007;7:268.

10. HIV and infant feeding. Revised principles and recommendations. Geneva: World Health Organization; 2009.

11. Report of the Ad Hoc Committee of the Whole of the Twenty-first Special Session of the General Assembly (General Assembly document, No. A/S-21/5/Add.1). New York: UN; 1999. Available at http://www.un.org/popin/unpopcom/32ndsess/gass/215a1e.pdf.

12. World Health Organization. Managing complications in pregnancy and childbirth: a guide for midwives and doctors. Available at: http://www.who.int/making_pregnancy_safer/survey/en/index.html. Accessed 10 May 2010.

14

Health providers pass knowledge and abilities acquired by training in obstetric emergencies to their peers: the average treatment on the treated effect of PRONTO on delivery attendance in Mexico

Jimena Fritz[1], Héctor Lamadrid-Figueroa[1]* (iD), Gustavo Angeles[2], Alejandra Montoya[1] and Dilys Walker[3]

Abstract

Background: A significant proportion of newborn and maternal deaths can be prevented through simple and cost-effective strategies. The main aim of this study was to evaluate the impact of the PRONTO obstetric-emergency management training for improving evidence-based birth attendance practices among providers attending the training at 12 hospitals in three states of Mexico from 2010 to 2012, and to estimate dissemination of the training within the hospitals.

Methods: The average treatment on the treated effect of the PRONTO intervention for the probability of performing certain practices during birth attendance was estimated in a sample of 310 health providers. Impact estimates were obtained by performing provider-level matching using a mixed Mahalanobis distance one-to-one nearest-neighbor and exact matching approach. A secondary analysis estimated the positive externalities caused by the intervention in the treated hospitals using the same analytical approach. Provider-level fixed effects regression models were used to estimate the rate of decay of the probability of performing the examined practices.

Results: Providers attending the PRONTO training showed significant increases in the probability of performing the complete active management of the third stage of labor, especially the first and third steps, and skin-to-skin-contact. There was a negative and significant effect on the probability of performing uterine sweeping. Providers who did not attend the training in treated hospitals also showed marked significant changes in the same practices, except for uterine sweeping. There was no evidence of a significant decay of the probability of performing the routine practices over time among the treated providers.

Conclusions: PRONTO is efficacious in changing trained providers' behavior, but not on all practices, suggesting that some practices are deeply ingrained. The results also suggest that information on practices is effectively transmitted to peers within treated hospitals. Previous findings of the dilution of the effect of PRONTO on some practices seem to be more related to the rotation of personnel (mainly interns) rather than providers returning to their former habits.

Keywords: Program evaluation, Labor stage, First, Delivery, Obstetric, Mexico

---

* Correspondence: hlamadrid@insp.mx
[1]Division of Reproductive Health, Research Center for Population Health, National Institute of Public Health (INSP), Av. Universidad 655, Col. Santa María Ahuacatitlán, 62100 Cuernavaca, Morelos, Mexico
Full list of author information is available at the end of the article

Background

Cost-effective health strategies are known to save women's lives and to protect their newborns [1]. In fact, a significant proportion of newborn and maternal deaths can be prevented through simple and cost-effective strategies [1]. In Mexico, routine delivery practices are not necessarily based on World Health Organization (WHO) recommendations, but rather on convention and out-of-date information [2–4]. Several of these practices are actually potentially harmful to women but are routinely used because of the hierarchical organization of clinical teams in Mexican hospitals [5]. At hospitals in Mexico, medical authorities are generally not questioned, and the implementation of evidence-based practices is lacking [6].

Maternal and newborn care is dependent on effective multiprofessional teams of health care providers. The current challenge for training programs is to increase the capacity and experience of these multidisciplinary teams [7]. Obstetric care in Mexico is provided primarily in health institutions [8], underscoring the importance of improving the quality of care through the appropriate training of health provider teams attending deliveries. The complexity of training these teams requires multifunctional systems that go beyond organizational divisions to facilitate communication, accountability, and the maintenance of supplies and equipment [9].

Many studies on maternal mortality have indicated that the quality of obstetric services, as well as the provision of timely and adequate care for obstetric emergencies, is key in reducing institutional maternal morbidity and mortality [9–12]. Models of traditional training, didactic sessions, and the introduction of guidelines and protocols have failed to show the expected results on relevant indicators and have not yielded an increase in the performance of evidence-based practices [13]. There is an urgent need to update the skills of professionals who do not currently have the competencies required to provide emergency obstetric care as a team [14].

An overview of interventions aimed at improving the performance of health professionals in low-income countries suggests that the simple dissemination of written guidelines is often ineffective, whereas educational outreach visits and audits with feedback are generally effective [14, 15]. Additionally, multifaceted interventions might be more effective than single interventions [14]. A previous impact evaluation showed that PRONTO, an obstetric emergency-management training intervention for health providers based on highly realistic simulation and team training, had a significant effect on several routinely performed obstetric practices in Mexican hospitals. However, an important issue left unexplored by this past work involves the magnitude of the spillover or positive externality of the intervention: Only 20% of the

eligible health providers were actually trained, but it was hypothesized that they would transmit their newly acquired knowledge and abilities to their peers, cascading the impact. Moreover, this evaluation also raised new questions about sustainability, because a marked dilution of the effect was observed over the course at one year [16]. This dilution may be explained by the rotation of trained health providers, the abandonment of newly learned practices by trained providers, or a combination of these two factors.

The present study built on the previous report of the average treatment effect (ATE) of PRONTO on routine practices. We sought to deepen the understanding of the mechanisms explaining the dilution of the effect by incorporating newly obtained information and a different analytical strategy. Instead of comparing practices performed in treated vs. untreated hospitals as a whole, we focused on the participants who actually received the treatment (i.e., participated in the training) to estimate the average treatment on the treated (ATT) effect. The ATT estimation allowed us to approximate how large the total ATE would be if a larger proportion of personnel had taken the training. Additionally, by comparing the effect on the trainees to the effect observed on those who did not actually attend the training but there were working side by side who those who did indeed attend (Average Treatment effect on the Non-Treated or ATNT), it can also provide insights on how well the competencies acquired through training are transmitted among peers in health institutions.

Our analysis addressed two key questions left unanswered by the previous ATE analysis of the impact of PRONTO on routine practices during delivery [16]: 1) What is the magnitude of the positive externalities of the intervention in terms of the transmission of knowledge and behavior changes within the treated hospitals among those providers who did not receive the training? and 2) What is the reason for the dilution of the effect of PRONTO on some of the outcomes?

Methods

Intervention

The PRONTO simulation-based training, a training course on the management of obstetric emergencies, was developed and piloted in Mexico in 2009. Although the training is not oriented toward the management of normal deliveries, that topic is included in several sessions of the curriculum [17]. A cluster randomized controlled trial was conducted in 24 hospitals in three Mexican states to evaluate the impact of PRONTO. A total of 450 participants (54% physicians and 46% nurses) received the PRONTO training at the 12 intervention hospitals. The selection of these participants was carried out by the authorities in the selected health

Health providers pass knowledge and abilities acquired by training in obstetric emergencies...

125

facilities, but the main selection criterion was that the trainees were personnel who attended deliveries or worked in emergency or delivery rooms [16]. For the original study, hospitals were matched one-to-one based on similar characteristics and incidence of obstetric complications; one member of the hospital pair was then randomly assigned to receive the training. Further details on the original impact evaluation study and the methods used in the training have been previously published [18].

Data collection: Observation of deliveries

Data collection began in August 2010, and the follow-up concluded in March 2013 in the 24 participating hospitals. Five field workers were instructed to conduct a structured observation of births from the beginning of the second stage of labor until 10–20 min after the third stage was completed, using a paper-based checklist to collect the data. During each data collection period (the baseline and follow-ups at 4, 8, and 12 months after the intervention), the goal was to observe at least 10 vaginal births attended by different providers on different shifts at each hospital over a maximum 5-day observation period. Prior to the observation of births, both the health provider and the laboring woman provided oral consent. The observers were not blinded to the treatment allocation, but they were blinded to the treatment status of individual providers. A more detailed explanation is provided elsewhere [16].

Retrieval of additional information

The original dataset analyzed by Fritz, et al. (2017) was a set of 641 observed deliveries [16]. However, to estimate the ATT effect, it was necessary to create a unique identifier for each health provider and to distinguish those providers who were trained using PRONTO from those who were not. Because the original study design was not planned to allow for analysis at the provider level, no unique provider identifier was recorded. Rather, the names of delivery attendants were recorded in an informal, non-standardized fashion. Consequently, there was vast heterogeneity in the way these names were written, which made it impossible to create unique identifiers in a straightforward manner. An additional problem was that the gender of the provider was not recorded. In some cases, we were able to infer gender from the name. However, this was not always possible, especially for interns, who were usually referred to in hospital notes only by the prefix MIP and their family name (e.g., "MIP Perez," which means "Undergraduate Intern Medic Perez" and is a gender-neutral expression in Spanish).

A uniformization of the providers' names was performed using the Stata command STRGROUP [19], which matches similar names of providers within each hospital and profession. The algorithm for the matching between all pairwise

combinations of strings into the "provider name" variable considered the estimation of the Levenshtein distance, defined as the minimum number of single-character edits (i.e., insertions, deletions, or substitutions) required to change one string into the other [20]. A normalization was then performed by dividing the distance by the length of the shorter string in the comparison. Subsequently, we matched a string pair if the names' normalized distance was less than or equal to a threshold of 0.25, which corresponded to the 10th percentile of the distribution of Levenshtein distances. The algorithm was also applied to identify name similarities among the list of participants in the training, which were stored in a different dataset. Finally, each set of matches was assigned a unique provider identification number, and this was manually re-checked prior to analysis. The health provider's gender was inferred from their name or from clues such as the use of "Dr." or "Dra." as prefixes for the name. We were unable to retrieve information on the name of the provider for 3% of the observed deliveries, and we were unable to identify the gender of the provider for 12% of cases. We were able to ascertain gender for 100% of the treated providers. The study protocol for the original study (Reference 845), as well as for additional data gathering and analysis on individual providers (Reference 733) were reviewed and approved by the Ethics and Research Committees of the National Institute of Public Health in Cuernavaca, Mexico.

Analytic sample

The original dataset of 641 observed deliveries was collapsed by hospital and stage (4, 8, and 12 months following the training) to a dataset of 310 providers who attended at least one delivery after the time of the training. We summarized the outcomes as the proportion of attended deliveries in which routine practice was followed. The unit of analysis was the ith provider at the tth stage of the study, for a final analytic sample size of 356 observations, of which 50 corresponded to observations of trained providers, 141 were observations of non-trained providers in treated hospitals, and 165 were potential controls (providers observed in control hospitals). The study flow chart is included as supplementary material [see Additional file 1].

Variable definitions

The main outcomes were the routine practices performed during delivery. Three practices can improve patient outcomes and prevent significant childbirth complications, according to the WHO [9]: 1) Active management of the third stage of labor (AMTSL), defined as (1st Step) applying 10 international units of oxytocin in the first minute after the birth of the baby, (2nd Step) traction and countertraction of the umbilical cord, and (3rd Step) uterine massage immediately after the birth of the placenta; 2) use of delayed cord clamping (DCC), defined as a delay in the clamping of the umbilical cord of at least 60 s after the birth of the baby; and 3) Skin-to-skin contact (SSC), defined as immediate contact or attachment between mother and child after birth. Three unsubstantiated and harmful practices that can worsen patient outcomes if used routinely, according to the WHO [9] are as follows: 1) episiotomy, defined as the performance of a surgical incision in the woman's perineum, including the skin, muscular plane, and vaginal mucosa; 2) fundal uterine pressure (the Kristeller maneuver), defined as the application of manual pressure on the upper part of the uterus directed toward the birth canal; and 3) uterine sweeping, defined as the introduction of a hand or a gauze-wrapped instrument into the fundus of the uterus after the birth of the placenta.

The main explanatory variable was participation in the PRONTO training (yes/no). Important covariates at the individual level were the health provider's gender, shift, and profession.

Statistical analysis

The following equation is the mathematical approach used to estimate the ATT effect of the PRONTO training (δ_1), which can be understood as the expected difference on the performance of routine practices (AMTSL, DCC, SSC, episiotomy, fundal pressure, and uterine sweeping) between those in the intervention group and those who were trained:

$$\delta_1 = E(y_1 - y_0 | t = 1) \qquad (1)$$

In this equation, y_1 is the probability of a trained provider performing a routine practice and y_0 is the probability of practice performance with no training (counterfactual), given that the participant was actually trained. The ATT impact estimators were obtained by comparing the prevalence of practices performed by participants with the prevalence among non-participants who would have taken the training had they been offered the opportunity to do so, the prevalence among this non-participants serves as a proxy of the counterfactual: the prevalence on those who were indeed trained in the hypothetical situation were the training never took place. To accomplish this, and because participants in the training were not randomly selected within the treated hospitals, we matched each trained provider with a non-trained provider from the control hospitals, this procedure relies on the assumption that that conditional on the matched covariates, the trained providers and non-trained providers are exchangeable [21]. We performed the matching using one-to-one nearest-neighbor matching in terms of the minimum Mahalanobis distance [22], which was defined using the following covariates: matched hospital pair, state, gender, shift, and profession. Additionally, to control for trends in the probability of performing the practices, we matched exactly on time elapsed

since the training (4, 8, or 12 months). Because the accuracy of the estimators depended on the comparability of the treatment groups, we performed a sensitivity analysis using matching to the one, two, and three nearest neighbors with the *tebalance* Stata routine. We chose the one-to-one matching procedure, because it provided more than twice the bias reduction (in terms of the average difference in covariates between the groups) yielded by the use of two or more neighbors.

To estimate the possible effect of PRONTO on those who were not directly trained (positive externality), we performed an estimation of the ATE for non-treated providers (ATNT), matching those who did not attend the training but were working in treated hospitals to those working in control hospitals, otherwise following the same approach described above. Finally, to test for possible decay (linear trend) of the probability of treated providers performing the examined practices in the post-training period, we fitted a provider-level fixed effects regression model with robust standard errors and clustering correction at the hospital level, including time after training as a continuous variable with time units of four months (time elapsed between observation rounds). All analyses were performed with Stata 14.0 (StataCorp LP, College Station, TX, USA). All relevant data is included in anonymized form as a supplementary file [see Additional file 2].

Results

Descriptive statistics on providers who attended the training, providers who did not attend but who worked in treated hospitals, and providers working in control hospitals are presented in Table 1. The providers who took the training are not representative of the composition of providers attending deliveries, because the training attendees were not randomly selected.

Approximately 46% of the health providers who attended deliveries in the control hospitals were interns, whereas interns comprised only 10% of the providers attending the training. Most providers taking the training and attending deliveries were either general practitioners (66%) or obstetricians (20%). The proportion of treated providers who were obstetricians was very similar to the overall proportion of delivery-attending providers made up by obstetricians in the control hospitals. No treated residents attended deliveries, whereas 5.5% of the providers attending deliveries in control hospitals were residents. The proportion of treated providers who were nurses was quite low, but it was higher than the proportion of providers attending deliveries who were nurses in the control hospitals (4 vs. 1.2%).

We found that providers trained by PRONTO showed significant increases in the probability of performing the complete AMTSL (21 percentage point (p.p.) increase) and especially the first and third steps (28 and 29 p.p.

Table 1 Descriptive statistics on providers attending deliveries in studied hospitals

Variable	Number	Percent	Number	Percent	Number	Percent
Gender	Treated		Non-Treated		Controls	
Male	29	58.0	66	46.8	83	50.3
Female	21	42.0	61	43.3	61	37.0
missing	0	0.0	14	9.9	21	12.7
Total	50	100	141	100	165	100
Profession						
Interns	5	10.0	48	34.0	75	45.5
Social service practitioners	0	0.0	7	4.9	8	4.8
General Practitioners	33	66.0	55	39.0	32	19.4
Residents	0	0.0	8	5.7	9	5.5
Ob-Gyns	10	20.0	17	12.1	39	23.6
Nurses	2	4.0	5	3.6	2	1.2
missing	0	0.0	1	0.7	0	0.0
Total	50	100	141	100	165	100
Shift						
Morning	16	32.0	53	37.6	50	30.3
Afternoon	25	50.0	57	40.4	84	50.91
Night	8	16.0	28	19.9	29	17.6
missing	1	2.0	3	2.1	2	1.2
Total	50	100	141	100	165	100

increase, respectively), as well as skin-to-skin-contact (26 p.p. increase). We also found a negative and significant effect of the PRONTO training on the probability of performing uterine sweeping (26 p.p. decrease) (Table 2).

We found that non-trained providers working in treated hospitals (Table 3) also showed marked and significant changes in the same practices, except for uterine sweeping, and there was a significant impact on the performance of delayed cord clamping (15 p.p.). No significant changes in the performance of episiotomy or the Kristeller maneuver were found in any of the models. As expected, the effect on the treated providers was substantially larger, on average,

Table 2 Average treatment effect on treated[a] for probability of performing routine delivery practices among trained providers

Practice	N[c]	β	95% CI		p-value
Complete AMTSL[b]	48	0.21	0.06	0.35	0.005
1st step of AMTSL	48	0.28	0.09	0.46	0.003
2nd step of AMTSL	49	0.08	−0.04	0.20	0.198
3rd step of AMTSL	49	0.29	0.10	0.48	0.003
Skin-to-skin contact	49	0.26	0.14	0.38	< 0.001
Delayed cord clamping	24	0.21	−0.07	0.49	0.148
Episiotomy	49	−0.06	−0.27	0.16	0.592
Fundal pressure (Kristeller maneuver)	49	0.10	−0.04	0.23	0.157
Uterine sweeping	48	−0.26	−0.44	−0.08	0.004

[a]Impact estimates were obtained by Mahalanobis distance nearest-neighbor matching in terms of the following covariates: matched hospital pair, state, gender, work shift, and profession, with exact matching on time elapsed since the training
[b]AMTSL: active management of the third stage of labor
[c]Number of trained providers

Table 3 Average treatment effect on non-treated[a] for probability of performing routine delivery practices among untrained providers

Practice	N[c]	β	95% CI		p-value
Complete AMTSL[b]	118	0.20	0.08	0.32	0.001
1st step of AMTSL	124	0.21	0.07	0.36	0.005
2nd step of AMTSL	123	0.07	−0.03	0.17	0.160
3rd step of AMTSL	118	0.15	0.02	0.28	0.021
Skin-to-skin contact	124	0.10	0.03	0.17	0.004
Delayed cord clamping	50	0.15	0.02	0.28	0.027
Episiotomy	123	−0.04	−0.18	0.10	0.611
Fundal pressure (Kristeller maneuver)	123	−0.04	−0.13	0.05	0.363
Uterine sweeping	123	−0.08	−0.20	0.04	0.184

[a]Impact estimates were obtained by Mahalanobis distance nearest-neighbor matching in terms of the following covariates: matched hospital pair, state, gender, work shift, and profession, with exact matching on time elapsed since the training
[b]AMTSL: active management of the third stage of labor
[c]Number of untrained providers working in treated hospitals

than the effect on non-treated providers working in treated hospitals (Fig. 1).

Finally, we did not find evidence of a significant decay of the probability of performing any of the routine practices (or of an increase in the performance of harmful practices) over time among the treated providers. Most time trend coefficients indicated very close to zero change, except for two practices: uterine sweeping and 1st step of AMTSL, in which changes (non-significant) occurred in the expected direction (negative and positive respectively) (Table 4).

Discussion

In this study, we used a matching procedure to estimate the ATT impact of receiving the intervention (PRONTO training) on the probability of performing routine practices. This approach may allow us to estimate the effect of the intervention if all providers at the trained facilities had attended the program. In a previous impact evaluation of PRONTO, significant changes in the probability of routine practices being performed were found, but it was not known if these were diluted because of the relatively small fraction of eligible health providers who were trained or to what extent there was a spillover effect [16]. Our analysis concludes that the spillover effect is about 53% as large, on average, as the effect on the treated providers.

That no effect was observed for several of the practices, namely episiotomy and fundal pressure, reflects how deeply engrained these practices are in the culture of care and underscores the importance of interventions designed to impact the use of these practices earlier in the providers' careers, even during medical school. The results also suggest that the previously observed dilution of the effect of the intervention might be more related to the rotation of personnel than to providers returning

Table 4 Linear time trend of probability[a] of performing routine delivery practices among trained providers

Practice	N[c]	β[a]	95% CI		p-value
Complete AMTSL[b]	48	0.03	−0.18	0.24	0.768
1st step of AMTSL	48	0.15	−0.28	0.57	0.462
2nd step of AMTSL	49	0.00	(non estimable)		
3rd step of AMTSL	49	−0.09	−0.42	0.24	0.571
Skin-to-skin contact	49	0.00	(non estimable)		
Delayed cord clamping	24	−0.03	−0.33	0.27	0.835
Episiotomy	49	0.03	−0.36	0.42	0.872
Fundal pressure (Kristeller maneuver)	49	−0.06	−0.20	0.08	0.384
Uterine sweeping	48	−0.21	−0.47	0.06	0.120

[a]Fixed effects linear model with robust standard errors and clustering correction at the hospital level. □ coefficients are changes in probability per 4 elapsed months
[b]AMTSL: active management of the third stage of labor
[c]Number of trained providers working in treated hospitals

to their old habits. This suggestion is supported by more than 40% of deliveries being attended by interns, who only spend 2–4 months on the obstetrics rotation.

Several previous studies have estimated the treatment effects of a program evaluation approach associated with maternal health outcomes. Kaul et al. used propensity score matching to estimate ATT associated with deliveries at health care institutions for women in India [23]. Habibov et al. used probit models to estimate the effects of delivering in health care facilities on the probability of child survival, taking into account self-selection into the treatment, with nonrandomized data from a cross-sectional survey in Azerbaijan [24]. Wang et al. used propensity score matching to estimate the impact of health insurance status on the use of antenatal care and facility-based delivery care in eight countries of sub-Saharan Africa, West Asia, and South and Southeast Asia [25].

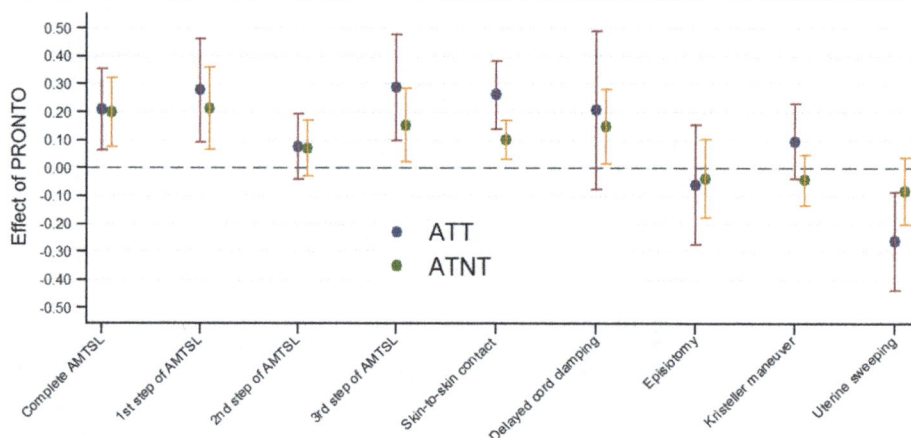

ATT: Average Treatment Effect on the Treated; ATNT: Average Treatment Effect on the Non-Treated
AMTSL: Active Management of the Third Step of Labor

Fig. 1 Average treatment effects for probability of performing routine delivery practices among providers in treated hospitals

Renfrew and colleagues established a comprehensive list of beneficial and harmful practices during intrapartum care [26]. Included in this list are those practices that can be easily addressed within the context of a simulation training program, such as PRONTO, with the primary focus of improving obstetric and neonatal emergency care. Harmful delivery practices in Mexico are likely contributing to the country's high rate of caesarean sections [2–4]. This may be because of a tendency to practice traditional authority-based medicine instead of applying new evidence-based practices [27].

A group of researchers who conducted a study in Latin America reported that, within institutions, interventions founded in evidence-based medicine were generally underused, while ineffective or even harmful practices continue to be used. This study showed that the intervention, carried out within a randomized trial and relying on a combination of practice and knowledge was significant in terms of changing delivery practices in favor of those based on evidence [15].

Several study limitations related to our analysis must be acknowledged. As the study was not originally designed to examine providers, we were only able to match on a limited number of available covariates. Data on provider gender was missing for a sizeable fraction of the original sample of observed deliveries. We were unable to identify gender in 12% of the original sample, although most of these providers were interns, who constituted only a small proportion of the treated providers. Gender was identified for 100% of the trained sample. In addition, the sample size of providers who actually received the training was quite small, which reduced the power of the study. Nonetheless, this sample size was large enough for us to detect significant effects for most of the indicators examined.

Conclusions

The analysis of the impact of PRONTO training on providers yields new insights on the true efficacy of this approach and, through comparing the estimated effect on the treated vs. that on the non-treated providers, the extent to which knowledge and abilities acquired through this training are disseminated within hospitals. It also further highlights the importance of continuous, ongoing training to counter the dilution effect, which is probably caused by the rotation of personnel within health institutions in Mexico, to ensure the provision of quality maternal and newborn care.

Abbreviations

AMTSL: active management of the third stage of labor; ATE: average treatment effect; ATT: average treatment on the treated; DCC: delayed cord clamping; p.p.: percentage points; PRONTO: Programa de Rescate Obstétrico y Neonatal: Tratamiento Óptimo y Oportuno; SSC: skin-to-skin contact; WHO: World Health Organization

Acknowledgements

We would like to acknowledge the Secretaries of Health in the states of Chiapas, Mexico, and Guerrero for logistical and organizational support for the study and for providing observer access. We extend a special acknowledgement to INMUJERES for their financial and political support of this project. The authors would also like to make a special acknowledgement to the MEASURE Evaluation project for their invaluable support.

Funding

The funder for this project was the Mexican National Institute of Women (Instituto Nacional de las Mujeres, INMUJERES), under agreement number 274, with additional funding from the Bill and Melinda Gates Foundation. The funders had no input in the design, implementation, or evaluation of this trial.

Authors' contributions

JF contributed substantially to the conception, design, implementation, analysis, interpretation of results, and drafting of this article. HLF contributed substantially to the design, analysis, interpretation of results, and drafting of this article. GA contributed to the analysis, interpretation of results, and drafting of this article. AM contributed to the analysis, interpretation of results, and drafting of this article. DW contributed substantially to the conception, design, implementation, and interpretation of results presented in this article. All authors have read and approved the final version of this manuscript

Competing interests

Dilys Walker is on the board of PRONTO International, a nongovernmental organization that offers PRONTO training courses. The other authors declare that they have no competing interests.

Author details

[1]Division of Reproductive Health, Research Center for Population Health, National Institute of Public Health (INSP), Av. Universidad 655, Col. Santa María Ahuacatitlán, 62100 Cuernavaca, Morelos, Mexico. [2]Department of Maternal and Child Health, University of North Carolina at Chapel Hill (UNC), Chapel Hill, North Carolina, USA. [3]Department of Obstetrics, Gynecology and Reproductive Sciences, Bixby Center for Global Reproductive Health, University of California in San Francisco, (UCSF), San Francisco, California, USA.

References

1. Deliver W. Focus on 5: Women's health and the MDGs. United Nations Population Fund. 2009; https://www.unfpa.org/sites/default/files/pub-pdf/Focus-on-5.pdf. Accessed 4 Jan 2017
2. Sachse-Aguilera M, Sesia PM, García-Rojas M. Calidad de la atención durante el parto normal en establecimientos públicos de salud en el estado de Oaxaca. Revista de Investigación Médica de Oaxaca. 2013;1(1):17–36.
3. Valdez Santiago R, Hidalgo Solórzano E, Mojarro Iñiguez M, Arenas Monreal LM. Nueva evidencia a un viejo problema: el abuso de las mujeres en las salas de parto. Revista CONAMED. 2013;18(1):14–20.
4. Walker D, DeMaria LM, Suarez L, Cragin L. Skilled birth attendants in Mexico: how does care during normal birth by general physicians, obstetric nurses, and professional midwives compare with World Health Organization evidence-based practice guidelines? J Midwifery Womens Health. 2012; 57(1):18–27.
5. Consejo C, Viesca-Treviño C. Ética y relaciones de poder en la formación de médicos residentes e internos: algunas reflexiones a la luz de Foucault y Bourdieu. Bol Mex His Fil Med. 2008;11(1):16–20.

6.   Gutiérrez-Alba G, González-Block MA, Reyes-Morales H. Desafíos en la implantación de guías de práctica clínica en instituciones públicas de México: estudio de casos múltiple. Salud Publica Mex. 2015;57:547–54.

7.   Walker D, Cohen S, Estrada-Márquez F, Sosa-Rubí SG. PRONTO Programa de Rescate Obstétrico y Neonatal: tratamiento óptimo y oportuno. Ensayo aleatorizado para una evaluación de impacto. Protocolo del proyecto de investigación. Instituto Nacional de Salud Pública: Cuernavaca, México; 2009.

8.   Gutierrez JP, Rivera-Dommarco J, Shamah-Levy T, Villalpando-Hernandez S, Franco A, Cuevas-Nasu L, et al. Encuesta Nacional de Salud y Nutricion 2012. In: Resultados nacionales. Cuernavaca, Mexico: Instituto Nacional de Salud Publica (MX); 2012.

9.   Hamman WR. The complexity of team training: what we have learned from aviation and its applications to medicine. Qual Saf Health Care 2004; 13(Supplement 1):i72–i79; https://doi.org/10.1136/qshc.2004.009910.

10. Mathai M, Sanghvi H, Guidotti RJ. Managing complications in pregnancy and childbirth: a guide for midwives and doctors. Geneva: Reproductive Health and Research, World Health Organization; 2000.

11. Graham WJ, Filippi VG, Ronsmans C. Demonstrating programme impact on maternal mortality. Health Policy Plann. 1996;11(1):16–20.

12. Hussein J, Clapham S. Message in a bottle: sinking in a sea of safe motherhood concepts. Health Policy. 2005;73:294–302.

13. Frenk J, Chen L, Bhutta ZA, Cohen J, Crisp N, Evans T, et al. Health professionals for a new century: transforming education to strengthen heath systems in an interdependent world. Lancet. 2010;10:61854–5.

14. Dumont A, Fournier P, Abrahamowicz M, Fraser WD, Beaudoin F, Haddad S, et al. Quality of care, risk management, and technology in obstetrics to reduce hospital-based maternal mortality in Senegal and Mali (QUARITE): a cluster-randomised trial. Lancet. 2013;382:146–57.

15. Althabe F, Buekens P, Bergel E, Belizán JM, Campbell MK, Moss N, et al. A behavioral intervention to improve obstetrical care. New Engl J Med. 2008; 358(18):1929–40.

16. Fritz J, Walker D, Cohen S, Angeles G, Lamadrid-Figueroa H. Can a simulation-based training program impact the use of evidence based routine practices at birth? Results of a hospital-based controlled trial in Mexico. PLoS One. 12(3): e0172623. https://doi.org/10.1371/journal.pone.0172623.

17. Walker DM, Cohen SR, Estrada F, Monterroso ME, Jenny A, Fritz J, et al. PRONTO training for obstetric and neonatal emergencies in Mexico. Int J Gynaecol Obstet. 2012;116(2):128.

18. Walker DM, Cohen SR, Fritz J, Olvera-García M, Zelek ST, Fahey JO, et al. Impact evaluation of PRONTO Mexico: a simulation-based program in obstetric and neonatal emergencies and team training. Simul Healthc 2016; 11(1):1–9.

19. Reif J. STRGROUP: Stata module to match strings based on their Levenshtein edit distance. Stat Softw Components. 2012. https://ideas.repec. org/c/boc/bocode/s457151.html. Accessed 4 Jan 2017.

20. Levenshtein distance. In. Black PE, editor. Dictionary of algorithms and data structures. U.S. In: National Institute of Standards and Technology; 2008. https://xlinux.nist.gov/dads/HTML/Levenshtein.html. Accessed 4 Jan 2017.

21. Wang A, Nianogo RA, Arah OA. G-computation of average treatment effects on the treated and the untreated. BMC Med Res Methodol. 2017 Jan 9; 17(1):3.

22. Abadie A, Imbens GW. Large sample properties of matching estimators for average treatment effects. Econometrica. 2006;74:235–67.

23. Kaul S, You W, Boyle KJ. Delivery at home versus delivery at a health care facility – a case study of Bihar, India. Paper presented at the Agricultural & Applied Economics Association's 2012 Annual meeting, Seattle, Washington, August 12–14, 2012.

24. Habibov N, Fan L. The effect of maternal healthcare on the probability of child survival in Azerbaijan. Biomed Res Int. 2014;2014:1–7.

25. Wang W, Temsah G, Mallick L. Health insurance coverage and its impact on maternal health care utilization in low- and middle-income countries. DHS Analytical Studies No. 45. Rockville: ICF International; 2014.

26. Renfrew MJ, McFadden A, Bastos MH, Campbell J, Channon A, Cheung N, et al. Midwifery and quality care: findings from a new evidence-informed framework for maternal and newborn care. Lancet. 2014; https://doi.org/10. 1016/S0140-6736(14)60789-3.

27. Faveau V, Bernis L. 'Good obstetrics' revisited: too many evidence-based practices and devices are not used. Int J Gynaecol Obstet. 2006;94:179–84.

15

Are women with history of pre-eclampsia starting a new pregnancy in good nutritional status in South Africa and Zimbabwe?

Gabriela Cormick[1,2]*, Ana Pilar Betrán[3], Janetta Harbron[2], Tina Dannemann Purnat[4], Catherine Parker[5,6,7], David Hall[8], Armando H. Seuc[9], James M. Roberts[10], José M. Belizán[1], G. Justus Hofmeyr[5,6,7] and on behalf of the Calcium and Pre-eclampsia Study Group

Abstract

Background: Maternal nutritional status before and during pregnancy is an important contributor to pregnancy outcomes and early child health. The aim of this study was to describe the preconceptional nutritional status and dietary intake during pregnancy in high-risk women from South Africa and Zimbabwe.

Methods: This is a prospective observational study, nested to the CAP trial. Anthropometric measurements before and during pregnancy and dietary intake using 24-h recall during pregnancy were assessed. The Intake Distribution Estimation software (PC-SIDE) was used to evaluate nutrient intake adequacy taking the Estimated Average Requirement (EAR) as a cut-off point.

Results: Three hundred twelve women who had pre-eclampsia in their last pregnancy and delivered in hospitals from South Africa and Zimbabwe were assessed. 73.7 and 60.2% women in South Africa and Zimbabwe, respectively started their pregnancy with BMI above normal (BMI ≥ 25) whereas the prevalence of underweight was virtually non-existent. The majority of women had inadequate intakes of micronutrients. Considering food and beverage intake only, none of the micronutrients measured achieved the estimated average requirement. Around 60% of pregnant women reported taking folic acid or iron supplements in South Africa, but almost none did so in Zimbabwe.

Conclusion: We found a high prevalence of overweight and obesity and high micronutrient intake inadequacy in pregnant women who had the previous pregnancy complicated with pre-eclampsia. The obesity figures and micronutrient inadequacy are issues of concern that need to be addressed. Pregnant women have regular contacts with the health system; these opportunities could be used to improve diet and nutrition.

Keywords: Nutrient intake, Weight, Pregnancy, Supplement, Obesity, BMI

* Correspondence: gabmick@yahoo.co.uk
[1]Instituto de Efectividad Clínica y Sanitaria (IECS-CONICET), Emilio Ravignani, 2024 Buenos Aires, Argentina
[2]Division of Human Nutrition, Department of Human Biology, Faculty of Health Sciences, University of Cape Town, Cape Town, South Africa
Full list of author information is available at the end of the article

Background

Nutrition status of women before and during pregnancy is one of the main contributors to pregnancy outcomes and early child health [1]. In many low and middle-income countries undernutrition and overnutrition coexist in the same population [2]. Obesity is increasing while micronutrient deficiencies still persist, particularly in the most vulnerable groups such as women and children [3]. Consequently, women start pregnancy with higher risks to develop complications such as pre-eclampsia, gestational diabetes mellitus, gestational hypertension, depression, fetal macrosomia, stillbirth, preterm birth, birth by caesarean section and infant mortality [4–9]. In addition, high maternal body mass index (BMI) has also been associated with delayed breastfeeding, weight retention and in women with gestational diabetes, a higher risk of developing chronic diseases [5]. Inter-pregnancy interval is also an important factor that may influence maternal availability of nutrients, especially in those populations with existing micronutrient deficiencies [10].

Interest in pre-conceptional interventions to reduce risk factors during pregnancy is growing, although their effectiveness on pregnancy outcomes is less certain [11]. Current WHO Guidelines on antenatal care recommend supplementation with iron and folic acid to all pregnant women, and with calcium and vitamin A to women in specific areas with a high prevalence of deficiency [12]. In populations where calcium intake is low, the WHO recommends supplementation with 1.5–2.0 g elemental calcium/day from 20 weeks´ gestation until the end of pregnancy for the prevention of pre-eclampsia. The WHO Guidelines also report that women receiving counselling on diet and/or exercise are less likely to experience excess weight gain during pregnancy, although the evidence on the impact of other pregnancy outcomes is less certain [12].

In South Africa, the National Health and Nutrition Examination Survey (SANHANES-1) reported a prevalence of overweight (BMI ≥ 25 kg/m2) and obesity (BMI ≥ 30) in women of 24.8 and 39.2%, respectively in 2012 [13]. Data from Zimbabwe in 2000 shows a prevalence of overweight and obesity in women of 17.4 and 5.7% respectively [14]. However information on overweight and obesity rates as well as dietary intake during pregnancy is scarce in these countries. Nutrient and supplement intake information would be important to better plan and tailor interventions to improve pregnancy outcomes [10].

We conducted a randomized controlled trial to evaluate the effect of pre-pregnancy calcium supplementation on the incidence of recurrent pre-eclampsia (Calcium and Pre-eclampsia: CAP trial) [15]. This was a multi-country trial conducted in South Africa, Zimbabwe and Argentina. This manuscript presents the results of a sub-analysis of the CAP trial with the aim of describing the nutritional status of women from South Africa and Zimbabwe that became pregnant during the CAP trial. More specifically, we aimed to describe levels of overweight and obesity before and during pregnancy, and the adequacy of macronutrient and micronutrient intake during pregnancy.

Participants and methods

This is a nested prospective observational study of women from South Africa and Zimbabwe recruited in the CAP trial [15]. The CAP trial is a multi-centre randomized, double-blind placebo-controlled clinical trial with the objective to determine whether calcium supplementation before conception and during the first half of pregnancy reduces the incidence of recurrent pre-eclampsia more effectively than supplementation starting at 20 weeks, which is the current WHO recommendation. In the CAP trial, non-pregnant women with history of pre-eclampsia or eclampsia in their most recent pregnancy were invited to participate as they are at higher risk of developing pre-eclampsia in subsequent pregnancies. Once admitted in the trial, participants were required to attend study sites every 12 weeks for follow up until pregnancy occurred. Pregnant women were followed up throughout their pregnancy and trial visits were scheduled at 8, 20 and 32 weeks´ gestation. Eligible women were randomized to receive either 500 mg of elemental calcium daily or placebo from recruitment and blinded supplementation continued while participants were non-pregnant or until 20 weeks' gestation. From 20 weeks' gestation, all participants received calcium supplements in compliance with WHO guidelines [16]. The CAP trial started in 2011 and recruitment was completed in September 2016.

Settings and study population

Participants were recruited from government secondary or tertiary urban referral hospitals with large obstetric units serving urban and rural populations. The maternity and obstetric units included in the CAP trial were located in Cape Town (1), East London (2) and Johannesburg (1) in South Africa; and in Harare (2), Zimbabwe. Women were eligible for the CAP trial if they had pre-eclampsia or eclampsia in their most recent pregnancy, if they were not pregnant but in a sexual relationship, not using contraception and if they gave informed consent. For admission we reviewed the participant clinical records and accepted the clinical evaluation of pre-eclampsia or eclampsia reported there. Exclusion criteria included: less than 18 years of age; chronic hypertension with persistent proteinuria; calcium supplement intake; and history or symptoms of urolithiasis, renal disease or parathyroid disease [15]. For a complete list of eligible criteria please refer to the published protocol [15]. In this analysis, we included women recruited in the CAP trial who became pregnant and reached 20 weeks´ gestation between March 2013 to March 2016.

Anthropometric assessment and clinical data collection

Variables used for this sub-study included: age, height, pre-pregnancy weight, number of previous pregnancies and date of birth of last pregnancy complicated with pre-eclampsia. This data were collected at admission. For women who became pregnant, weight during pregnancy was recorded at 8, 20 and 32 weeks´ gestation during the scheduled trial follow-up visits. Research nurses specially trained for the CAP trial assessed all anthropometric, clinical and dietary variables at admission and during follow up visits at each participating site.

Body weight was measured to the nearest 0.1 kg in light clothing and without shoes. Height was measured to the nearest 0.1 cm and without shoes using a stadiometer. Scales and stadiometers were those provided by each hospital and remained the same throughout the study. The Manual of Operations and the Standard Operating Procedures (SOPs) provided clear instructions on how women should be weighted and measured.

Pre-pregnancy BMI was calculated as weight (kg) divided by the square of the body height (m) using measurements recorded at admission. Women were classified according to the WHO BMI standards for adults, defined as underweight (BMI < 18.5), normal (18.5 ≤ BMI < 25), overweight (BMI ≥ 25), or obese (BMI ≥ 30) [17].

Gestational weight gain was calculated by subtracting the weight at 8 weeks´ gestation from the weight at 32 weeks´ gestation, since the participant's weight at delivery was not assessed.

Dietary assessment

The dietary intake of participants was assessed at 20-weeks' gestation using a triple pass 24-h dietary recall adapted from the method developed by Nelson M. team from the King's College London after it was piloted in South Africa and Zimbabwe [18]. The 24-h recall is a guided interview to assess food intake of the previous day. CAP trial research nurses were trained in-site in March 2013 to administer the triple pass 24-h recalls and to use the Dietary Assessment Education Kit (DAEK) to assist with the portion size estimation [19]. Xhosa and Zulu translators were trained at the sites that required them.

Reported food intakes from the 24-h recall were entered and analysed using the Food Finder III computer program, provided by the South African medical research council (SAMRC) to obtain daily energy and nutrient intakes for each participant. If properly conducted, a single day 24-h dietary recall is a reliable method to assess individual intake on one day and can be used to estimate a population mean [20]. However, as food and nutrient intakes have a wide day-to-day variability, data obtained from one single day is not sufficient to describe the usual intake or to assess the proportion of individuals with intakes below certain thresholds (e.g. below requirements). Statistical models have been developed to better estimate usual nutrient intakes in a population by adjusting for within-individual intake variability [21]. Therefore, in order to estimate the proportion of women with intakes below requirements we used the Intake Distribution Estimation software (PC-SIDE, version 1.0, 2003; Department of Statistics, Iowa State University, Ames) that requires a sample of at least 50 dietary assessments that are repeated on a non-consecutive day to the first assessment [22]. For these purposes, a second 24-h dietary recall assessment was administered in a subsample of women on a non-consecutive day after the first 24-h recall. Energy and nutrient intake distributions from the single 24-h recall were thus adjusted by within-person variance obtained from the second 24-h recall assessment and by interview weekday to estimate usual nutrient intake and to calculate the proportion of women with intakes below requirements.

The Estimated Average Requirement (EAR) of carbohydrates and each micronutrient as recommended by the Institute of Medicine (IOM) for pregnant women was used as the cut-off point to assess adequacy of nutrient intake [23]. The Estimated Energy Requirement (EER) for pregnant women during the second trimester was calculated for each participant using the age, weight and height at admission and according to the Dietary Reference Intake (DRI) formula for adult women [23]. As data of physical activity was not collected the value for sedentary lifestyle was used conservatively. Energy intake obtained from the first 24-h recall assessment was divided by the EER then normalized using PC-SIDE [23, 24]. The 80% of EER during pregnancy suggested by Goldberg was used to calculate the plausibility of energy intake [25]. Protein adequacy was calculated using the EAR of 0.88 g per kg of body weight, using weight at 20 weeks´ gestation [23].

A specific questionnaire was also included to investigate supplement intake during pregnancy. Women were asked about frequency and dose of the supplements and medicines. Trial supplementation was not computed in the dietary assessment of this sub-study as it was the intervention being tested and not, otherwise, part of the diet of this group of women.

Statistical analysis

Categorical values were described using percentages and numerical variables using means and standard deviations (SD). Statistical data analyses were performed using the SPSS 23.0 software package (IBM, New York, NY, USA). Dietary intake variables were log transformed and tested for normality using the Anderson-Darling statistical test using the PC-SIDE software. The software performs three steps: adjustments for weekday; transformation to normality using power transformation; and estimation of within-person variance using an error measurement model.

Ethics

Ethical approval was obtained from appropriate national and institutional ethics review bodies as applicable for each study site, and all participants provided informed written consent. The study was approved by the Research Project Review Panel of the UNDP/UNFPA/UNICEF/WHO/World Bank Special Programme of Research, Development and Research Training in Human Reproduction at the Department of Reproductive Health and Research of WHO, and the WHO Research Ethics Review Committee, Geneva, Switzerland.

Data management procedures were compliant with good clinical practice (GCP) [26].

Results

A total of 2187 women were screened in South Africa and Zimbabwe during the sub-study period (March 2013 to March 2016) and 1101 (50.3%) were eligible and accepted to participate (Fig. 1). Of the 1101 participants randomized, 541 (49.1%) became pregnant of whom, 55 (10.0%) had a miscarriage or a pregnancy termination

before 20 weeks' gestation, 34 did not attend to the pregnancy visit at 20 weeks' gestation, and 102 (18.8%) completed the visits at 20 weeks' gestation outside the sub-study period. A total of 350 women were eligible for this sub-study, however 38 (10.8%) missed the dietary assessment interview. Thus, we present the results of 312 women that completed the dietary assessment at the 20 weeks' gestation visit. Of these women 224 (71.8%) were from South Africa and 88 (28.2%) from Zimbabwe. Repeated dietary assessments were obtained from 107 (34.3%) women, 79 from South Africa and 28 from Zimbabwe.

At the time of the assessment, women from South Africa had been in the study an average of 12.5 (SD ±7.4) months and women from Zimbabwe 13.1 (SD ±7.4) months. Their inter-pregnancy interval was 24.5 (SD ± 22.5) months in South Africa and 30.3 (SD ±23.7) months in Zimbabwe (Table 1).

Clinical characteristics

At recruitment, the mean age of women in this sub-study was 29.2 years (SD ± 5.2) in South Africa and 29.3 (SD ± 4.8) in Zimbabwe. Parity was three or more in about 25% of the women (22.8 and 31.8% in South Africa and Zimbabwe, respectively). The mean height was 159.9 cm (SD ±6.4) in South Africa and 161.1 cm (SD ±6.4) in Zimbabwe; and the mean weight before

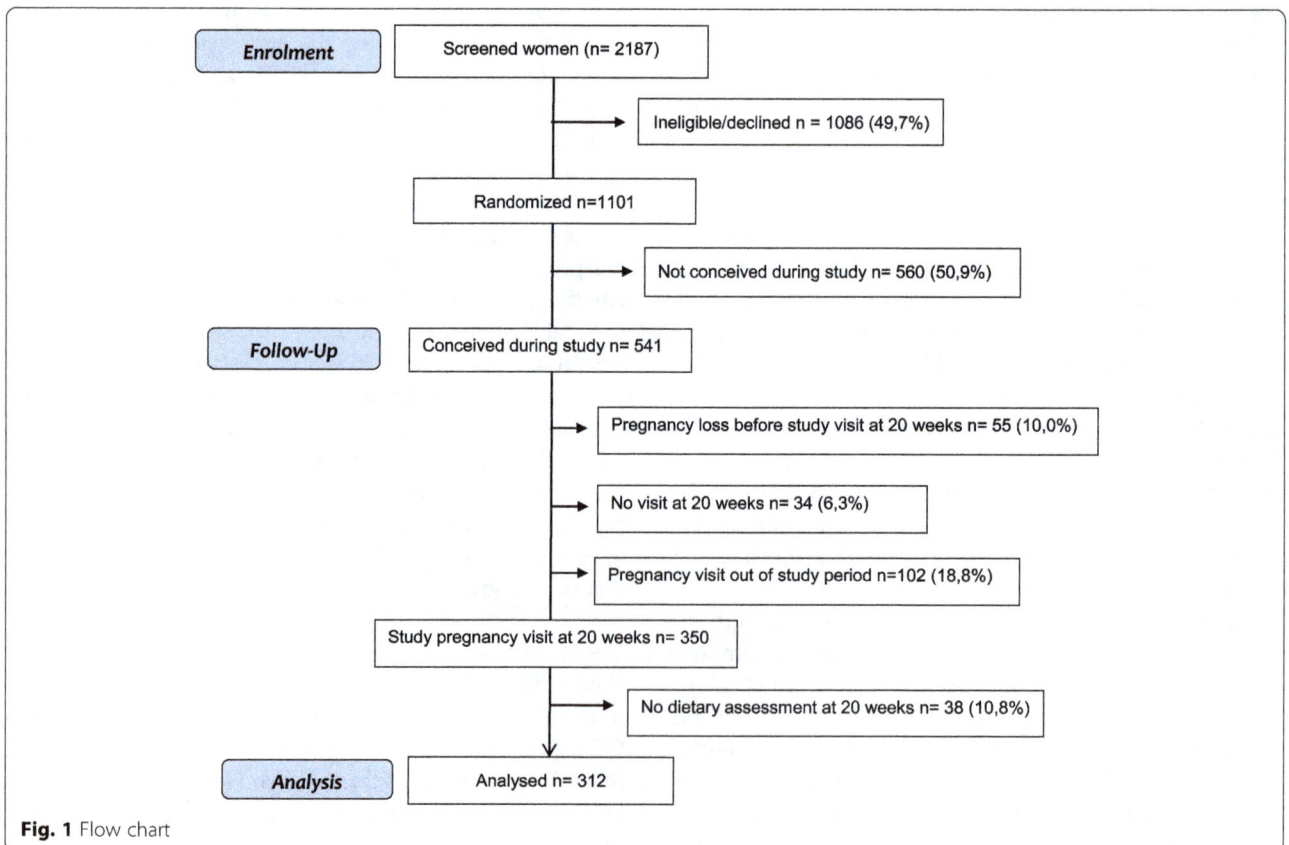

Fig. 1 Flow chart

Table 1 Participant Characteristics

	All		South Africa		Zimbabwe	
	n = 312	%	n = 224	%	n = 88	%
Age (years)						
Less than 20	1	0.3	0	0	1	1.1
20 to less than 35	255	81.7	182	81.3	73	83
35 and older	56	17.9	42	18.8	14	17.9
Parity						
1	121	38.8	93	41.5	28	31.8
2	111	35.6	79	35.3	32	36.4
3 or more	79	25.3	51	22.8	28	31.8
Missing	1	0.3	1	0.4	0	0
Months in study from admission to 20 weeks' gestation						
Mean (sd)	312	12.5 (7.4)	224	13.1 (7.4)	88	11.0 (7.4)
Less than 6 month	94	30.1	60	26.8	34	38.6
6 to less than 12 month	88	28.2	59	26.3	29	33.0
12 to less than 24 month	97	31.1	79	35.3	18	20.5
24 or more month	32	10.3	25	11.2	7	8.0
Missing	1	0.3	1	0.4	0	0
Months since last birth with PE to 20 weeks' gestation						
Mean (sd)	312	24.5 (22.5)	224	30.3 (23.7)	88	27.4 (19.0)
Less than 6 month	9	2.9	7	3.1	2	2.3
6 to less than 12 month	54	17.3	39	17.4	15	17.0
12 to less than 24 month	94	30.1	62	27.7	32	36.4
24 or more month	135	43.3	102	45.5	33	37.5
Missing	20	6.4	14	6.3	6	6.8
Anthropometric variables						
Height at admission - mean (sd)	286	160.3 (6.4)	202	159.9 (6.4)	84	161.1 (6.4)
Weight at admission - mean (sd)	302	76.1 (17.4)	217	78.9 (18.2)	85	69.0 (12.6)
Weight at week 8 of gestation - mean (sd)	251	77.1 (16.9)	173	80.2 (17.7)	78	70.2 (12.4)
Weight at week 20 of gestation - mean (sd)	300	80.2 (17.5)	215	83.5 (18.1)	85	71.9 (12.6)
Weight at week 32 of gestation - mean (sd)	224	84.0 (17.0)	158	88.2 (17.5)	66	74.0 (10.1)
Mean BMI at admission - mean (sd)	283	29.6 (6.3)	201	30.7 (6.6)	82	26.8 (4.5)
Body Mass Index at admission						
Underweight (BMI < 18.5 kg/m2)	3	1.0	2	0.9	1	1.1
Normal (18.5 BMI < 25 kg/m2)	62	19.9	34	15.2	28	31.8
Overweight (25 BMI < 30 kg/m2)	95	30.4	62	27.7	33	37.5
Obesity I (30 BMI 35 kg/m2)	75	24.0	58	25.9	17	19.3
Obesity II (35 BMI 40 kg/m2)	32	10.3	30	13.4	2	2.3
Obesity III (BMI > 40 kg/m2)	16	5.1	15	6.7	1	1.1
Missing	29	9.3	23	10.3	6	6.8

pregnancy was 78.9 kg (SD ±18.2) in South Africa and 69.0 kg (SD ±12.6) in Zimbabwe. The prevalence of overweight was 27.7% in South Africa and 37.5% in Zimbabwe while the prevalence of any degree of obesity was 46.0% in South Africa and 22.7% in Zimbabwe (Table 1). In total, 73.7 and 60.2% women in South Africa and Zimbabwe, respectively entered the trial with BMI above normal. On the other hand, the prevalence of underweight was virtually non-existent in both countries.

Gestational weight gain

We found that women who were initially classified according to their BMI as normal weight had gained from 8 to 32 weeks' gestation an average 8.9 kg (SD ± 4.4) in South Africa and 7.4 kg (SD ± 3.3) in Zimbabwe. Those classified as overweight had gained 7.8 kg (SD ± 4.5) in South Africa and 5.8 kg (SD ±3.8) in Zimbabwe and those classified as obese had gained 5.9 kg (SD ± 6.2) in South Africa and 3.1 kg (SD ± 4.1) in Zimbabwe.

Diet

Macronutrients

The average total daily energy intake was 1765.6 kcal (SD ±346.6) in South Africa and 1827.9 (SD ±303.9) in Zimbabwe. Average daily carbohydrate, fat and protein intakes were 230.8 (SD ± 57.5) grams, 59.1 (SD ± 6.4) grams and 54.7 (SD ±7.8) grams in South Africa and 213.6 (SD ± 22.3) grams, 76.4 (SD ± 24.8) grams and 52.9 (SD ± 25.8) grams in Zimbabwe, respectively (Table 2). Most (54.4%) of total energy intake came from carbohydrates, 27.8% from fats and 12.6% from proteins in South Africa while the percentages in Zimbabwe were 48.0, 36.38 and 11.26% respectively.

Average daily intake of total sugars was 45.6 (SD ± 40.9) grams in South Africa and 34.5 (SD ±26.0) grams in Zimbabwe representing 10.6 and 7.5% of the total energy intake. The majority of women in both countries had lower than recommended protein intake and a higher intake of carbohydrates (Table 2).

Micronutrients

Adjusted usual nutrient intakes (from food and beverage, excluding supplements) are presented in Table 2. Micronutrient inadequacy was highly prevalent in both countries. Almost all women in South Africa had inadequate intakes of folate, calcium, iron and selenium, while the majority also had inadequate intakes of magnesium, zinc, niacin and vitamin E. More than half of the women had inadequate intakes of riboflavin while less than half had inadequate intake of vitamin C. All women in Zimbabwe had inadequate dietary intakes of iron and folate; the majority also had inadequate intakes of calcium, magnesium, zinc, selenium and riboflavin. The intake of vitamin C and E was however, adequate in the majority of women from Zimbabwe. (Table 2).

Supplements

In South Africa, 62.9% of women (141) reported taking 5 mg of folic acid supplements, 57.1% (128) reported taking iron supplements with doses ranging between 75 to 400 mg; 24.1% (54) reported taking vitamin C with doses ranging between 100 to 250 mg daily and 9.8%

Table 2 Usual intake from foods and beverages, excluding supplements, estimated using repeated 24-h recalls in 312 women and repeated in a sub-sample of 107 women, and percentage of women with usual intake below Estimated Average Requirement (EAR)

Estimated Daily Usual Intake[b]	South Africa	Zimbabwe	EAR[a]	% women with intakes below EAR	
	n = 224	n = 88		South Africa	Zimbabwe
Energy (kcal)	1765.6 (346.6)	1827.9 (303.9)	NA[c]	NA	NA
EER Estimated Energy Requirement (%)	0.88 (0.20)	0.93 (0.14)	0.8	37.7	19.1
Protein (g)	54.7 (7.8)	52.9 (25.8) [d]	NA	NA	NA
Protein (g/kg)	0.82 (0.43)	0.79 (0.04)	0.88	71.1	98.3
Carbohydrates (g)	230.8 (57.5)	213.6 (22.3)	135	02.9	0.00
Total Sugars (g)	45.4 (19.4)	35.4 (10.7)	NA	NA	NA
Fats (g)	59.1 (6.4)	76.4 (24.8)	NA	NA	NA
Calcium (mg)	441.0 (97.7)	360.5 (171.4)	800	99.9	97.6
Iron (mg)	9.9 (5.3)	7.9 (1.7)	22	96.9	100.0
Folate (mcg)	253.2 (69.1)	240.6 (46.2)	520	99.9	100.0
Mg (mg)	239.6 (51.1)	262.5 (38.8)	290	83.9	77.3
Zn (mg)	7.3 (1.7)	6.4 (1.6)	9.5	90.4	95.7
Se (mcg)	37.9 (4.3)	37.5 (11.8)	49	99.1	83.7
Riboflavin (mg)	1.3 (0.6)	0.8 (0.5)	1.2	54.0	84.0
Niacin (mg)	13.0 (3.8)	13.0 (3.7)	14	63.8	64.9
Vitamin C (mg)	82.4 (45.1)	109.80 (41.8)	70	46.6	15.6
Vitamin E (mg)	10.1 (3.8)	26.4 (9.1)	12	73.5	03.7

[a]EAR Estimated average requirement
[b]Usual intake was obtained using the IOWA methodology
[c]NA not applicable)
[d]This value represents the mean of the first interview

(22) reported taking vitamin B complex. At 20 weeks of pregnancy, women reported taking these supplements for a mean period of 2.1 to 2.7 months. Other supplements reported include calcium gluconate, magnesium sulphate and copper sulphate. Most of the supplements were provided by the hospital. On the other hand, a total of 29 (12.9%) women reported taking multivitamins for a mean period of 1 to 2 months, which are not provided by the hospitals.

In Zimbabwe, only one woman reported taking iron supplements during pregnancy. No other types of supplements intake were reported what so ever.

Discussion

This study shows that a high proportion of women whose previous pregnancy was complicated by pre-eclampsia in hospitals from South Africa and Zimbabwe started their subsequent pregnancy overweight or obese (73.7% in South Africa and 60.2% in Zimbabwe). In fact, obesity affected about 1 in 4 women in Zimbabwe, and as many as 1 in 2 women in South Africa were obese. Furthermore, at 20 weeks' gestation more than 90% of these women had intakes of micronutrients, like iron, calcium, folate and zinc below requirements.

Overweight and obesity problems have already been reported in these countries. The prevalence of overweight or obese women found in our study is higher than the 64% that has been reported for South Africa by the SANHANES-1 and the 54.9 and 25% that the WHO Global Database on Body Mass Index reports for South Africa in 2004 and Zimbabwe in 2006 respectively, but in line with other studies conducted in South Africa that reported 69% [27–29]. The fact that we only included women who had a previous pregnancy complicated with pre-eclampsia could contribute to the higher overweight or obesity prevalence in our study population [14, 15]. A link between obesity and hypertensive disorders of pregnancy has been reported in the literature. A systematic review concluded that for every 5 to 7 kg/m^2 increase in BMI, the risk of developing pre-eclampsia doubles which confirms the relevance and critical importance of developing and implementing special efforts to control the BMI of these women before they become pregnant [30].

We found that women with normal BMIs' at 8 weeks' gestation, compared to those with higher BMI, gained more weight at 32 weeks, which is in accordance to recommendations [31]. However, as we only assessed weight up to 32 weeks' gestation and most gestational weight gain occurs after 20 weeks' gestation, we would expect that many of these women would exceed the Institute of Medicine recommendations. In our study, women classified as normal weight gained from 8 to 32 weeks' gestation an average 8.9 kg (SD ± 4.4) in South Africa and 7.4 kg (SD ± 3.3) in Zimbabwe of the 11.5 to 16 kg recommended for this group. Those classified as overweight gained 7.8 kg (SD ± 4.5) in South Africa and 5.8 kg (SD ±3.8) in Zimbabwe of the 7 to 11.5 kg recommended for this group and those classified as obese gained 5.9 kg (SD ± 6.2) in South Africa and 3.1 kg (SD ± 4.1) in Zimbabwe of the 5 to 9 kg recommended for this group [12]. Programmes and interventions to reduce obesity before pregnancy and control weight gain during pregnancy would be advisable in view of the findings of this analysis.

The energy intake we report is similar to those reported for women in the US National Health and Nutrition Survey in 2010–2011 where the prevalence of overweight and obesity are also higher than 70% [32, 33]. According to Goldberg, if the estimated usual intake is below 80% of the estimated average requirement for a person, this would imply under-reporting. In our study this would imply 37.7% of underreporting in South Africa and 19.1% in Zimbabwe [25]. Fat intake as a percentage of total energy was within the recommended range of 20 to 35% of total energy in South Africa (27.8%), but slightly higher than recommended in Zimbabwe (36.4%). The high fat intake in Zimbabwe was due to a higher intake of polyunsaturated fats. In both countries, carbohydrates and protein intake as a percentage of total energy were within the recommended ranges of 46–65% and 10–35% respectively [23]. However, the intake of sugar in South Africa was slightly above the recommended maximum of 10% of total energy. Considering recommended grams of macronutrients, the women from both countries had mostly adequate total grams of carbohydrate intakes, but the majority had inadequate grams per kilograms of protein intake. It is thus important that interventions should focus on increasing the intake of affordable protein sources and decreasing sugar intake.

The prevalence of inadequate micronutrient intake from food sources was high in both countries. For the most basic micronutrients like iron, calcium, folate and zinc, the percentage of women below requirements was above 90% in both countries. The most common supplements taken in South Africa were folic acid, ferrous sulphate, and vitamin C, all issued by the hospital. There is a policy in South Africa to supplement pregnant women with 5 mg of folic acid and 200 mg of ferrous sulphate (equivalent to 40 mg elemental iron) daily, which allowed those women taking the supplements to reach the recommendations [34, 35]. The elemental iron supplementation provided by this policy is in accordance with the WHO guidelines for antenatal care, however folic acid supplementation is more than 10 times the recommended amount [12]. On the other hand, vitamin C is not recommended, as there is no evidence of an impact on birth outcomes. In contrast, only one woman in Zimbabwe reported taking supplements and this may be due to the fact that there is no policy to provide supplements during pregnancy in Zimbabwe and very few women bought commercial supplements. The inadequate intakes are worrying as iron and folic acid supplementation are known to prevent anaemia, puerperal sepsis, low birth weight and preterm birth; folate to prevent neural tube defects, calcium supplementation in areas with low calcium intake in order to reduce risk of pre-eclampsia; vitamin A in deficient areas to prevent night blindness. Regarding the diet a higher intake of vitamin E is usually related to higher intakes of oils and fats whereas vitamin C indicates an increased intake of fruits and vegetables [36, 37].

Strengths
Strengths of this study include the standardised procedures used throughout the trial in all sites. Women in this study had close follow up from the same research team before and during pregnancy.

The 24-h recall dietary assessment method used is subject to less recall bias than other dietary assessment methods, such as diet histories or food frequency checklists [38]. Major advantages of using 24-h recalls are that high literacy of the respondent is not required and that inter-observer differences are minimised [18]. On the other hand, food frequency questionnaires usually require use of generic memory and higher numeracy skills in the population interviewed to quantify average food intakes over a period of time [39].

Limitations
We did not use the same scales to measure weight across sites, as weight was not the main outcome of this trial. However, women were assessed with the same scale throughout the study at each participating site.

We did not use any technique to corroborate energy intake, however under-reporting has been described in the literature in women especially in those with high BMI [40].

Food data from both countries was analysed using the SAMRC-Food composition database as there is not a local food composition database in Zimbabwe. There were a few cases where foods reported during the assessment were not found in the database, and they were added as the most similar item in terms of macronutrients and calcium content. Nevertheless, this was only in a few cases and we believe it cannot affect the main results of this sub-study. Although not having a database for Zimbabwe might be a limitation, it prevents showing differences that are related to errors of the food composition tables rather than of the nutrient intake [41].

The IOWA methodology to estimate usual intake requires at least 50 repeated interviews, we obtained repeated 24-h recall for 107 women, however we obtained

fewer than 50 repeated interview for Zimbabwe so the estimation might not be as accurate as for South Africa.

Conclusion
We found a high prevalence of overweight and obesity and high prevalence of inadequate intakes of protein and micronutrients in pregnant women who had a previous pregnancy complicated with pre-eclampsia. Although this group is not representative of the general population of pregnant woman, taking into account the increasing prevalence of overweight and obesity worldwide among young age groups, the obesity and micronutrient inadequacy figures reported in this study are issues of concern that need to be addressed so that maternal and perinatal outcomes are improved [42, 43]. Noticing the differences found in both countries regarding BMI and nutrient intake it would be interesting to explore the reasons behind as it could help to tackle the problem.

Supplement intakes during pregnancy seem to be essential for these groups of women to achieve requirements of key micronutrients. Policies should be reinforced and reviewed according to the most recent evidence. Pregnancy is a period when women may have more regular contacts with the health system and, if health care services were integrated for mothers and babies, these regular contacts could be maintained after delivery to improve maternal health [44]. These opportunities could be used to deliver dietary and nutritional interventions to high-risk women to improve the outcomes of future pregnancies [45]. Furthermore, taking into account that women with a history of pre-eclampsia are at higher risk of developing cardiovascular disease later in life, pregnancy and postnatal periods could be an ideal time for preventing future health complication from a young age.

Abbreviations
BMI: Body mass index; CAP: The calcium and pre-eclampsia study; DRI: Dietary reference intake; EAR: Estimated average requirement; EER: Estimated energy requirement; IOM: Institute of Medicine; SAMRC: South African Medical Research Council; SANHANES-1: National Health and Nutrition Examination Survey; WHO: World Health Organization

Acknowledgements
We thank the CAP trial researchers at the sites: Emilia Makaza, Eunice Tahuringana and Bothwell Guzha (Harare, Zimbabwe); Catherine Parker and Gift Phoramphai (Johannesburg, South Africa); Patience Moloi, Annemarie Greef and Saadiqa Alie (Cape Town, South Africa); Xoliswa Williams and Pamela Njikelana (East London, South Africa); Erika von Papendorp (Stellenbosch, South Africa) and Nicole Minckas, Ricardo López and Paula Rubinstein. We especially thank all women in South Africa and Zimbabwe who took part in the trial.

Funding
The Calcium and Pre-eclampsia (CAP) study is part of the PRE-EMPT (Pre-eclampsia- Eclampsia, Monitoring, Prevention and Treatment) study and is supported by the University of British Columbia, a grantee of the Bill & Melinda Gates Foundation; United Nations Development Programme (UNDP) - United Nations Population Fund (UNFPA) - United Nations Children"s Emergency Fund (UNICEF) • World Health Organization (WHO) • World Bank Special Programme of Research, Development and Research Training in Human Reproduction, Department of Reproductive Health and Research; and the

Argentina Fund for Horizontal Cooperation of the Argentinean Ministry of Foreign Affairs. The Research Council of Norway, through its Centers of Excellence scheme and the University of Bergen (UiB), Norway, and the Centre for Intervention Science in Maternal and Child Health, supported this sub-study (CISMAC; project number 223269). The funders of the study had no role in study design, data collection, data analysis, data interpretation, or writing of the report.

Authors' contributions
GC, APB, GJH, CP, TDP and JB designed the substudy and interpreted the data; GC and JH performed statistical analysis; GC, APB, JB and JH drafted the manuscript with contributions from DH, AHS, JR, GJH. All named authors critically reviewed and approved the final version.

Ethics approval and consent to participate
Ethical approval was obtained from appropriate national and institutional ethics review bodies as applicable for each study site, and all participants provided informed written consent. The study was approved by the Research Project Review Panel of the United Nations Development Programme (UNDP) - United Nations Population Fund (UNFPA) - United Nations Children's Emergency Fund (UNICEF) - World Health Organization (WHO) - World Bank Special Programme of Research, Development and Research Training in Human Reproduction at the Department of Reproductive Health and Research of World Health Organization, and the World Health Organization Research Ethics Review Committee, Geneva, Switzerland. Approval has been obtained from the Health Sciences Faculty, Human Research Ethics Committee (HREC) of University of Cape Town (No HREC 457/2010), Health Research Ethics Committee 1, University of Stellenbosch, Cape Town, South Africa, Medical Research Council of Zimbabwe and the Human Research Ethics Committee (Medical), University of the Witwatersrand, Johannesburg, South Africa.

Competing interests
The authors declare that they have no competing interests.

Author details
[1]Instituto de Efectividad Clínica y Sanitaria (IECS-CONICET), Emilio Ravignani, 2024 Buenos Aires, Argentina. [2]Division of Human Nutrition, Department of Human Biology, Faculty of Health Sciences, University of Cape Town, Cape Town, South Africa. [3]HRP – UNDP/UNFPA/UNICEF/WHO/World Bank Special Programme of Research, Development and Research Training in Human Reproduction, Department of Reproductive Health and Research, World Health Organization, Geneva, Switzerland. [4]WHO Regional Office for Europe, World Health Organization, Copenhagen, Denmark. [5]Effective Care Research Unit, University of the Witwatersrand, Johannesburg, South Africa. [6]Effective Care Research Unit, Eastern Cape Department of Health Walter Sisulu University, Mthatha, South Africa. [7]Effective Care Research Unit, University of Fort Hare, East London, South Africa. [8]Department of Obstetrics and Gynaecology, Stellenbosch University and Tygerberg Hospital, Cape Town, South Africa. [9]Epidemiología y Microbiología La Habana, Instituto Nacional de Higiene, Havana, Cuba. [10]Magee-Womens Research Institute, Department of Obstetrics and Gynecology, University of Pittsburgh, Pittsburgh, USA.

References
1. Young MF, Nguyen PH, Addo OY, Hao W, Nguyen H, Pham H, Martorell R, Ramakrishnan U. The relative influence of maternal nutritional status before and during pregnancy on birth outcomes in Vietnam. Eur J Obstet Gynecol Reprod Biol. 2015;194:223–7.
2. Popkin BM. Nutrition in transition: The changing global nutrition challenge. Asia Pac J Clin Nutr. 2001;10:Suppl S13–8.
3. Lindsay KL, Gibney ER, McAuliffe FM. Maternal nutrition among women from sub-Saharan Africa, with a focus on Nigeria, and potential implications for pregnancy outcomes among immigrant populations in developed countries. J Hum Nutr Die. 2012;25(6):534–46.
4. Mission JF, Marshall NE, Caughey AB. Pregnancy risks associated with obesity. Obstet Gynecol Clin N Am. 2015;42(2):335–53.
5. Black RE, Victora CG, Walker SP, Bhutta ZA, Christian P, de Onis MUR. Maternal and child undernutrition and overweight in low-income and middle-income countries. Lancet. 2013;382(9890):427–51.
6. Marchi J, Berg M, Dencker A, Olander EK, Begley C. Risks associated with obesity in pregnancy, for the mother and baby: a systematic review of reviews. Obes Rev. 2015;16(8):621–38.
7. Spradley FT, Palei AC, Granger JP. Increased risk for the development of preeclampsia in obese pregnancies: weighing in on the mechanisms. Am J Physiol Regul Integr Comp Physiol. 2015;309(11):R1326–43.
8. Ramakrishnan U, Grant F, Goldenberg T, Zongrone A, Martorell R. Effect of women's nutrition before and during early pregnancy on maternal and infant outcomes: a systematic review. Paediatr Perinat Epidemiol. 2012;26(Suppl 1):285–301.
9. Dean SV, Lassi ZS, Imam AM, Bhutta ZA. Preconception care: nutritional risks and interventions. Reprod Health. 2014;11(Suppl 3):S3.
10. Abu-Saad K, Fraser D. Maternal nutrition and birth outcomes. Epidemiol Rev. 2010;32:5–25.
11. Temel S, van Voorst SF, Jack BW, Denktaş S, Steegers EA. Evidence-based preconceptional lifestyle interventions. Epidemiol Rev. 2014;36:19–30.
12. World Health Organization. WHO recommendations on antenatal care for a positive pregnancy experience. 2016. http://apps.who.int/iris/bitstream/10665/250796/1/9789241549912-eng.pdf. Accessed 29 May 2018.
13. Shisana O, Labadarios D, Rehle T, Simbayi L, Zuma K, Dhansay A, Reddy P, Parker W, Hoosain E, Naidoo P, Hongoro C, Mchiza Z, Steyn NP, Dwane N, Makoae M, Maluleke T, Ramlagan S, Zungu N, Evans MG, Jacobs L, Faber M, the SANHANES-1 Team. South African National Health and nutrition examination survey (SANHANES-1): edition. Cape Town: HSRC Press; 2014.
14. Martorell R, Khan LK, Hughes ML, Grummer-Strawn LM. Obesity in women from developing countries. EurJClinNutr. 2000;54:247–52.
15. Hofmeyr GJ. Protocol 11PRT/4028: Long term calcium supplementation in women at high risk of pre-eclampsia: a randomised, placebo-controlled trial (PACTR201105000267371). Lancet. 2011 [http://www.thelancet.com/protocol-reviews/11PRT-4028]. Accessed 29 May 2018.
16. WHO: World Health Organization. In Guideline: Calcium supplementation in pregnant women. Edited by World Health Organization. Geneva: Geneva, World Health Organization, 2013. [http://apps.who.int/iris/bitstream/10665/85120/1/9789241505376eng.pdf]. Accessed 29 May 2018.
17. WHO Consultation on Obesity. Obesity: preventing and managing the global epidemic: report of a WHO consultation. Geneva: World Health Organization; 1999.
18. Dietary assessment and physical activity measurements toolkit. 2017. http://dapa-toolkit.mrc.ac.uk. Accessed 29 May 2016.
19. Steyn NP, Senekal M. A Guide for the use of the Dietary Assessment and Education Kit (DAEK). Cape Town: South African Medical Research Council; 2004.
20. Dodd KW, Guenther PM, Freedman LS, Subar AF, Kipnis V, Midthune D, Tooze JA. Statistical methods for estimating usual intake of nutrients and foods: a review of the theory. J Am Diet Assoc. 2006;106(10):1640–50.
21. Allen LH, De Benoist B, Dary O, Hurrell R, editors. Guidelines on food fortification with micronutrients. Geneva: World Health Organization; 2006.
22. Boon N, Hul GB, Stegen JH, Sluijsmans WE, Valle C, Langin D, Viguerie N, Saris WH. An intervention study of the effects of calcium intake on faecal fat excretion, energy metabolism and adipose tissue mRNA expression of lipid-metabolism related proteins. Int J Obes. 2007;31(11):1704–12.
23. IOM (Institute of Medicine) and NRC (National Research Council). Weight gain during pregnancy: Reexamining the Guidelines. Washington: The National Academies Press; 2009.
24. Nusser SM, Carriquiry AL, Dodd KW, et al. A semi- parametric transformation approach to estimating usual daily intake distributions. J Am Stat Assoc. 1996;91:1440–9.
25. Goldberg GR, Black AE, Jebb SA, Cole TJ, Murgatroyd PR, Coward WA, Prentice AM. Critical evaluation of energy intake data using fundamental

principles of energy physiology: 1. Derivation of cut-off limits to identify under-recording. Eur J Clin Nutr. 1991;45:569–81.

26. WHO Technical Report Series. Guidelines for Good Clinical Practice (GCP) for Trials on Pharmaceutical Products, vol. 850. Geneva: World Health Organization; 1995. p. 97–137.

27. World Health Organisation. BMI classifications. Geneva: WHO; 2006. http://apps.who.int/bmi/index.jsp?introPage=intro_3.html. Accessed 29 May 2016.

28. Ng M, Fleming T, Robinson M, Thomson B, Graetz N, Margono C, et al. Global, regional, and national prevalence of overweight and obesity in children and adults during 1980-2013: a systematic analysis for the global burden of disease study 2013. Lancet. 2014;384:766–81.

29. Nieuwoudt M, van der Merwe JL, Harvey J, Hall DR. Pregnancy outcomes in super-obese women - an even bigger problem? A prospective cohort study. S Afr J OG. 2014;20(2):54–9.

30. O'Brien TE, Ray JG, Chan WS. Maternal body mass index and the risk of preeclampsia: a systematic overview. Epidemiology. 2003;14(3):368–74.

31. Rasmussen KM, Catalano PM, Yaktine AL. New guidelines for weight gain during pregnancy: What obstetrician/gynecologists should know. Curr Opin Obstet Gynecol. 2009;21(6):521–6.

32. Trends in energy intake among adults in the United States: findings from NHANES. Am J Clin Nutr. 2013;97(4):848–53.

33. Fryar C, Carrol MD, Ogden CL. Prevalence of Overweight, Obesity, and Extreme Obesity Among Adults: United States, 1960–1962 Through 2011–2012. Atlanta: National Center for Health Statistics; 2016. Accessed 29 May 2016

34. Standard Treatment Guidelines and Essential Medicines List for South Africa. Hospital Level, Adults. 4th ed. Pretoria: The National Department of Health; 2015.

35. National Department of Health, South Africa. Guidelines for Maternity Carein South Africa A Manual for Clinics, Community Dent HealthCommunity Health Centres and District Hospitals, vol. 172. 4th ed. Pretoria: NDoH; 2015. http://www.health.gov.za/index.php/2014-03-17-09-09-38/policies-and-guidelines/category/230-2015p#. Accessed 29 May 2016

36. Zhao Y, Monahan FJ, McNulty BA, Gibney MJ, Gibney ER. Effect of vitamin E intake from food and supplement sources on plasma α- and γ-tocopherol concentrations in a healthy Irish adult population. Br J Nutr. 2014;112(9): 1575–85.

37. Olza J, Aranceta-Bartrina J, González-Gross M, Ortega RM, Serra-Majem L, Varela-Moreiras G, Gil Á. Reported dietary intake and food sources of zinc, selenium, and vitamins A, E and C in the Spanish population: findings from the ANIBES Study. Nutrients. 2017;9(7):697.

38. Rush D, Kristal AR. Methodologic studies during pregnancy: the reliability of the 24-hour dietary recall. Am J Clin Nutr. 1982;35(5 Suppl):1259–68.

39. Holmes B, Dick K, Nelson M. A comparison of four dietary assessment methods in materially deprived households in England. Public Health Nutr. 2007;11(05)

40. Scagliusi F. Underreporting of energy intake in Brazilian women varies according to dietary assessment: a cross-sectional study using doubly labeled water. J Am Diet Assoc. 2008;108(12):2031–40.

41. Merchant AT, Dehghan M. Food composition database development for between country comparisons. Nutr J. 2006;19(5):2.

42. Kleinerta S, Hortona R. Rethinking and reframing obesity. Lancet. 2015; 385(14):61746–3.

43. Lobstein T, Jackson-Leach R, Moodie ML, Hall KD, Gortmaker SL, Swinburn BA, et al. Child and adolescent obesity: part of a bigger picture. Lancet. 2015;385(9986):2510–20.

44. Thomas M, Hutchison M, Castro G, Nau M, Shumway M, Stotland N, Spielvogel A. Meeting women where they are: integration of care as the Foundation of Treatment for at-risk pregnant and postpartum women. Matern Child Health J. 2017;21(3):452–7.

45. Craici IM, Wagner SJ, Hayman SR, Garovic VD. Pre-eclamptic pregnancies: an opportunity to identify women at risk for future cardiovascular disease. Womens Health (Lond). 2008;4(2):133–5.

16

Assessing the sensitivity of placental growth factor and soluble fms-like tyrosine kinase 1 at 36 weeks' gestation to predict small-for-gestational-age infants or late-onset preeclampsia

Teresa M. MacDonald[1,2,3]* (iD), Chuong Tran[4], Tu'uhevaha J. Kaitu'u-Lino[2,3], Shaun P. Brennecke[2,5], Richard J. Hiscock[2], Lisa Hui[1,2,3], Kirsten M. Dane[1], Anna L. Middleton[1,2], Ping Cannon[2,3], Susan P. Walker[1,2,3] and Stephen Tong[1,2,3]

Abstract

Background: Fetal growth restriction is a disorder of placental dysfunction with three to four-fold increased risk of stillbirth. Fetal growth restriction has pathophysiological features in common with preeclampsia. We hypothesised that angiogenesis-related factors in maternal plasma, known to predict preeclampsia, may also detect fetal growth restriction at 36 weeks' gestation. We therefore set out to determine the diagnostic performance of soluble fms-like tyrosine kinase 1 (sFlt-1), placental growth factor (PlGF), and the sFlt-1:PlGF ratio, measured at 36 weeks' gestation, in identifying women who subsequently give birth to small-for-gestational-age (SGA; birthweight <10th centile) infants. We also aimed to validate the predictive performance of the analytes for late-onset preeclampsia in a large independent, prospective cohort.

Methods: A nested 1:2 case-control study was performed including 102 cases of SGA infants and a matched group of 207 controls; and 39 cases of preeclampsia. We determined the diagnostic performance of each angiogenesis-related factor, and of their ratio, to detect SGA infants or preeclampsia, for a predetermined 10% false positive rate.

Results: Median plasma levels of PlGF at 36 weeks' gestation were significantly lower in women who subsequently had SGA newborns (178.5 pg/ml) compared to normal birthweight controls (326.7 pg/ml, $p < 0.0001$). sFlt-1 was also higher among SGA cases, but this was not significant after women with concurrent preeclampsia were excluded. The sensitivity of PlGF to predict SGA infants was 28.8% for a 10% false positive rate. The sFlt-1:PlGF ratio demonstrated better sensitivity for preeclampsia than either analyte alone, detecting 69.2% of cases for a 10% false positive rate.

Conclusions: Plasma PlGF at 36 weeks' gestation is significantly lower in women who subsequently deliver a SGA infant. While the sensitivity and specificity of PlGF currently limit clinical translation, our findings support a blood-based biomarker approach to detect late-onset fetal growth restriction. Thirty-six week sFlt-1:PlGF ratio predicts 69.2% of preeclampsia cases, and could be a useful screening test to triage antenatal surveillance.

Keywords: Biomarker, Fetal growth restriction, Late-onset, Placental growth factor, Preeclampsia, Small-for-gestational-age, Soluble fms-like tyrosine kinase 1

* Correspondence: teresa.mary.macdonald@gmail.com
[1]Mercy Perinatal, Mercy Hospital for Women, Melbourne, VIC, Australia
[2]Department of Obstetrics and Gynaecology, University of Melbourne, Melbourne, VIC, Australia
Full list of author information is available at the end of the article

Background

Fetal growth restriction (FGR) due to placental insufficiency [1] is a major risk factor for stillbirth [2]. Small-for-gestational-age (SGA, birthweight <10th centile) fetuses, a common surrogate classification for FGR, have three to four-fold increased stillbirth risk at every gestation [2–4]. A large prospective cohort study demonstrated that when SGA fetuses are detected and appropriately managed, the rate of stillbirth is halved compared to pregnancies where a SGA fetus remains undiagnosed [2].

Improved identification of FGR has been listed as a top 10 priority to reduce the global burden of stillbirth [5]. Measuring symphysis-fundal height is current practice for detecting the SGA fetus, despite low sensitivity, reported at 17–58% over the last decade [6–8]. While universal third trimester ultrasound improves detection of SGA fetuses beyond that of selective ultrasound, its sensitivity is only 57%, with 35% positive predictive value [9]. A blood test able to detect the SGA fetus with better accuracy would provide clinicians with a valuable screening tool that may reduce the incidence of stillbirth.

Preeclampsia is associated with disordered release of angiogenesis-related factors into the maternal circulation – reduced pro-angiogenic placental growth factor (PlGF) and increased anti-angiogenic soluble fms-like tyrosine kinase 1 (sFlt-1) [10–12]. A high sFlt-1:PlGF ratio is associated with preeclampsia, performs as a better predictor than either analyte alone [13, 14] and demonstrates high negative predictive value [15, 16].

Like preeclampsia, FGR is characterised by placental dysfunction which can lead to aberrant release of angiogenesis-related factors into the maternal circulation. The sFlt-1:PlGF ratio has been shown to be significantly higher in cases of ultrasound-diagnosed SGA fetuses [17], and in women where SGA fetuses have failed to be detected by routine third trimester ultrasound [18]. A nested case-control study specifically including pregnant women with ultrasound estimated fetal weight > 10th centile at 32–36 weeks' gestation, demonstrated significantly higher sFlt-1:PlGF ratios (at the same gestation as the ultrasound) among 80 cases of a term SGA infant compared to 80 controls, but with just 30% sensitivity at a 10% false positive rate (FPR) [18]. While a relationship between elevated sFlt-1:PlGF ratios and SGA fetuses has been described, the predictive value of the ratio at a single point in late pregnancy to identify the SGA, without ultrasound, has not been established.

Given that sFlt-1 and PlGF are placenta-derived proteins, we hypothesised that measuring their levels at 36 weeks' gestation may be able to detect late-onset placental dysfunction to identify the SGA fetus, and to predict preeclampsia. We performed this nested case-control study from a large prospective cohort of 1000 pregnant women who had blood sampled at 36 weeks' gestation. We examined the performance of sFlt-1, PlGF and the sFlt-1:PlGF ratio at 36 weeks' gestation in the identification of women who subsequently gave birth to a SGA infant, or who developed preeclampsia.

Methods

This analysis is part of the Fetal Longitudinal Assessment of Growth (FLAG) study at the Mercy Hospital for Women, a tertiary maternity hospital in Melbourne with approximately 6000 births annually. The FLAG study (https://mercyperinatal.com/project/fetal-studies), designed to identify biomarkers to detect SGA fetuses, included prospective collection of 2015 blood samples from pregnant women at 36 weeks' gestation.

We performed a 1:2 nested case-control study using samples chosen from the first 1000 FLAG participants. We compared the 36 week sFlt-1, PlGF and sFlt-1:PlGF ratio values from women who delivered a SGA infant, to the analyte levels from a cohort of appropriate-for-gestational-age (AGA, birthweight ≥10th centile) controls, matched for maternal age, booking body mass index (BMI), smoking status, gestational diabetes mellitus (GDM), and parity. While a cohort study utilising all 1000 samples would be more powerful, and while case-control studies can be subject to overfitting, we used this nested case-control design to minimise costs. We made an a priori plan to proceed to a validation study utilising the remaining 1015 samples (from the subsequent FLAG study participants), which would mitigate the effects of any overfitting in the initial case-control study, if any analyte(s) demonstrated good diagnostic performance in predicting SGA infants.

This study was approved by the Mercy Health Research Ethics Committee (Ethics Approval Number R14/12) and written informed consent was obtained from all participants.

English-speaking women aged over 18 years, carrying a singleton pregnancy with normal mid-trimester morphology ultrasound were eligible to participate. Women booked to attend the Mercy Hospital for Women for their oral glucose tolerance test, offered around 28 weeks' gestation to diagnose GDM, were screened for eligibility and invited to participate between January 2015 and September 2016. Women who consented formed a convenience series of participants. Samples from women where a SGA fetus or preeclampsia were suspected at the time of blood sampling were not excluded. Whole blood was collected in a 10 ml ethylenediaminetetraacetic acid tube at 35^{+0} to 37^{+0} weeks' gestation inclusive. Plasma was stored at $-80\ °C$ until the time of PlGF and sFlt-1 measurement.

Outcomes and diagnostic criteria

Maternal characteristics and pregnancy outcomes were obtained from review of each participant's medical record, investigation results and hospital database entry, by a single clinician blinded to sFlt-1 and PlGF levels. Similarly, scientists performing the measurement of sFlt-1 and PlGF levels were blinded to the clinical characteristics and birthweight centiles of the participants. All sFlt-1 and PlGF levels were measured for research purposes only, and were not made available to any clinician involved in participants' obstetric care. Therefore there was no possibility of intervention bias.

Infant birthweights were assigned a customised centile using the GROW software [19] (http://www.gestation.net/), which generates a 'term optimal weight' based on an optimised fetal weight standard. We adjusted for the following non-pathological factors: maternal height, weight and parity; infant sex; and exact gestational age. Coefficients for the Australian dataset of GROW were informed by a local dataset; the multiple regression model has a constant to which weight is added or subtracted for each of the adjusted variables. SGA was defined as customised birthweight <10th centile.

Preeclampsia was diagnosed according to The American College of Obstetricians and Gynecologists' Taskforce on Hypertension in Pregnancy definition [20]: new onset hypertension (blood pressure ≥ 140 mmHg systolic, or ≥ 90 mmHg diastolic on two occasions ≥ 4 h apart after 20 weeks' gestation); plus one of new-onset: proteinuria, thrombocytopaenia, renal insufficiency, impaired liver function, pulmonary oedema or cerebral symptoms.

We analysed the differences in sFlt-1, PlGF and sFlt-1:PlGF ratio values between the control group and three different case groups: (i) 'All SGA' – all cases where the infant was SGA, including cases of concurrent preeclampsia; (ii) 'SGA only' – cases of concurrent preeclampsia were excluded; (iii) 'Preeclampsia' – all cases of preeclampsia, regardless of birthweight centile.

For cases of birthweight <10th centile, we also searched hospital ultrasound records to see which cases (i) were referred for a clinically-indicated third trimester ultrasound scan which included biometry to estimate fetal weight, and (ii) which cases were identified by a third trimester ultrasound as SGA on the basis of EFW or abdominal circumference < 10th centile. This allowed us to compare the sensitivities of the analytes to detect SGA to that of current clinical practice – selective ultrasound – in our institution.

Assessment of plasma analyte levels

Maternal plasma levels of sFlt-1 and PlGF were measured with a commercial electrochemiluminescence immunoassay platform (Roche Diagnostics). Analysis of change in sFlt-1 and PlGF values over gestational age in days was made using LOWESS smooth and regression techniques of both mean and median values (Additional file 1: S2). There was no significant trend for either sFlt-1 or PlGF values seen across the gestational weeks where sampling

was performed (35^{+0}–37^{+0} weeks), hence adjustment for gestational age was not performed.

Statistical analysis

Maternal characteristics and birth outcome data were compared for all women who delivered SGA infants, and for all cases of preeclampsia, against controls using unpaired t-test or rank-sum test for continuous data, according to distribution; and Chi-squared test for categorical data. Statistical analyses were performed using GraphPad Prism version 6 (GraphPad Software Inc., San Diego, CA) and Stata v14 (College Station, TX: StataCorp LP). Two-sided significance level was set at 0.05.

We determined the sensitivities, at a predetermined 10% FPR, of sFlt-1, PlGF, and the sFlt:PlGF ratio for the detection of: (i) SGA <10th centile, with and without concurrent preeclampsia, (ii) SGA <3rd centile, with and without concurrent preeclampsia, and (iii) Preeclampsia. Overall discrimination of the analytes for each disease group was assessed with area under the Receiver Operating Characteristic (ROC) curve analysis. In this nested case-control study positive predictive value (PPV) and negative predictive value (NPV) were calculated using the sampling fraction adjustment based upon the number of controls in this study compared to the original cohort and associated 95% confidence limits were calculated using a logit based standard error [21].

We chose 10% FPR as the cut-off as this is the FPR of universal ultrasound biometry at 36 weeks' gestation, as determined by the large, prospective, blinded Pregnancy Outcome Prediction study [9]. We chose to assess for SGA <10th centile, as this is considered by many to be an important threshold clinically [22]. In addition, customised birthweight <10th centile was the threshold used to define FGR in the large population study of over 92,000 births that demonstrated a halving of stillbirth risk when fetuses below this threshold were detected antenatally [2]. We also evaluated the performance of the analytes to predict infants destined to be born at <3rd centile as this was a cut-off agreed upon by recent Delphi procedure as a consensus definition of FGR [23].

Results

Baseline characteristics

Between March 2015 and February 2016 the first 1000 36 week FLAG study plasma samples were obtained. 105 (10.5%) participants delivered a SGA infant, including seven with co-existent preeclampsia. There were 28 (2.8%) cases of infant birthweight <3rd centile (one with concurrent preeclampsia). There were 32 cases of preeclampsia among women with AGA newborns (39 (3.9%) total preeclampsia cases). We matched the 105 women with SGA infants to 210 controls. Due to instrument error sFlt-1 values were not available for two SGA cases, and three controls (Fig. 1).

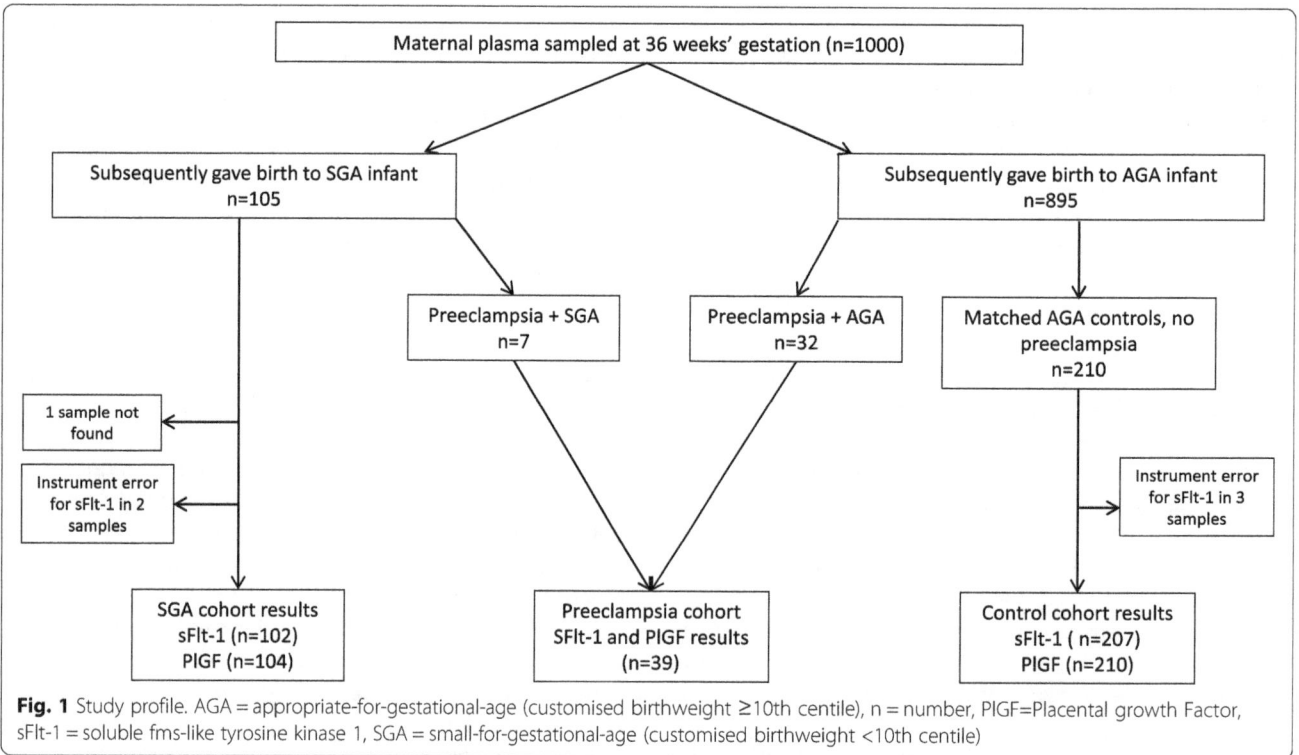

Fig. 1 Study profile. AGA = appropriate-for-gestational-age (customised birthweight ≥10th centile), n = number, PlGF=Placental growth Factor, sFlt-1 = soluble fms-like tyrosine kinase 1, SGA = small-for-gestational-age (customised birthweight <10th centile)

Maternal characteristics and birth outcomes for participants with complete sample analysis results are summarised in Table 1. There were no significant differences between controls and SGA cases except for birthweight, birthweight centiles and gestation at delivery: SGA infants were a mean 864 g and 46.8 centiles smaller, and were born 5 days' gestation earlier than control infants. Participants who developed preeclampsia had significantly higher booking BMI than controls (mean 27.4 vs 25.4 kg/m^2); and significantly higher emergency caesarean section rate. Infants of preeclamptic mothers were also significantly smaller than those of controls, and were born 5 days' gestation earlier.

Angiogenesis factor levels in cases compared to controls
Analysis was performed according to three case groups: (i) 'All SGA' – concurrent preeclampsia cases included; (ii) 'SGA only' – concurrent preeclampsia cases excluded; (iii) 'Preeclampsia' – all preeclampsia cases included, regardless of birthweight centile. Each case group was independently compared to controls (AGA infant, no preeclampsia).

(i) **'All SGA' vs controls**

The angiogenesis factors were all significantly altered in cases of SGA infants compared to controls (Fig. 2a, c, e, Table 2). When comparing 'All SGA' to controls, the median sFlt-1 level was significantly higher and the median PlGF level was significantly lower. Correspondingly, the median sFlt-1:PlGF ratio of the 'All SGA' cohort was significantly higher than that of controls (14.24 vs 7.11 respectively, $P < 0.0001$).

(ii) **'SGA only' vs controls**

When the angiogenesis factor levels were compared between controls and cases of 'SGA only' (excluding cases of co-existent preeclampsia) the differences between the groups became less pronounced (Fig. 2, Table 2). The median PlGF level remained significantly lower in 'SGA only' cases compared to controls, but there was no significant difference in sFlt-1 levels. The median sFlt-1:PlGF ratio of the 'SGA only' cases remained significantly higher than that of the controls (13.00 vs 7.11 respectively, $p = 0.0006$).

(iii) **Preeclampsia versus controls**

The levels of the angiogenesis factors were all significantly different in cases of preeclampsia compared to controls (Fig. 3, Table 2). When comparing preeclampsia cases to controls, the median sFlt-1 level was significantly higher, and median PlGF was significantly lower. The median sFlt-1:PlGF ratio of the preeclampsia cohort was correspondingly significantly higher than that of the control group (54.25 vs 7.11 respectively, $P < 0.0001$).

Table 1 Participant characteristics compared between controls and: (i) those with a SGA infant; (ii) women who developed preeclampsia

	Controls (n = 207)	All SGA (n = 102)	P	Preeclampsia (n = 39)	P
Age (years)	32.1 (4.7)	31.9 (4.2)	0.72	33.1 (4.7)	0.27
Booking Body Mass Index (kg/m^2)	25.4 (4.6)	25.4 (5.8)	0.45	27.6 (6.0)	0.02
Smoking status					
Current smoker	17 (8.2%)	8 (7.8%)	0.98	2 (5.1%)	0.80
Ex-smoker	51 (24.6%)	26 (25.5%)		10 (25.6%)	
Never	139 (67.1%)	68 (66.7%)		27 (69.2%)	
Gestational diabetes mellitus	38 (18.4%)	18 (17.6%)	1.00	9 (23.1%)	0.51
Parity					
0	118 (57.0%)	58 (56.9%)	0.97	28 (71.8%)	0.20
1	65 (31.4%)	33 (32.4%)		9 (23.1%)	
> 1	24 (11.6%)	11 (10.8%)		2 (5.1%)	
Onset of delivery					
Induction of labour	88 (42.5%)	47 (46.1%)	0.08	19 (48.7%)	0.25
Spontaneous labour	96 (46.4%)	36 (35.3%)		13 (33.3%)	
No labour	23 (11.1%)	19 (18.6%)		7 (17.9%)	
Mode of delivery					
Normal vaginal delivery	102 (49.3%)	45 (44.1%)	0.64	11 (28.2%)	0.01
Instrumental delivery	42 (20.3%)	22 (21.6%)		7 (17.9%)	
Emergency caesarean	42 (20.3%)	20 (19.6%)		17 (43.6%)	
Elective caesarean	21 (10.1%)	15 (14.7%)		4 (10.3%)	
Birthweight (g)	3547 (444)	2683 (333)	< 0.0001	3308 (640)	0.005
Birthweight centile	52.1 (26.1)	5.3 (3.0)	< 0.0001	42.8 (30.4)	0.049
Gestational age at delivery (weeks^{+days})	39^{+5} (1^{+1})	39^{+0} (1^{+4})	< 0.0001	39^{+0} (1^{+4})	0.03

Data represented as mean (standard deviation), or number (%). *g* grams, *kg* kilograms, *m* metres, *n* number, *PlGF* placental growth factor, *sFlt-1* soluble fms-like tyrosine kinase 1, *SGA* small-for-gestational-age (birthweight <10th centile). Note: some percentages do not sum to 100% due to rounding to one decimal place

Sensitivity of the analytes to detect the SGA and preeclampsia

The sensitivities of the analytes at a fixed 10% FPR (90% specificity) to predict birth of a SGA infant, or preeclampsia, are presented in Table 3. In Fig. 4 we have also presented the area under the ROC curve as a measure of overall discrimination for the analyte that had the greatest sensitivity for each of 'All SGA', 'SGA only' and 'Preeclampsia'.

For 'All SGA' and 'SGA only', at both <10th and < 3rd centile definitions, sFlt-1 had sensitivities below 23%. PlGF was the most sensitive analyte to detect both 'All SGA' and 'SGA only', but with sensitivities less than 33%. For 'All SGA' and 'SGA only' at both <10th and < 3rd centile definitions, the sFlt-1:PlGF ratio demonstrated less than 29% sensitivity (Table 3). For PlGF, the area under the ROC curve was only 0.66 for 'All SGA'; with a similarly modest result for 'SGA only' (Fig. 4a & b). Given these very modest performances for the detection of SGA fetuses, we did not think it would be cost-effective or valuable to proceed with the validation step in our second 1015 samples, so we did not perform it.

Seventy four (70.4%) of the 105 cases of a SGA infant were referred for a third trimester ultrasound to estimate fetal weight (41 were performed between 35^{+0} and 37^{+0} weeks – the same gestation range as our blood samples). 24 (32.4%) of the 74 third trimester ultrasound scans detected a SGA fetus with an EFW or abdominal circumference measurement <10th centile. Therefore, the strategy of selective ultrasound, in practice in our institution, performed with a sensitivity for SGA of 22.9% (24 out of 105 cases identified) overall.

All three analytes demonstrated moderate sensitivity, at over 56% for a 10% FPR, for preeclampsia (Table 3). The sFlt-1:PlGF ratio had the highest sensitivity for preeclampsia, at 69.2% with a 10% FPR. The sFlt-1:PlGF ratio performed moderately well on ROC curve analysis, with an area under the curve of 0.86 (Fig, 4c).

Discussion

The central role of the placenta in preeclampsia and FGR suggests that these two clinical conditions may share common plasma biomarkers. We therefore investigated the

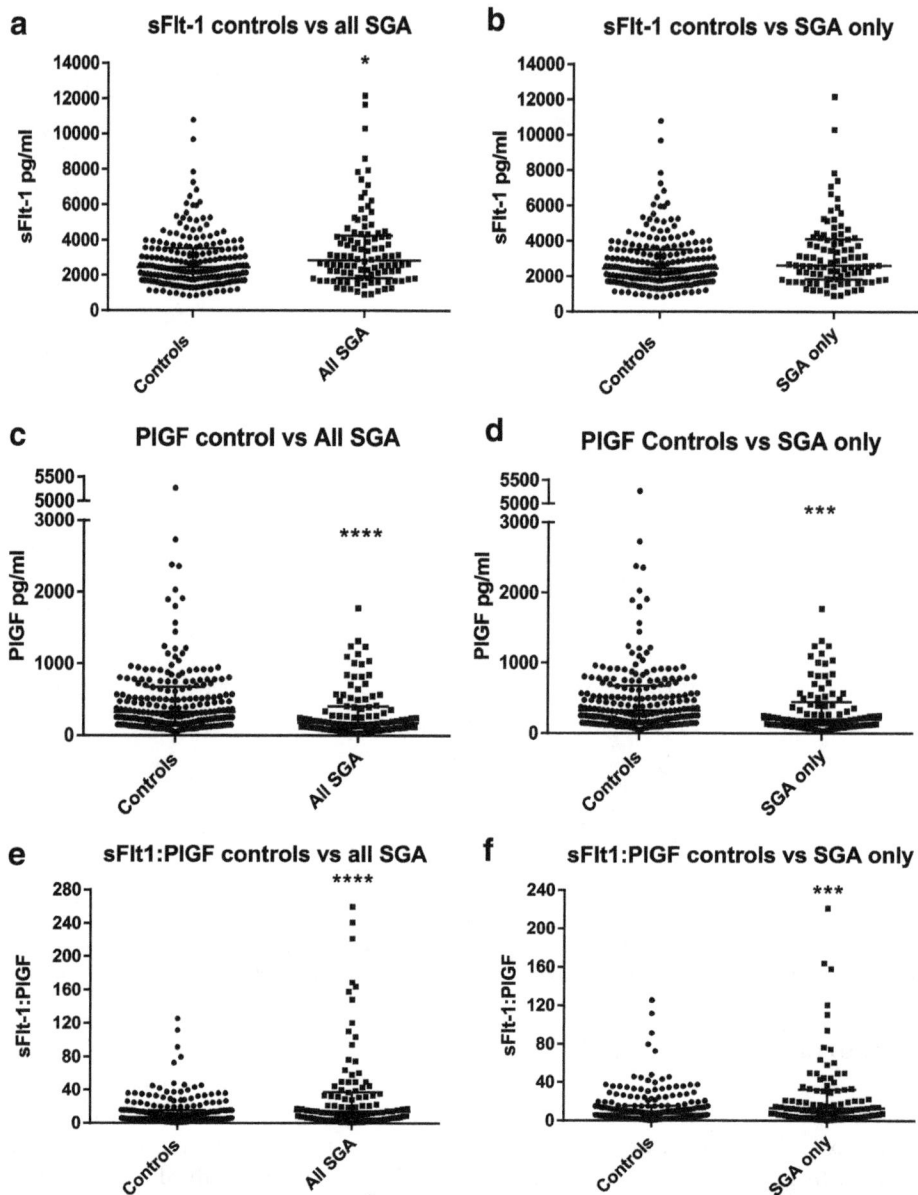

Fig. 2 Levels of angiogenesis-related factors in cases of small-for-gestational-age (SGA) fetuses compared to controls. **a.** soluble fms-like tyrosine kinase-1 (sFlt-1) levels in 'All SGA' cases and controls; **b.** sFlt-1 levels in 'SGA only' (excluding concurrent preeclampsia) cases and controls; **c.** Placental growth factor (PlGF) levels in 'All SGA' cases and controls; **d.** PlGF levels in 'SGA only' cases and controls; **e.** sFlt:PlGF ratios in 'All SGA' cases and controls; **f.** sFlt-1:PlGF ratios in 'SGA only' cases and controls. Medians and interquartile ranges shown. * = $P < 0.05$, *** = $P < 0.001$, **** = $P < 0.0001$

value of two known placenta-derived preeclampsia biomarkers (and their ratio), for the prediction of SGA infants in a large, independent, prospective cohort. Through analysis of samples obtained from a large unselected cohort, we found maternal plasma PlGF at 36 weeks' gestation to be significantly lower in women that subsequently gave birth to SGA infants compared to women with AGA newborns.

At a fixed 10% FPR, low PlGF identified 32.1% of women who subsequently gave birth to a newborn with birthweight <3rd centile, and 28.8% of those with a < 10th centile infant. Current tools for detection of late-onset FGR are poor. Significantly, a single PlGF level, even at the modest detection rates reported here, may still outperform the traditional methods of symphysis-fundal height [6], and selective ultrasound [9]. Indeed in our cohort, a strategy of selective ultrasound, the current clinical practice in our institution, predicted only 22.9% of SGA infants – comparatively less than PlGF would have. While the

Table 2 sFlt-1, PlGF and sFlt-1:PlGF ratios compared between controls and: (i) cases with a SGA infant; (ii) preeclampsia cases

	Controls	All SGA	P	SGA only	P	Preeclampsia	P
sFlt-1 (pg/ml)	2446 [1795–3503]	2837 [1850–4250]	0.02	2620 [1835–4099]	0.10	4857 [3777–6941]	< 0.001
PlGF (pg/ml)	326.7 [173.1–675.4]	178.5 [106.4–404.8]	< 0.001	199.9 [118.1–448.6]	< 0.001	99.73 [61.99–158.6]	< 0.001
sFlt-1:PlGF ratio	7.11 [3.08–15.58]	14.24 [6.00–37.37]	< 0.001	13.00 [5.27–32.44]	< 0.001	54.25 [26.81–114.5]	< 0.001

Data presented as median [25th–75th percentile]. "All SGA" = Cases with a SGA fetuses including cases with co-existent preeclampsia; "SGA only" = Cases with SGA fetuses with cases of co-existant preeclampsia excluded; pg/ml = picogram/millilitre, *PlGF* placental growth factor, *sFlt-1* soluble fms-like tyrosine kinase-1, *SGA* small-for-gestational-age (birthweight <10th centile). For sFlt-1 and sFlt-1:PlGF ratio results n = 207 for controls, n = 102 for 'All SGA', n = 39 for 'Preeclampsia'. For PlGF results $n = 210$ for controls, $n = 104$ for 'All SGA', and $n = 39$ for 'Preeclampsia'

predictive performance of PlGF alone is not sufficient to warrant adoption into clinical practice, our data supports the potential of a multi-biomarker approach. We also report that sFlt-1 is not significantly altered in pregnancies with a SGA fetus unless preeclampsia is present, suggesting sFlt-1 to be a biomarker more specific to preeclampsia.

Our study also validated the diagnostic performance of the sFlt-1:PlGF ratio at 36 weeks' gestation for late-onset preeclampsia. When we applied the same ratio cut-off (≥38 pg/ml) as used in the PROGNOSIS study [15] to our cohort, 66.7% sensitivity and 94.2% specificity were achieved (Table 4), surpassing the performance reported in the original trial for preeclampsia within 4 weeks of testing [15]. Application of the ≥38 pg/ml cut-off did not perform as well to predict SGA infants however, displaying sensitivities of 24.5% and 25.0% for <10th and < 3rd centile birthweight respectively (Table 4). Overall, the data from our study acts to validate some of the results from the PROGNOSIS study in an independent cohort, strengthening the potential clinical utility of the ratio for detecting late-onset preeclampsia.

The strength of this study was our large prospective cohort of 1000 singleton pregnancies from which

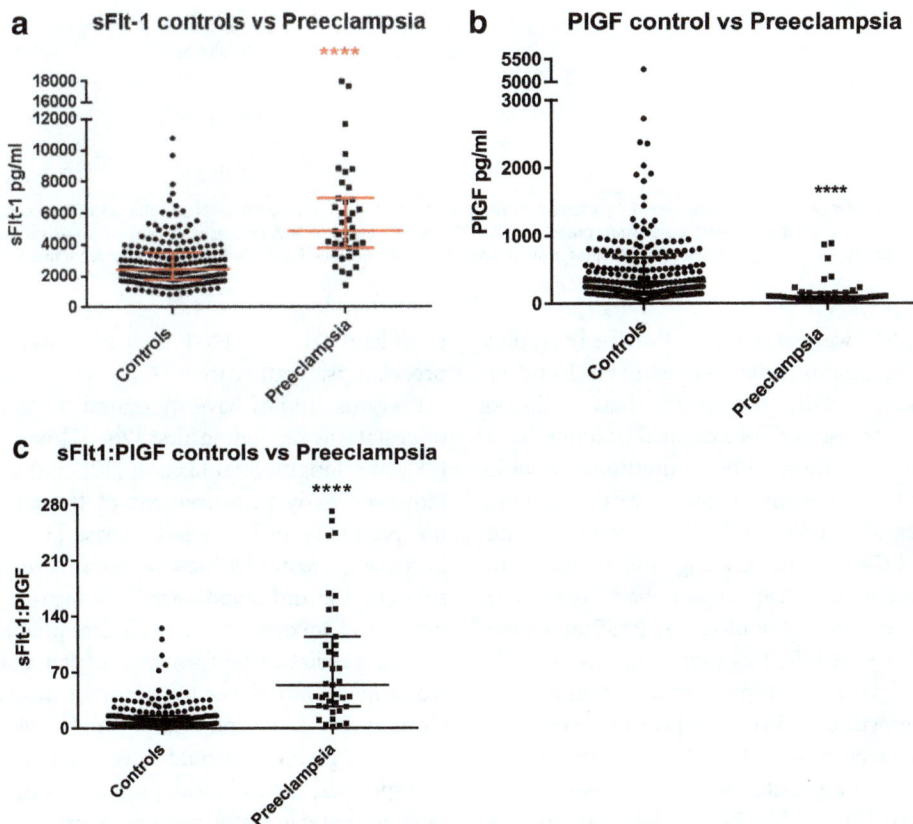

Fig. 3 Levels of angiogenesis-related factors in cases of preeclampsia compared to controls. **a.** soluble fms-like tyrosine kinase-1 (sFlt-1) levels in preeclampsia cases and controls; **b.** Placental growth factor (PlGF) levels in preeclampsia cases and controls; **c.** sFlt-1:PlGF ratios in preeclampsia cases and controls. Medians and interquartile ranges shown. **** = $P < 0.0001$

Table 3 Diagnostic performance of each analyte to predict <10th and < 3rd centile infants, and preeclampsia

Outcome	Analyte and cut-point	Sensitivity	Specificity	PPV	NPV
Birthweight < 10th centile (All SGA)	sFlt-1 > 4570 pg/ml	19.6% [12.4–28.6%]	89.9% [84.9–93.6%]	18.0% [11.1–27.9%]	90.8% [89.8–91.6%]
	PlGF < 117.3 pg/ml	28.8% [20.4–38.6%]	89.5% [84.6–93.3%]	24.2% [16.3–34.5%]	91.6% [90.5–92.5%]
	sFlt-1:PlGF > 33.4	26.5% [18.2–36.1%]	89.9% [84.9–93.6%]	22.9% [15.0–33.2%]	91.5% [90.5–92.4%]
Birthweight < 10th centile (SGA only)	sFlt-1 > 4570 pg/ml	16.8% [9.9–25.9%]	89.9% [84.9–93.6%]	14.8% [8.7–24.2%]	91.1% [90.3–91.9%]
	PlGF < 117.3 pg/ml	24.7% [16.5–34.5%]	89.5% [84.6–93.3%]	20.2% [13.0–30.0%]	91.7% [90.7–92.6%]
	sFlt-1:PlGF > 33.4	22.1% [14.2–31.8%]	89.9% [84.9–93.6%]	18.6% [11.6–28.5%]	91.7% [90.7–92.5%]
Birthweight < 3rd centile (All SGA)	sFlt-1 > 4570 pg/ml	21.4% [8.3–41.0%]	87.5% [83.1–91.2%]	4.7% [2.2–9.7%]	97.5% [96.9–97.9%]
	PlGF < 117.3 pg/ml	32.1% [15.9–52.4%]	85.0% [80.3–88.9%]	5.8% [3.3–10.1%]	97.8% [97.1–98.3%]
	sFlt-1:PlGF > 33.4	28.6% [13.2–48.7%]	85.8% [81.1–89.6%]	5.5% [2.9–10.0%]	97.7% [97.0–98.1%]
Birthweight < 3rd centile (SGA only)	sFlt-1 > 4570 pg/ml	22.2% [8.6–42.3%]	88.7% [84.4–92.2%]	5.2% [2.4–10.7%]	97.6% [97.1–98.1%]
	PlGF < 117.3 pg/ml	29.6% [13.8–50.2%]	86.4% [81.9–90.2%]	5.7% [3.1–10.4%]	97.8% [97.2–98.3%]
	sFlt-1:PlGF > 33.4	25.9% [11.1–46.3%]	87.3% [82.7–91.0%]	5.4% [2.7–10.3%]	97.7% [97.1–98.2%]
Preeclampsia	sFlt-1 > 4570 pg/ml	56.4% [39.6–72.2%]	89.9% [84.9–93.6%]	18.4% [12.1–26.9%]	98.1% [97.3–98.6%]
	PlGF < 117.3 pg/ml	64.1% [47.2–78.8%]	89.5% [84.6–93.3%]	19.9% [13.6–28.2%]	98.4% [97.6–98.9%]
	sFlt-1:PlGF > 33.4	69.2% [52.4–83.0%]	89.9% [84.9–93.6%]	21.7% [14.9–30.4%]	98.6% [97.8–99.1%]

Data presented with [95% Confidence Interval]. *determined by a false positive rate of 10% in the birthweight ≥10th centile and no preeclampsia control group. "All SGA" = Cases of SGA fetuses including cases with co-existent preeclampsia; "SGA only" = Cases of SGA fetuses with cases of co-existant preeclampsia excluded; NPV Negative Predictive value, pg/ml = pictogram/millilitre, PlGF placental growth factor, PPV Positive Predictive Value, sFlt-1 soluble fms-like tyrosine kinase-1, SGA small-for-gestational-age

case-control samples were selected. Previous studies have investigated the relationships between sFlt-1 and/or PlGF and late-onset FGR, but most have utilized methods not readily translated into clinical practice for a general antenatal population. These methods include placental rather than plasma protein analysis [24]; multi-modality integrated models [25, 26]; prior ultrasound diagnosis of SGA [27–33]; and investigation confined to cases of preterm infants [32]. Our large cohort specifically enabled us to compare the utility of sFlt-1, PlGF, and their ratio, in all cases of a SGA infant as well as in a 'SGA only' cohort, actively removing the impact of participants with concurrent preeclampsia. Our results add clarity where previous findings have been inconsistent. Prior to this study, elevated sFlt-1 had been associated with FGR in some animal [34], and human [31, 32, 35, 36] studies with cases of preeclampsia excluded, but not in others [18, 33]. The large numbers in our study and the ability to test levels in both 'All SGA' and 'SGA only' cohorts have allowed us to

confidently define sFlt-1 as a biomarker more specific to preeclampsia, rather than FGR.

Previous studies have measured the analytes at a variety of gestations, including first [26, 37] and second trimesters [38], in a longitudinal fashion [12], and at delivery [31, 39]. However, early measurement of the angiogenic factors is not predictive of late-onset disease [38], except if included in a complex model incorporating several maternal, ultrasonographic and blood-based risk factor assessments [26] – difficult to incorporate into clinical practice. In preeclampsia, the predictive performance of the analytes is improved when measured closer to the onset of disease [15]. Future biomarkers requiring only single blood sampling at 36 weeks' gestation would have the potential to be rapidly incorporated into clinical practice, with the availability of safe, acceptable interventions (surveillance and planned timely delivery) to reduce stillbirth risk for SGA fetuses.

While the predictive potential of a single measurement of the sFlt-1:PlGF ratio at 36 weeks' gestation has been

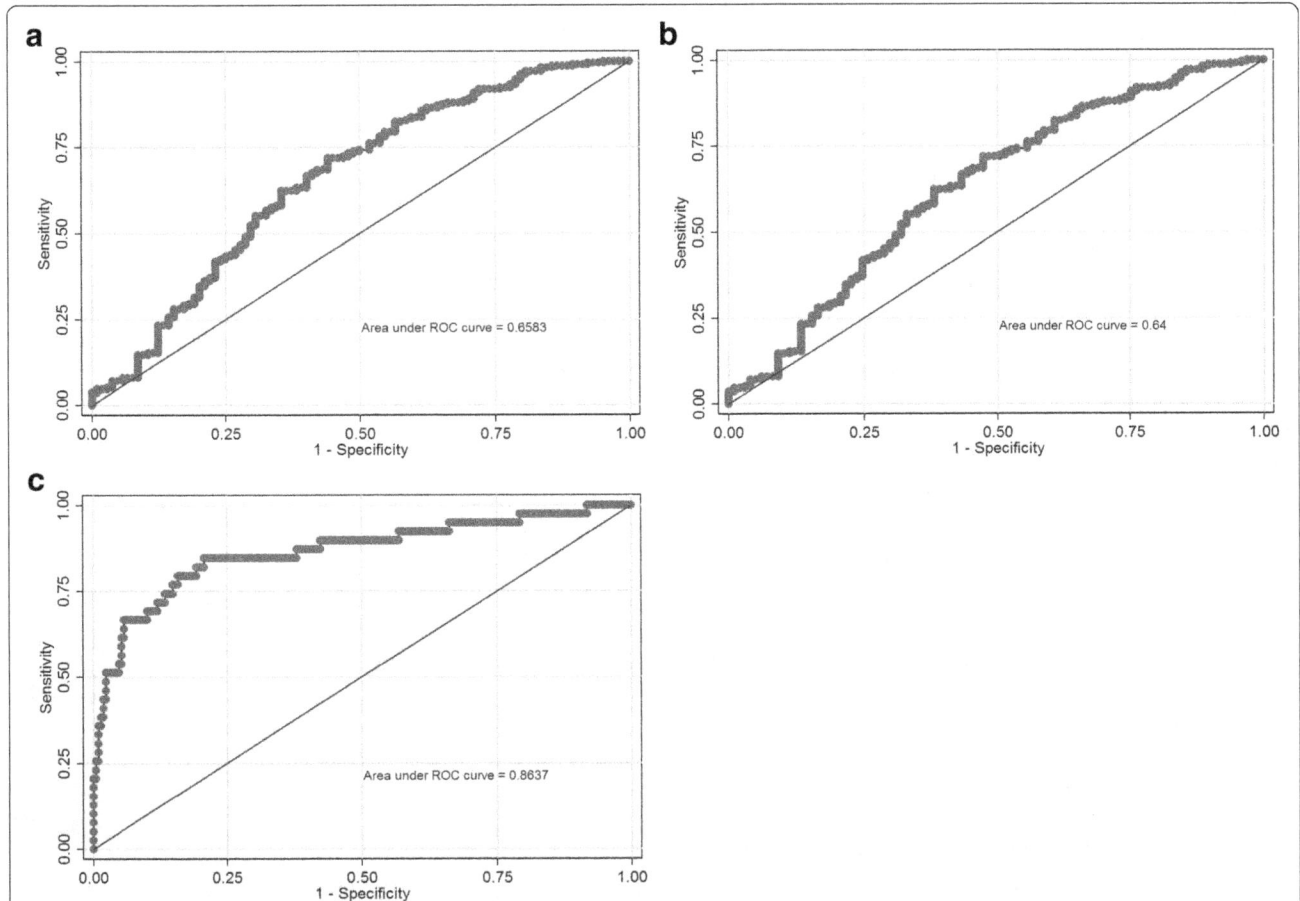

Fig. 4 Receiver operating characteristic curves for most sensitive analytes to detect small-for-gestational-age (SGA) infants, or preeclampsia. **a.** ROC curve for the performance of placental growth factor (PlGF) in detecting 'All SGA' – including cases of concurrent preeclampsia; **b.** ROC curve for the performance of PlGF in detecting 'SGA only' – excluding cases of concurrent preeclampsia; **c.** ROC curve for the performance of the soluble fms-like tyrosine kinase 1:PlGF ratio in detecting preeclampsia

assessed for preeclampsia [16], only the Pregnancy Outcome Prediction (POP) study has previously analysed the sFlt-1:PlGF ratio specifically at 36 weeks' gestation for FGR [40]. This study defined FGR as birthweight <10th centile plus perinatal morbidity and/or preeclampsia and found the combination of sFlt-1:PlGF ratio > 38 and ultrasound EFW <10th centile – both present together in just 3% of participants – to demonstrate a higher PPV (21.6%) and specificity (98%) than either parameter alone, but with lower sensitivity (only 38%) compared to either test alone. In this study, a 36 week PlGF value among the lowest decile performed with almost exactly the same diagnostic accuracy as the highest decile of the sFlt-1:PlGF ratio to identify FGR. Both tests performed with 43.1% sensitivity, 90.6% specificity, 6.7% PPV and 99% NPV for the definition of FGR in use [40].

Table 4 Diagnostic performance of sFlt-1:PlGF ratio ≥ 38 for preeclampsia, and < 10th and < 3rd centile infants

Outcome	Sensitivity	Specificity	PPV	NPV
Preeclampsia	66.7% [49.8–80.9%]	94.2% [90.1–97.0%]	31.8% [20.5–45.8%]	98.6% [97.8–99.1%]
Birthweight < 10th centile (All SGA)	24.5% [16.5–34.0%]	94.2% [90.1–97.0%]	32.4% [20.1–47.8%]	91.7% [90.7–92.5%]
Birthweight < 3rd centile (All SGA)	25.0% [10.7–44.9%]	89.3% [85.1–92.7%]	6.3% [3.2–12.3%]	97.6% [97.1–98.1%]

Data presented with [95% Confidence Interval]. *NPV* Negative Predictive value, *PlGF* placental growth factor, *PPV* Positive Predictive Value, *sFlt-1* soluble fms-like tyrosine kinase-1, *SGA* small-for-gestational-age

This mirrors the finding in our study, that the addition of sFlt-1 to PlGF in the form of the ratio at 36 weeks' gestation adds no value. It is also not surprising that the sensitivities reported for the analytes alone were higher in the POP study compared to ours – as the POP definition of FGR occurred in only 1.5% of the population. Interestingly, in the POP cohort, sFlt-1:PlGF ratio > 38 demonstrated 37.2% sensitivity for birth weight < 3rd centile. This was much higher than the 25% sensitivity seen in our study. However, the POP study utilised a large cohort study in comparison to our nested case-control design; and used a population reference to define birthweight centile in contrast to customised birth weight centiles.

One other previous study measured sFlt-1 and PlGF at 35–37 weeks' gestation and reported their ability, in combination with ultrasound biometry and maternal characteristics, to predict SGA infants in the absence of preeclampsia, but did not assess the sFlt-1:PlGF ratio [36]. Again, similar to our findings, while addition of PlGF to biometry and maternal characteristics marginally improved the detection of SGA fetuses, addition of sFlt-1 did not [36]. Measurement of the analytes at a single time-point in late pregnancy was a strength of our study, adding to this body of evidence, as was our direct comparison of the sFlt-1:PlGF ratio to its constituent analytes.

The generalisability of our data is supported by the incidence of both preeclampsia and SGA infants among our participants, in keeping with expected rates [9, 41–43]. We present a well-characterised cohort, featuring a control group carefully matched for factors known to influence fetal growth. We used GROW software [19] to customise birthweight centiles, as this customised standard has stronger associations with adverse perinatal outcomes attributable to placental insufficiency than population references [44]. Additionally, the Elecsys immunoassays used for sFlt-1 and PlGF (Roche Diagnostics) have received Conformité Européene marking for use as in vitro medical devices.

One potential reason that PlGF displayed relatively low detection of SGA infants is that 'SGA' is not a functional diagnosis, and therefore may include infants who are constitutionally, rather than pathologically, small. Constitutionally small fetuses would not be expected to exhibit a low PlGF, as they are not suffering placental insufficiency. This in part may explain why PlGF levels, although significantly different, were not able to differentiate between cases and controls with both high sensitivity and specificity. However, PlGF was also not able to predict <3rd centile infants, those largely regarded to be growth restricted [23], with great accuracy which suggests that while low PlGF is associated with placental insufficiency, the strength of association is not strong enough for its use as a biomarker in isolation.

Overall, our study demonstrates that PlGF may be a useful component of a multi-biomarker predictive blood test for SGA, which we aim to develop. Our sFlt-1 results highlight that FGR and preeclampsia do not share the same plasma biomarker profile, such that future studies dedicated to FGR-specific biomarkers are needed. However, there are many challenges to performing well-conducted prospective studies, including the large numbers of participants required, and substantial associated costs. Despite this, we believe that future biomarkers requiring only single blood sampling at 36 weeks' gestation would have the potential to be rapidly incorporated into clinical practice, with the availability of safe, acceptable interventions (surveillance and planned timely delivery) to reduce stillbirth risk for SGA fetuses.

Conclusions

Thirty-six week plasma PlGF is significantly lower in women who subsequently deliver a SGA infant, but its diagnostic performance limits clinical translation as an individual biomarker. Further research is required to identify other biomarkers for FGR that together may perform with high sensitivity and specificity. The sFlt-1:PlGF ratio at 36 weeks however predicts preeclampsia with 69.2% sensitivity for 90% specificity, and therefore may be useful in triaging antenatal surveillance.

Abbreviations
AGA: Appropriate-for-gestational-age (birthweight ≥10th centile); BMI: Body Mass Index; FGR: Fetal growth restriction; FLAG: Fetal Longitudinal Assessment of Growth; FPR: False positive rate; g: Grams; GDM: Gestational Diabetes Mellitus; kg: Kilograms; m: Metres; n: Number; NPV : Negative Predictive Value; PlGF : Placental growth factor; PPV : Positive Predictive Value; ROC: Receiver Operating Characteristic; sFlt-1: Soluble fms-like tyrosine kinase 1; SGA : Small-for-gestational-age (birthweight <10th centile)

Acknowledgments
We wish to thank the pathology, health information services, and antenatal clinic staff at the Mercy Hospital for Women for their assistance in conducting this research.

Funding
National Health and Medical Research Council Grant #1065854, and Stillbirth Foundation Grant to SW; Australian Government Research Training Program Scholarship, and RANZCOG Taylor Hammond Scholarship to TM; National Health and Medical Research Council Early Career Fellowship #1105603 to LH; Norman Beischer Medical Research Foundation to TK, TM and SW. Funding sources had no involvement in study design, collection or analysis of data, or in the writing or submission of this manuscript.

Authors' contributions
ST conceived the study. ST, SPW, TMM, LH, KMD, SPB and TJK designed the study. TMM, KMD and ALM recruited participants and performed sample

collection. TMM characterised the cohort, and matched the control cohort. CT, TJK, PC and SPB performed sample preparation and analyte measurement processes. RJH, TMM and TJK performed data analysis. TMM wrote the first draft of the paper and all authors provided input and approved the final manuscript.

Consent for publication
Not applicable.

Competing interests
The authors declare that they have no competing interests.

Author details
[1]Mercy Perinatal, Mercy Hospital for Women, Melbourne, VIC, Australia. [2]Department of Obstetrics and Gynaecology, University of Melbourne, Melbourne, VIC, Australia. [3]Translational Obstetrics Group, University of Melbourne, Melbourne, VIC, Australia. [4]Department of Laboratory Services, Royal Children's Hospital, Melbourne, VIC, Australia. [5]Department of Maternal-Fetal Medicine, Royal Women's Hospital, Melbourne, VIC, Australia.

References
1. Flenady V, Koopmans L, Middleton P, Froen JF, Smith GC, Gibbons K, Coory M, Gordon A, Ellwood D, McIntyre HD, et al. Major risk factors for stillbirth in high-income countries: a systematic review and meta-analysis. Lancet. 2011; 377:1331–40.
2. Gardosi J, Madurasinghe V, Williams M, Malik A, Francis A. Maternal and fetal risk factors for stillbirth: population based study. BMJ. 2013;346:f108.
3. Vashevnik S, Walker S, Permezel M. Stillbirths and neonatal deaths in appropriate, small and large birthweight for gestational age fetuses. Aust N Z J Obstet Gynaecol. 2007;47:302–6.
4. Mendez-Figueroa H, Truong VT, Pedroza C, Khan AM, Chauhan SP. Small-for-gestational-age infants among uncomplicated pregnancies at term: a secondary analysis of 9 maternal-fetal medicine units network studies. Am J Obstet Gynecol. 2016;215:628.e621–7.
5. Pattinson R, Kerber K, Buchmann E, Friberg IK, Belizan M, Lansky S, Weissman E, Mathai M, Rudan I, Walker N, Lawn JE. Stillbirths: how can health systems deliver for mothers and babies? Lancet. 2011;377:1610–23.
6. Sparks TN, Cheng YW, McLaughlin B, Esakoff TF, Caughey AB. Fundal height: a useful screening tool for fetal growth? J Matern Fetal Neonatal Med. 2011;24:708–12.
7. Hargreaves K, Cameron M, Edwards H, Gray R, Deane K. Is the use of symphysis-fundal height measurement and ultrasound examination effective in detecting small or large fetuses? J Obstet Gynaecol. 2011;31:380–3.
8. Goto E. Prediction of low birthweight and small for gestational age from symphysis-fundal height mainly in developing countries: a meta-analysis. J Epidemiol Community Health. 2013;67:999–1005.
9. Sovio U, White IR, Dacey A, Pasupathy D, Smith GC. Screening for fetal growth restriction with universal third trimester ultrasonography in nulliparous women in the pregnancy outcome prediction (POP) study: a prospective cohort study. Lancet. 2015;386:2089–97.
10. Kwiatkowski S, Dolegowska B, Kwiatkowska E, Rzepka R, Marczuk N, Loj B, Torbe A. Maternal endothelial damage as a disorder shared by early preeclampsia, late preeclampsia and intrauterine growth restriction. J Perinat Med. 2016;
11. Crispi F, Dominguez C, Llurba E, Martin-Gallan P, Cabero L, Gratacos E. Placental angiogenic growth factors and uterine artery Doppler findings for characterization of different subsets in preeclampsia and in isolated intrauterine growth restriction. Am J Obstet Gynecol. 2006;195:201–7.
12. Romero R, Nien JK, Espinoza J, Todem D, Fu W, Chung H, Kusanovic JP, Gotsch F, Erez O, Mazaki-Tovi S, et al. A longitudinal study of angiogenic (placental growth factor) and anti-angiogenic (soluble endoglin and soluble vascular endothelial growth factor receptor-1) factors in normal pregnancy and patients destined to develop preeclampsia and deliver a small for gestational age neonate. J Matern Fetal Neonatal Med. 2008;21:9–23.
13. Villa PM, Hamalainen E, Maki A, Raikkonen K, Pesonen AK, Taipale P, Kajantie E, Laivuori H. Vasoactive agents for the prediction of early- and late-onset preeclampsia in a high-risk cohort. BMC Pregnancy Childbirth. 2013;13:110.
14. Verlohren S, Herraiz I, Lapaire O, Schlembach D, Moertl M, Zeisler H, Calda P, Holzgreve W, Galindo A, Engels T, et al. The sFlt-1/PlGF ratio in different types of hypertensive pregnancy disorders and its prognostic potential in preeclamptic patients. Am J Obstet Gynecol. 2012;206(58):e51–8.
15. Zeisler H, Llurba E, Chantraine F, Vatish M, Staff AC, Sennstrom M, Olovsson M, Brennecke SP, Stepan H, Allegranza D, et al. Predictive value of the sFlt-1:PlGF ratio in women with suspected preeclampsia. N Engl J Med. 2016;374:13–22.
16. Sovio U, Gaccioli F, Cook E, Hund M, Charnock-Jones DS, Smith GC. Prediction of preeclampsia using the soluble fms-like tyrosine kinase 1 to placental growth factor ratio: a prospective cohort study of unselected nulliparous women. Hypertension. 2017;69:731–8.
17. Schoofs K, Grittner U, Engels T, Pape J, Denk B, Henrich W, Verlohren S. The importance of repeated measurements of the sFlt-1/PlGF ratio for the prediction of preeclampsia and intrauterine growth restriction. J Perinat Med. 2014;42:61–8.
18. Triunfo S, Parra-Saavedra M, Rodriguez-Sureda V, Crovetto F, Dominguez C, Gratacos E, Figueras F. Angiogenic factors and Doppler evaluation in normally growing fetuses at routine third-trimester scan: prediction of subsequent low birth weight. Fetal Diagn Ther. 2016;40:13–20.
19. Customised Weight Centile Calculator-GROW-Centile v.5.12/6.2. http://www.gestation.net/.
20. The American College of Obstetricians and Gynecaologists. Task force on hypertension in pregnancy. Hypertension in pregnancy. Pp. 100. Acog.Org; 2013. p. 100.
21. van Zaane B, Vergouwe Y, Donders AR, Moons KG. Comparison of approaches to estimate confidence intervals of post-test probabilities of diagnostic test results in a nested case-control study. BMC Med Res Methodol. 2012;12:166.
22. The Royal College of Obstetricians and Gynaecologists. The investigation and management of the small-for-gestational-age fetus. In: RCOG Green-top Guideline No 31, 2nd edition; 2013.
23. Gordijn SJ, Beune IM, Thilaganathan B, Papageorghiou A, Baschat AA, Baker PN, Silver RM, Wynia K, Ganzevoort W. Consensus definition of fetal growth restriction: a Delphi procedure. Ultrasound Obstet Gynecol. 2016;48:333–9.
24. Rajakumar A, Jeyabalan A, Markovic N, Ness R, Gilmour C, Conrad KP. Placental HIF-1 alpha, HIF-2 alpha, membrane and soluble VEGF receptor-1 proteins are not increased in normotensive pregnancies complicated by late-onset intrauterine growth restriction. Am J Physiol Regul Integr Comp Physiol. 2007;293:R766–74.
25. Miranda J, Rodriguez-Lopez M, Triunfo S, Sairanen M, Kouru H, Parra-Saavedra M, Crovetto F, Figueras F, Crispi F, Gratacos E. Prediction of fetal growth restriction using estimated fetal weight versus a combined screening model at 32-36 weeks of gestation. Ultrasound Obstet Gynecol. 2016;
26. Crovetto F, Triunfo S, Crispi F, Rodriguez-Sureda V, Roma E, Dominguez C, Gratacos E, Figueras F. First-trimester screening with specific algorithms for early- and late-onset fetal growth restriction. Ultrasound Obstet Gynecol. 2016;48:340–8.
27. Triunfo S, Lobmaier S, Parra-Saavedra M, Crovetto F, Peguero A, Nadal A, Gratacos E, Figueras F. Angiogenic factors at diagnosis of late-onset small-for-gestational age and histological placental underperfusion. Placenta. 2014;35:398–403.
28. Margossian A, Boisson-Gaudin C, Subtil F, Rudigoz RC, Dubernard G, Allias F, Huissoud C. Intra-uterine growth restriction impact on maternal serum concentration of PlGF (placental growth factor): a case control study. Gynecol Obstet Fertil. 2016;44:23–8.
29. Herraiz I, Droge LA, Gomez-Montes E, Henrich W, Galindo A, Verlohren S. Characterization of the soluble fms-like tyrosine kinase-1 to placental growth factor ratio in pregnancies complicated by fetal growth restriction. Obstet Gynecol. 2014;124:265–73.
30. Benton SJ, McCowan LM, Heazell AE, Grynspan D, Hutcheon JA, Senger C, Burke O, Chan Y, Harding JE, Yockell-Lelievre J, et al. Placental growth factor as a marker of fetal growth restriction caused by placental dysfunction. Placenta. 2016;42:1–8.
31. Wallner W, Sengenberger R, Strick R, Strissel PL, Meurer B, Beckmann MW, Schlembach D. Angiogenic growth factors in maternal and fetal serum in pregnancies complicated by intrauterine growth restriction. Clin Sci (Lond). 2007;112:51–7.

32. Borras D, Perales-Puchalt A, Ruiz Sacedon N, Perales A. Angiogenic growth factors in maternal and fetal serum in pregnancies complicated with intrauterine growth restriction. J Obstet Gynaecol. 2014;34:218–20.

33. Semczuk-Sikora A, Krzyzanowski A, Stachowicz N, Robak J, Kraczkowski J, Kwiatek M, Semczuk M. Maternal serum concentration of angiogenic factors: PlGF, VEGF and VEGFR-1 and placental volume in pregnancies complicated by intrauterine growth restriction. Ginekol Pol. 2007;78:783–6.

34. Kuhnel E, Kleff V, Stojanovska V, Kaiser S, Waldschutz R, Herse F, Plosch T, Winterhager E, Gellhaus A. Placental-specific overexpression of sFlt-1 alters trophoblast differentiation and nutrient transporter expression in an IUGR mouse model. J Cell Biochem. 2016;

35. Zamarian AC, Araujo Junior E, Daher S, Rolo LC, Moron AF, Nardozza LM. Evaluation of biochemical markers combined with uterine artery Doppler parameters in fetuses with growth restriction: a case-control study. Arch Gynecol Obstet. 2016;294:715–23.

36. Fadigas C, Peeva G, Mendez O, Poon LC, Nicolaides KH. Prediction of small-for-gestational-age neonates: screening by placental growth factor and soluble fms-like tyrosine kinase-1 at 35-37 weeks. Ultrasound Obstet Gynecol. 2015;46:191–7.

37. Smith GC, Crossley JA, Aitken DA, Jenkins N, Lyall F, Cameron AD, Connor JM, Dobbie R. Circulating angiogenic factors in early pregnancy and the risk of preeclampsia, intrauterine growth restriction, spontaneous preterm birth, and stillbirth. Obstet Gynecol. 2007;109:1316–24.

38. Crispi F, Llurba E, Dominguez C, Martin-Gallan P, Cabero L, Gratacos E. Predictive value of angiogenic factors and uterine artery Doppler for early-versus late-onset pre-eclampsia and intrauterine growth restriction. Ultrasound Obstet Gynecol. 2008;31:303–9.

39. Schlembach D, Wallner W, Sengenberger R, Stiegler E, Mortl M, Beckmann MW, Lang U. Angiogenic growth factor levels in maternal and fetal blood: correlation with Doppler ultrasound parameters in pregnancies complicated by pre-eclampsia and intrauterine growth restriction. Ultrasound Obstet Gynecol. 2007;29:407–13.

40. Gaccioli F, Sovio U, Cook E, Hund M, Charnock-Jones DS, Smith GCS. Screening for fetal growth restriction using ultrasound and the sFLT1/PlGF ratio in nulliparous women: a prospective cohort study. The Lancet Child & Adolescent Health. 2018;2:569–81.

41. Hernandez-Diaz S, Toh S, Cnattingius S. Risk of pre-eclampsia in first and subsequent pregnancies: prospective cohort study. Bmj. 2009;338:b2255.

42. Ananth CV, Keyes KM, Wapner RJ. Pre-eclampsia rates in the United States, 1980-2010: age-period-cohort analysis. Bmj. 2013;347:f6564.

43. Duley L. The global impact of pre-eclampsia and eclampsia. Semin Perinatol. 2009;33:130–7.

44. Gardosi J, Francis A. Adverse pregnancy outcome and association with small for gestational age birthweight by customized and population-based percentiles. Am J Obstet Gynecol. 2009;201(28):e21–8.

17

Ten years of simulation-based shoulder dystocia training-impact on obstetric outcome, clinical management, staff confidence, and the pedagogical practice

Johanna Dahlberg[1], Marie Nelson[2], Madeleine Abrandt Dahlgren[3] and Marie Blomberg[1,2*]

Abstract

Background: To assess the impact of 10 years of simulation-based shoulder dystocia training on clinical outcomes, staff confidence, management, and to scrutinize the characteristics of the pedagogical practice of the simulation training.

Methods: In 2008, a simulation-based team-training program (PROBE) was introduced at a medium sized delivery unit in Linköping, Sweden. Data concerning maternal characteristics, management, and obstetric outcomes was compared between three groups; prePROBE (before PROBE was introduced, 2004–2007), early postPROBE (2008–2011) and late postPROBE (2012–2015). Staff responded to an electronic questionnaire, which included questions about self-confidence and perceived sense of security in acute obstetrical situations. Empirical data from the pedagogical practice was gathered through observational field notes of video-recordings of maternity care teams participating in simulation exercises and was further analyzed using collaborative video analysis.

Results: The number of diagnosed shoulder dystocia increased from 0.9/1000 prePROBE to 1.8 and 2.5/1000 postPROBE. There were no differences in maternal characteristics between the groups. The rate of brachial plexus injuries in deliveries complicated with shoulder dystocia was 73% prePROBE compared to 17% in the late postPROBE group ($p > 0.05$). The dominant maneuver to solve the shoulder dystocia changed from posterior arm extraction to internal rotation of the anterior shoulder between the pre and postPROBE groups. The staff questionnaire showed how the majority of the staff (48–62%) felt more confident when handling a shoulder dystocia after PROBE training. A model of facilitating relational reflection adopted seems to provide ways of keeping the collaboration and learning in the interprofessional team clearly focused.

Conclusions: To introduce and sustain a shoulder dystocia training program for delivery staff improved clinical outcome. The impaired management and outcome of this rare, emergent and unexpectedly event might be explained by the learning effect in the debriefing model, clearly focused on the team and related to daily clinical practice.

Keywords: Team training, Simulation, Debriefing, Shoulder dystocia, Brachial plexus injury

* Correspondence: marie.blomberg@regionostergotland.se
[1]Department of Clinical and Experimental Medicine, Linköping University, Linköping, Sweden
[2]Department of Obstetrics and Gynecology, Linköping University, Linköping, Sweden
Full list of author information is available at the end of the article

Background

Emergent obstetrical events are rare but will always occur. It is critical for staff to be well trained and coordinated and confident when a complication appears, even when it happens so seldom that staff members will not gain experience by frequent clinical work. One way to tackle the dilemma is to introduce different types of skills and simulation training programs for the staff team. Research evidence supports that team training and simulation exercises improve technical skills, team communication, coordination, and documentation [1–3]. It is also well described how staff confidence increases after team-based obstetric skills and simulation exercises [4–6]. When it comes to improved obstetric and neonatal outcomes, only a small percentage of reports primarily addresses clinical outcomes and results are inconsistent [7]. One multicenter randomized control trial from the Netherlands showed how a one-day, off-site, simulation-based team training did not reduce obstetric complications (low Apgar score, severe postpartum hemorrhage, trauma due to shoulder dystocia, eclampsia, hypoxic ischemic encephalopathy) [8]. In contrast an Australian retrospective cohort study reported an overall improvement in some clinical outcomes (Apgar at 1 minute, umbilical cord lactate, and average length of infant's stay in clinic) after a single day of training for the trainers at eight different maternity units [9]. Crofts et al. found significant benefits of a long-term multiprofessional 1-day training course with improvements in clinical outcomes, including the prevalence of brachial plexus injury due to shoulder dystocia [10]. Comparable results concerning a decrease in obstetric brachial plexus injury was found after introduction of a shoulder dystocia training protocol [11, 12]. Others could not show a beneficial effect on the number of children injured due to shoulder dystocia after introducing simulation-based team training [13, 14].

When reflecting on the diverse picture of the impact of simulation training on clinical outcome previous studies share the fact that they do not provide detailed information of contextual factors and how the training was performed. This makes it difficult to compare and understand what pedagogical arrangements that support improvement of clinical outcomes. In general, simulation training traditionally follows a pedagogical model comprising three phases. In the introductory briefing phase, the participants are introduced to the scenario and receive information about the situation they are going to encounter as they start the simulation. The following phase is the practical enactments of the simulation, where the team members act in their professional role in collaboration to take care of the patient in the emerging situation. The final phase is the debriefing where the process and outcomes of the simulated scenario is discussed [15]. From a learning perspective, debriefing sessions are considered central for the participants' learning and provide the learner with the opportunity to reflect their understanding of the course of the scenario and their actions and interactions in the team [16]. However, the achieved level of reflection is interconnected with the questions posed by the facilitator and it is a challenging task for the instructor to facilitate reflection at a deep level in the participants [17]. It is reasonable to assume that different approaches to pedagogy in simulation also might influence clinical outcomes differently.

The aims of the present study were to evaluate the impact of 10 years of simulation-based shoulder dystocia training on clinical outcomes for the mother and the infant, on staff confidence, on management in the delivery room, and to scrutinize the characteristics of the pedagogical practice of the simulation training.

Methods

The present study applies a mixed method approach, combining quantitative obstetric outcome data with qualitative analyses of video-recorded simulation based training sessions. The use of a mixed methods research approach was claimed to gain a deeper and broader understanding than using only one research design, and to allow for contextualizing information that might provide richer insights into the phenomenon under study [18].

In a mixed methods approach, quantitative and qualitative data can be integrated through different study designs, methods and interpretations [19]. In the present study, an explanatory sequential design was applied, meaning that the researchers first collected and analyzed the quantitative data, and these data then informed the qualitative data collection and analysis. In our findings, we are presenting the quantitative and qualitative data in different but contiguous sections, in an attempt at integrating clinical outcomes with contextual factors and thereby develop a complementary picture, that examine process experiences along with outcomes [20].

The simulation program

In 2008, a simulation-based team-training program, Practical obstetric team-training (PROBE), was introduced in the delivery ward at the University Hospital, Linköping, Sweden. The objectives were to improve obstetric emergency skills and develop interprofessional teamwork, thus promoting better patient outcome. Participation in PROBE was mandatory for obstetricians, midwifes and nurse assistants who worked at the delivery ward. Participants were scheduled during working hours for simulation exercises at an interval of 1.5 years. To cover the need of staff's regular training, PROBE was organized six times each year. The PROBE sessions took place at the clinical training center, Clinicum, at the

University Hospital, a simulation center equipped with an obstetric skills laboratory. Each team session was scheduled for 3 hours, including two simulation scenarios and one practical skills training station. During the whole study period, PROBE included a 40-min shoulder dystocia scenario. Obstetric emergencies were simulated using actors, usually instructors, and/or mannequins, depending on the scenario.

All participants were prepared in advance by individually studying a theoretical management course specific for the complications to be trained. In each simulation, staff members worked in maternity care teams of one or two midwifes, one doctor, and one nurse assistant so that the simulations would be as realistic as possible.

The PROBE program is based on clinical skills suggested by Advanced Life Support in Obstetrics (ALSO®), but has been further developed since PROBE also had focus on team work and communication. Each scenario was led by certified and experienced instructors, both midwifes and obstetricians, who had participated in ALSO® training courses [21]. The aim of the simulation exercises was for the participants to recognize an emergency and use the subsequent standardized management methods and procedures established in the obstetric department's clinical guidelines. The mnemonic to remember in managing shoulder dystocia was HELPERR (H—call for Help, E—consider Episiotomy, Legs—McRobert's maneuver, Pressure—Suprapubic pressure externally, Enter—Enter the vagina using internal pressure to reduce impacted shoulder, finally using a Wood's screw maneuver to bring the shoulders into oblique diameter and 180 degrees rotation, and, if necessary, Remove—the posterior arm. Finally, the last R—Rotate the patient to her hands and knees.)

Instructors observed the team and made notes during the whole simulation. Immediately after each scenario, the team along with the instructors reflected upon how the team had performed. The reflection consisted of three parts: first, everyone reconfirmed what happened chronologically, thereafter everyone stated what they did well, and, finally, everyone summarized what they had learned and would bring to clinical practice. Questions and the notes of the instructor were used to support the discussion.

Quantitative data collection and statistics

To identify deliveries complicated with shoulder dystocia, all medical records with the ICD-10 diagnosis O66.0, obstructed labor due to shoulder dystocia, were extracted from the hospitals digital birth- and maternity care registration system Obstetrix® over the study period 2004–2015. Data were divided into three groups; prePROBE (before PROBE was introduced, 2004–2007), early postPROBE (2008–2011) and late postPROBE (2012–

2015). Data concerning maternal characteristics, management at delivery, and obstetric and neonatal clinical outcomes were collected and compared between the prePROBE and the two postPROBE groups. Data collected were maternal age, parity, body mass index (BMI), incidence of diabetes mellitus, gestational weight gain (defined as maternal weight at delivery minus maternal weight at booking gestational week 8–10), gestational age at delivery, if labor was induced, if contractions were augmented with oxytocin, delivery method (normal vaginal delivery or vacuum extraction), and the prevalence of acute anal sphincter injury. Additional management variables at delivery were extracted, when the shoulder dystocia was confirmed, according to HELPPER; whether oxytocin infusion was stopped, if internal rotation of the anterior shoulder was performed, and/or if posterior arm extraction was done before the delivery.

Three times during the postPROBE period (year 2011, 2013 and 2016) staff who had attended PROBE-sessions responded to an electronic questionnaire (Additional file 1), which included questions about self-confidence and perceived sense of security in acute obstetrical situations, specifically obstetric emergency situations including shoulder dystocia trained at PROBE. Only staff members who had attended PROBE received the questionnaire.

Continuous variables are presented as mean value and standard error of the mean (SEM). Means in the three groups were compared using an analysis of variance, and a p-value for similarity was given. Categorical variables are presented as numbers and frequencies. Group differences between prePROBE and postPROBE groups were for categorical variables analyzed by Fischer exact test using StatXact, Cytel software corp.

Qualitative data collection and analysis

For the purpose of this study, three maternity care teams participating in simulation exercises according to PROBE were video-recorded, both during the simulation exercise and the debriefing session. Empirical data from the pedagogical practice was gathered through observational field notes of the three video-recordings. The recordings and field notes were analyzed by the authors using collaborative video analysis [22]. Individual field notes were compared and consensus was negotiated through a constant comparative analysis [23]. Focus for the analysis was how the team members reconstructed the course of communication, individual actions and interactions in the team during the debriefing of the scenario. The researchers each contributed different professional background in healthcare work and in education, specifically medical education.

The Regional Ethical Review Board in Linköping, Sweden approved this study (Dnr 2016/177–31).

Results

Quantitative data

During the study period 2004–2015, there were 33,853 births in total distributed equally over the years, meaning about 3000 births each year. The number of non-instrumental vaginal deliveries increased from 73.8 to 82.4%, while the frequency of caesarean deliveries decreased from 17.0 to 11.3% (Table1). These dramatic changes in obstetric clinical practice could be explained by implementation of a nine-item list for organizational and cultural change, where PROBE is one of the nine items [24]. Among the deliveries, there was a statistically significant increase of diagnosed shoulder dystocia between the prePROBE and the early and late postPROBE periods, 0.9/1000 deliveries prePROBE compared to 1.8 and 2.5/1000 postPROBE (Table 1).

There were no significant differences in maternal age, parity, BMI, gestational weight gain, or prevalence of diabetes mellitus type 1 between deliveries complicated with shoulder dystocia in prePROBE compared to the postPROBE groups (Table 2).

No significant differences were found concerning induction of labor and the use of oxytocin infusion between the prePROBE and the postPROBE groups (Table 3).

Fewer infants diagnosed with a shoulder dystocia were delivered instrumentally in the postPROBE group compared with the prePROBE group. The risk of anal sphincter injury was similar before and after the introduction of PROBE training.

No significant difference between the groups was observed concerning Apgar score or umbilical artery pH (Table 4).

There was a significant decrease of infants born with a brachial plexus injury, or fracture of the clavicle or humerus, after the staff had attended PROBE training (Table 4). The rate of brachial plexus injuries in deliveries complicated with shoulder dystocia was 73% prePROBE compared to 17% in the late postPROBE group (Table 4), which was a significant reduction. There were a couple of persistent brachial plexus injuries in each group at 6 months of age.

The documentation in the medical records concerning maneuvers used after diagnosis of shoulder dystocia was significantly improved after PROBE training. When a shoulder dystocia is confirmed, the oxytocin infusion (if present) should be stopped, as further uterine contractions aggravate the entrapment of the infant. The oxytocin infusion was stopped significantly more often postPROBE compared to prePROBE (Table 5).

Internal rotation of the anterior shoulder was used in 54% of the deliveries postPROBE compared to 9% prePROBE, a significant favor over time of this maneuver instead of posterior arm extraction.

The results of the staff questionnaire showed how the majority of the staff (48–62%) felt more confident when a shoulder dystocia occurred at the delivery unit after they had participated in PROBE training. The rest, 32–39%, answered that they had never experienced shoulder dystocia in clinical practice (Table 6). The response rate was between 68 and 78%.

Qualitative data

The collaborative video analysis showed that attention was drawn to how the facilitators/instructors support team reflections, and still supporting individual reflection for learning. All through the reflection, the experience from the simulation exercise was also related to clinical practice at the delivery unit. For instance, as an obstetrician stated "-Being summoned to a delivery room, not knowing what to expect, the need of communication and time to reflect on this information is crucial" Even if the team in the room already was aware of the next step, the obstetrician in charge has to consider different options based on information provided, before making final decisions and share this with the team.

Interestingly, as a first phase of the reflection, each of the team members was invited in sequence to describe when and how they acted and interacted during the scenario. The emerging narrative was told from each individual perspective, but grew into a web as all individuals in the team also included how they related to each other, building the bigger picture in their narrative. The instructor utilized the notes taken during the observation

Table 1 The obstetric context during the study period, including all deliveries

	PrePROBE (2004–2007)	Early postPROBE (2008–2011)	Late postPROBE (2012–2015)	p-value
Number of deliveries	11,064	11,122	11,667	
Induction of labor, n (%)	1248 (11.3)	1411 (12.7)	1781 (15.2)	< 0.001
Non-instrumental vaginal delivery, n (%)	8169 (73.8)	8785 (79.0)	9620 (82.4)	< 0.001
Cesarean section, n (%)	1881 (17.0)	1560 (14.0)	1322 (11.3)	< 0.001
Vacuum extraction, n (%)	1014 (9.2)	777 (7.0)	725 (6.2)	< 0.001
Anal sphincter injury, n (%)	401 (3.6)	286 (2.6)	278 (2.4)	< 0.001
Number of shoulder dystocia, n (per 1000 deliveries)	11 (1.0)	20 (1.8)	29 (2.5)	0.005

Table 2 Maternal and pregnancy characteristics in deliveries complicated with shoulder dystocia

	PrePROBE (2004–2007) $n = 11$	Early postPROBE (2008–2011) $n = 20$	Late postPROBE (2012–2015) $n = 29$	p-value
Maternal age, mean (SEM)	29.8 (1.64)	31.9 (1.28)	30.4 (1.23)	0.60
Primiparous, n (%)	5 (45)	9 (45)	10 (34)	0.45
BMI, mean (SEM)	27.8 (1.64)	27.7 (1.39)	27.7 (1.10)	0.99
Diabetes mellitus type 1, n (%)	3 (27)	1 (5)	3 (10)	0.27
Gestational weight gain (kg), mean (SEM)	13.0 (1.50)	15.2 (1.19)	14.8 (1.22)	0.49
Gestational age at delivery (days), mean (SEM)	278 (2.15)	285 (1.84)	282 (1.60)	0.15

BMI Body Mass Index
SEM Standard error of the mean

of the simulation exercise to recall and describe a particular sequence of events, in which every single activity was integrated. This thorough recapitulation made the team aware of every step in the process and every individual confident to speak up and contribute to the collective narrative. The team reflections were also guided and facilitated by probing questions that recalled the emerging collaboration and actions, such as "In what sequence did things happen?", "Do everyone agree to this description?", "What help did you need?", "What happened when you arrived?", or "Who decided what to do next?". One example is when the obstetrician emphasized the value of the report from the coordinating midwife, and subsequently how the team agreed on the next action, and finally who would deliver the child.

In the second phase of the reflection, the instructor supported the identification of what each member did well and how this contributed to the teamwork. This is a technique that is commonly used in simulation-based training, but the typical feature of this phase in this case is that the instructors were building confidence in the participants through acknowledging that appreciating one's own actions as knowing in practice that can be difficult to verbalize. One example is when the importance and value of continuous documentation of the process was emphasized when the actions of the assisting nurse were discussed as being responsible for documentation and the technical support. Confidence building was also discernible in relation to the performance of the whole team; e.g., when the two midwifes in the scenario discussed the value of communication to facilitate the activities of the team. The instructor emphasized

and appreciated this by verbalizing how difficult can be for the whole team to see how they perform together.

Finally, each member of the team were invited to express personal insights that they identified as good procedures or improvements intended to be utilized in everyday practice. These statements were formulated individually and spontaneously and not imposed by the instructor or other team members. In parallel, during the debriefing, a discussion about medical and caring issues revealed deepened and insightful reflections. One example is an awareness of the need to include the woman in labor in the progress of the delivery, so that a sense of a collaborative effort, "We are doing this together" could be communicated, as well as the importance of communication to create a sense of security for the parents to be. This way, the debriefing sessions also addressed the professional's experiences from every day practice, which further strengthened the importance and sense of teamwork.

Discussion

When a delivery is progressing normally, the mother and the midwife create a team. However, if complications occur, the team suddenly grows in number and failure in communication or management could have devastating consequences. This cohort study is comparing clinical outcomes management, staff confidence before and after shoulder dystocia simulations were introduced. The results showed a significant decrease in infants born with a brachial plexus injury after the staff had attended PROBE training. The dominant maneuver to solve the shoulder dystocia changed from posterior

Table 3 Obstetric interventions and complications in deliveries with diagnosed shoulder dystocia

	PrePROBE (2004–2007) $n = 11$	Early postPROBE (2008–2011) $n = 20$	Late postPROBE (2012–2015) $n = 29$	p-value
Induction of labor, n (%)	4 (36)	3 (15)	9 (31)	0.94
Labor arrest, n (%)	4 (36)	12 (60)	19 (66)	0.12
Oxytocin infusion, n (%)	9 (82)	14 (70)	22 (76)	0.85
Instrumental delivery, n (%)	6 (54)	7 (35)	5 (17)	0.03
Anal sphincter injury n (%)	2 (18)	5 (25)	5 (17)	0.80

Table 4 Infant outcomes in deliveries complicated with shoulder dystocia

	PrePROBE (2004–2007) n = 11	Early postPROBE (2008–2011) n = 20	Late postPROBE (2012–2015) n = 29	p-value
Umbilical artery pH, mean	7.17	7.20	7.20	
Apgar score < 4 at 1 min, n (%)	2 (18)	7 (35)	9 (31)	0.56
Apgar score < 7 at 5 min, n (%)	1 (9)	6 (30)	8 (27)	0.33
No brachial plexus injury or fracture, n (%)	2 (18)	10 (50)	20 (69)	0.005
Brachial plexus injury at birth, n (%)	8 (73)	8 (40)	5 (17)	0.001
Fractured clavicle, n (%)	1 (9)	2 (10)	2 (7)	0.76
Fractured humerus, n (%)	1 (9)	3 (15)	2 (7)	0.65
Early neonatal death	0	0	1	
Brachial plexus injury at 6 months follow up, n (%)	1 (9)	1 (5)	2 (7)	0.89

arm extraction to internal rotation of the anterior shoulder between the pre and postPROBE groups. In Crofts' study, posterior arm extraction still dominated after 12 years of training [10], a difference that could be explained by a training program without the hierarchy proposed by HELPPER.

The number of diagnosed shoulder dystocia increased, 0.9/1000 deliveries prePROBE compared with 1.8 and 2.5/1000 in the early and late postPROBE group, respectively. These results are in accordance with findings in the UK, where the proportion was higher but increased over time [10]. There were no differences between the groups concerning potential risk factors for shoulder dystocia such as primiparity, maternal BMI gestational weight gain and diabetes mellitus. During the study period, the number of vaginal deliveries at the unit increased markedly in favor of cesarean sections [24]. The induction rate also increased significantly. This means that a fair amount of women with labor arrest disorders, a well-known risk factor for shoulder dystocia, were delivered vaginally postPROBE compared to prePROBE. This might have contributed to the increased rate of shoulder dystocia. The decreased rate of brachial plexus injury postPROBE persist when relating this complication to all vaginal deliveries which speaks against a higher proportion of milder cases postPROBE. At 6 months follow up, the number of cases with persistent injury was low (one case versus two cases each period) making interpretation difficult. Similar

to the present study, no statistically significant reduction in brachial plexus injury at six or 12 months follow up was found in the UK study although numbers declined [10]. Results concerning effects of simulation training on brachial plexus injury at birth differ. In an American setting, the implementation of a shoulder dystocia training protocol significantly reduced obstetric brachial plexus injury [12]. A reduction in brachial plexus injury at birth was also found at a unit with regular multi-professional training on shoulder dystocia management [10]. A cluster randomized controlled trial performed in the Netherlands allocated 24 obstetric units to team training or not and no decreased rate of brachial plexus injury at birth was found in the intervention group [8]. The follow up time in that study was 1 year compared with 8 years in the present study, which might explain the diverting results.

No differences in Apgar score or umbilical artery values among shoulder dystocia cases could be found in the present study, which is in accordance with results presented by Crofts and co-workers [10]. In an Australian study, evaluating the introduction of practical obstetric multi- professional training, an improvement in Apgar score at 1 minute and a decrease in cord lactate was found among all infants born but there were no specific data on shoulder dystocia cases [9]. We also evaluated the rate of maternal complications in terms of anal sphincter injury associated with shoulder dystocia and found no differences between the pre and postPROBE

Table 5 Shoulder dystocia management before and after introduction of PROBE

	PrePROBE (2004–2007) n = 11	Early postPROBE (2008–2011) n = 20	Late postPROBE (2012–2015) n = 29	p-value
Management well documented, n	7	20	27	0.03
Stop of oxytocin infusion, n (%)	0/9 (0)	4/10 (40)	12/22 (54)	0.007
Internal rotation of the anterior shoulder, n (%)	1 (9)	8 (40)	15 (52)	0.06[a]
Posterior arm extraction performed, n (%)	6 (54)	12 (60)	13 (45)	
Data on maneuver missing	4	0	1	

[a]Internal rotation versus posterior arm extraction

Table 6 Questionnaire-based follow up of staff confidence after attending PROBE training

Year	Response rate	Do you feel more confident in your daily practice managing an *obstetric emergency situation* after PROBE training?	Do you feel more confident in your daily practice managing a *shoulder dystocia* after PROBE training?		
	N/total (%)	Yes, n (%)	Yes, n (%)	No, n (%)	I have never been in the situation, n (%)
2011	52/67 (78)	48 (94)	26 (51)	5 (10)	20 (39)
2013	62/91 (68)	55 (95)	28 (48)	9 (15)	22 (37)
2016	63/90 (70)	59 (94)	39 (62)	4 (6)	20 (32)

groups. This is in accordance with results from van de Ven et al. who found no difference in risk of anal sphincter injury before and after introducing simulation-based team training [14].

The improved clinical results could apart from a change in shoulder dystocia management, be explained by an increased sense of confidence among staff, feeling safer in handling shoulder dystocia after participation in mandatory reoccurring PROBE training sessions. Another explanation of improvement might be found in the pedagogical practice during the simulation and debriefing session. Observation of how the instructors made use of notetaking during the simulation for commenting and analyzing of the interactions showed how the instructors facilitated individual professional reflections to be relationally linked to the work of the whole team during the simulation exercise. Each performance became in that way connected to a larger context than the individual perspective. The expansion to a larger context was accomplished through instructors commenting on an array of relational interactions, such as between the woman in labor and professionals, in relation to material arrangements of the delivery room, and how these interactions contributed to the delivery process. By keeping a relational focus of the actions in the scenario, the procedure of the whole team became outlined and highlighted against the backdrop of each individual participant. Nyström et al. identified recently two distinct patterns of debriefing sessions, one protocol-based and one more loosely structured collegial conversation [22]. However, neither the imposed structure of the debriefing, nor the lack of structure, ensured that interprofessional collaboration emerged as a salient topic for reflection. The model of facilitating relational reflection adopted in this study seem to provide ways of keeping the collaboration and learning in the interprofessional team clearly focused, and might be one of the factors leading to a successful outcome of simulation as a competence development activity over time.

This study has certain strengths and limitations. A strength is the long-term follow up of a constantly recurring obligatory simulation-based team-training program. Another strength is the different angles from which the effect of the program has been evaluated,

including maternal and infant outcome data, management data, staff confidence follow up and scrutinizing the scenario debriefing process from a learning perspective. Available data on deliveries over all made it possible to present rates of shoulder dystocia as well as brachial plexus injury related to number of births, both overall and among vaginal deliveries before and after introduction of PROBE. There has been no change in the management of shoulder dystocia (HELPERR) after the introduction of PROBE and the shoulder dystocia scenario has been part of every PROBE training event since it started. A putative important factor of adherence to PROBE training might have been that midwifes and doctors were scheduled for PROBE immediately from introduction without having any other tasks planned for these 3 hours as an integral part of their clinical work.

Conclusions

In conclusion this study showed that to introduce and sustain a shoulder dystocia training program for delivery staff increase the number of infants born after a diagnosed shoulder dystocia without a brachial plexus injury or fracture of the clavicle or humerus. The staff confidence on handling shoulder dystocia in daily clinical care increased after PROBE training. The analysis of the qualitative data showed that the main learning effect in the debriefing model used was that discussions concerned the team and related to daily clinical practice.

Abbreviations

ALSO®: Advanced Life Support in Obstetrics; BMI: Body mass index; HELPERR: H— call for Help, E—consider Episiotomy, Legs—McRobert's maneuver, Pressure—Suprapubic pressure externally, Enter—Enter the vagina using internal pressure to reduce impacted shoulder, finally using a Wood's screw maneuver to bring the shoulders into oblique diameter and 180 degrees rotation, and, if necessary, Remove—the posterior arm and the last R—Rotate the patient to her hands and knees; PROBE: Practical Obstetric team-training; SEM: Standard error of the mean

Funding

This study was supported by an unrestricted grant from the Östergötland County Council. The funding body had no involvement in the design of the study, the data collection, the analyses and interpretation or the manuscript preparation.

Authors' contributions

MB designed the study, interpreted the data, performed the statistical calculations and wrote the manuscript. MN collected all data concerning clinical management and outcome and staff confidence and wrote the manuscript. JD and MD performed the debriefing analyses from a pedagogical perspective and wrote the manuscript. All authors read and approved the final manuscript.

Competing interests

The authors declare that they have no competing interests.

Author details

[1]Department of Clinical and Experimental Medicine, Linköping University, Linköping, Sweden. [2]Department of Obstetrics and Gynecology, Linköping University, Linköping, Sweden. [3]Department of Medicine and Health Sciences, Linköping University, Linköping, Sweden.

References

1. Merién AE, van de Ven J, Mol BW, Houterman S, Oei SG. Multidisciplinary team training in a simulation setting for acute obstetric emergencies: a systematic review. Obstet Gynecol. 2010;115:1021–31.
2. Smith S. Team training and institutional protocols to prevent shoulder dystocia complications. Clin Obstet Gynecol. 2016;59:830–40.
3. Mannella P, Palla G, Cuttano A, Boldrini A, Simoncini T. Effect of high-fidelity shoulder dystocia simulation on emergency obstetric skills and crew resource management skills among residents. Int J Gynaecol Obstet. 2016; 135:338–42.
4. Sørensen JL, Løkkegaard E, Johansen M, Ringsted C, Kreiner S, McAleer S. The implementation and evaluation of a mandatory multi-professional obstetric skills training program. Acta Obstet Gynecol Scand. 2009;88: 1107–17.
5. Bullough AS, Wagner S, Boland T, Waters TP, Kim K, Adams W. Obstetric team simulation program challenges. J Clin Anesth. 2016;35:564–70.
6. Zech A, Gross B, Jasper-Birzele C, Jeschke K, Kieber T, Lauterberg J, et al. Evaluation of simparteam - a needs-orientated team training format for obstetrics and neonatology. J Perinat Med. 2017;45:333–41.
7. Satin AJ. Simulation in obstetrics. Obstet Gynecol. 2018;132:199–209.
8. Fransen AF, van de Ven J, Schuit E, van Tetering A, Mol BW, Oei SG. Simulation-based team training for multi-professional obstetric care teams to improve patient outcome: a multicentre, cluster randomised controlled trial. BJOG. 2017;124:641–50.
9. Shoushtarian M, Barnett M, McMahon F, Ferris J. Impact of introducing practical obstetric multi-professional training (PROMPT) into maternity units in Victoria, Australia. BJOG. 2014;121:1710–8.
10. Crofts JF, Lenguerrand E, Bentham GL, Tawfik S, Claireaux HA, Odd D, et al. Prevention of brachial plexus injury-12 years of shoulder dystocia training: an interrupted time-series study. BJOG. 2016;123:111–8.
11. Grobman WA, Miller D, Burke C, Hornbogen A, Tam K, Costello R. Outcomes associated with introduction of a shoulder dystocia protocol. Am J Obstet Gynecol. 2011;205:513–7.
12. Inglis SR, Feier N, Chetiyaar JB, Naylor MH, Sumersille M, Cervellione KL, et al. Effects of shoulder dystocia training on the incidence of brachial plexus injury. Am J Obstet Gynecol. 2011;204:322.
13. Walsh JM, Kandamany N, Ni Shuibhne N, Power H, Murphy JF, O'Herlihy C. Neonatal brachial plexus injury: comparison of incidence and antecedents between 2 decades. Am J Obstet Gynecol. 2011;204:324.
14. van de Ven J, van Deursen FJ, van Runnard Heimel PJ, Mol BW, Oei SG. Effectiveness of team training in managing shoulder dystocia: a retrospective study. J Matern Fetal Neonatal Med. 2016;29:3167–71.
15. Dieckmann P, Molin Friis S, Lippert A, Ostergaard D. The art and science of debriefing in simulation: ideal and practice. Med Teach. 2009;31:e287–94.
16. Jeffries PR, Dreifuerst KT, Aschenbrenner DS, Adamson KA, Schram AP. Clinical simulations in nursing education: overview, essentials, and the evidence. In: Oermann MH, editor. Teaching in nursing and role of the educator: the complete guide to best practice in teaching, evaluation, and curriculum development. New York, NY, US: Springer Publishing Co; 2015. p. 83–101.
17. Husebø D, Dieckmann P, Rystedt H, Friberg F. The relationship between facilitators' questions and the level of reflection in the post-simulation debriefing. Simul Healthc. 2013;8:135–42.
18. Hurmerinta-Peltomaki L, Nummela N. Mixed methods in international business research: a value-added perspective. Manag Int Rev. 2006;46: 439–59.
19. Fetters MD, Curry LA, Creswell JW. Achieving integration in mixed methods designs-principles and practices. Health Serv Res. 2013;48:2134–56.
20. Klassen A, Creswell J, Plano Clark V, Smith K, Meissner H. Best practices in mixed methods for quality of life research. Qual Life Res. 2012;21:377–80.
21. Reynolds A, Ayres-de-Campos D, Lobo M. Self-perceived impact of simulation-based training on the management of real-life obstetrical emergencies. Eur J Obstet Gynecol Reprod Biol. 2011;159:72–6.
22. Nyström S, Dahlberg J, Edelbring S, Hult H, Abrandt Dahlgren M. Debriefing practices in interprofessional simulation with students: a sociomaterial perspective. BMC Med Educ. 2016;16:148.
23. Boeije HA. Purposeful approach to the constant comparative method in the analysis of qualitative interviews. Qual Quant. 2002;36:391–409.
24. Blomberg M. Avoiding the first cesarean section-results of structured organizational and cultural changes. Acta Obstet Gynecol Scand. 2016;95: 580–6.

18

Spontaneous haemorrhagic stroke complicating severe pre-eclampsia in pregnancy: a case report in a resource-limited setting in Cameroon

Paul Nkemtendong Tolefac[1,2*] , Nkemnji Standley Awungafac[1] and Jacqueline Ze Minkande[1]

Abstract

Background: Spontaneous intracerebral haemorrhage is a rare complication of preeclampsia during pregnancy associated with a high morbidity and mortality. Compared with the non-pregnant women stroke rates are relatively rare during pregnancy.

Case presentation: We report the case of a 32-year-old female Cameroonian gravida 4 para 3 who presented at 34 weeks of gestation with sudden onset of right sided hemiplegia associated with headache, blurred vision and a blood pressure of 182/126. Cerebral CT scan confirmed a left parietal spontaneous haemorrhage. Emergency caesarean delivery was done and the recovery uneventful.

Conclusion: This case highlights the importance of good neurological examination in pregnant women presenting with neurological symptoms as well as the place of multidisciplinary management in severe life threatening conditions.

Keywords: Haemorrhagic stroke, Pre-eclampsia, Pregnancy, Severe preeclampsia, Case report

Background

Stroke is a clinical syndrome of rapidly developing clinical signs of focal (or global) disturbance of cerebral function, lasting more than 24 h or leading to death, with no apparent cause other than vascular origin [1], whereas intracerebral haemorrhage which is a type of stroke refers to rapidly developing clinical signs of neurological dysfunction attributable to a focal collection of blood within the brain parenchyma or ventricular system that is not caused by trauma [2]. Stroke being one of the major cause of disability has a higher impact on the society.

Stroke is an extremely rare event during pregnancy with the incidence ranging from 10 to 34/100,000 deliveries [3]. A recently conducted cohort in England showed that compared to non-pregnant women, stroke rates are lower during the antepartum period, 9-fold higher in the early peripartum period and 3-fold higher

in the early postpartum period [4]. While the epidemiology of stroke in pregnancy in Africa and Cameroon remained largely unknown, the case fatality of stroke in Douala, Cameroon was estimated at 26.8% in a recent study by Mapoure et al [5].

The authors reports a case of a 32 year old female Cameroonian gravida 4 para 3 who presented at 34 weeks of gestation with sudden onset of right sided hemiplegia associated with headache, blurred vision and stage 2 hypertension. Cerebral (computed tomography) CT scan confirmed a left parietal spontaneous haemorrhage. Emergency caesarean delivery was done and the recovery uneventful. The aim of the case is to highlight the importance of rapid history and examination including neurological examination in pregnant women presenting with raised blood pressure. The authors adhered to the CARE guidelines/methodology for reporting case reports [6].

Case presentation

A 32 year old female Cameroonian gravida 4 para 3 at 34 weeks of gestation presented to the labour and

* Correspondence: ptolefac15@gmail.com
[1]Faculty of Medicine and Biomedical Sciences, University of Yaoundé 1, Yaoundé, Cameroon
[2]Mbalmayo District Hospita, Mbalmayo, Cameroon

delivery unit of Mbalmayo district hospital with 8 h history of severe generalized headache, expressive aphasia and right sided paralysis in an afebrile context. This was associated with blurred vision but no convulsions. There was no epigastric pain and no difficulty breathing and no history of trauma or fall. For this current pregnancy, antenatal care (ANC) was started at 18 weeks with a booking blood pressure of 100/70 mmHg. She did four ANCs and all were uneventful. During her routine four ANCs here blood pressure was always less than 140/90 mmHg and her urine dipsticks done during the four ANCs were all negative for proteinuria. She refused neurological symptoms such as headache during pregnancy. She has a history of gestational hypertension in her third pregnancy. There was no family history of chronic hypertension, diabetes and chronic kidney diseases. On examination she was afebrile with a blood pressure of 182/126 mmHg and pulse of 112beats/minute. Neurological examination revealed Glasgow coma score of 13/15, right sided hemiparesis and expressive Broca's aphasia, no signs of meningeal irritation. The abdomen was distended by a gravid uterus with a fundal height of 35 cm, foetus in a longitudinal lie and cephalic presentation. The cervix was long, posterior, soft and closed with a station of − 1. We had a working diagnosis of severe pre-eclampsia complicated by stroke. Shown on Table 1 are laboratory investigations done and their results.

An emergency obstetric ultrasound showed a life foetus with an estimated foetal weight of 2300 g at 33 weeks of gestation. Emergency cerebral non contrast-CT scan showed a 3.2 cm hyperdense region in the left parietal lobe with surrounding hypodensity due to clot retraction as shown on Fig. 1. Emergency management by

Table 1 Results of initial laboratory investigations

Investigation	Result	Reference value
Plasma glucose	5.3 mmol/L	3.9–6.1 mmol/L
Urea	1.2 mmol/L	2.0–7.1 mmol/L
Creatinine	70 µmol/L	50–110 µmol/L
Sodium	132 mEq/L	135-145 mEq/L
Potassium	3.8 mEq/L	3.5–5.5 mEq/L
Chloride	109 mEq/l	98-112 mEq/L
Alanine amino transferase (ALAT)	17 IU/L	10-40 IU/L
Aspartate amino transferase (ASAT)	16 IU/L	10-35 IU/L
Alkaline phosphatase	57 IU/L	36-92 IU/L
Urine dipstick for protein	3+	Negative
Haemoglobin level	11.8 g/dl	12 -16 g/dl
White cell count	9.800 cells / mm³	4.000–10.000 cells / mm³
Platelet count	160.000cells/mm³	150.000–400.000 cells / mm³

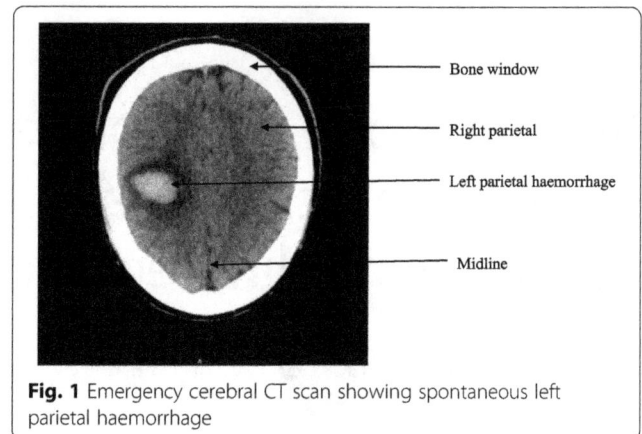

Fig. 1 Emergency cerebral CT scan showing spontaneous left parietal haemorrhage

the obstetrician consisted of MgSO4 using the Pritchard protocol [7], which consisted of 14 g loading dose then 5 g maintenance every 6 h until 24 h after caeserean section; bethamethasone 12 mg intramuscular and reduction of blood pressure with nicardipine 5 mg/h. Four hours later an emergency caesarean section was done by the obstetrician under spinal anaesthesia and it let to the extraction of a life female with APGAR 8 and 10 at the 1st and 5th minute respectively and weight 2200 g. The management after caesarean section consisted of hospitalization in the intensive care unit with nicardipine titrated in an electric syringe at 2.5 mg/hour, ceftriaxone 2 g intravenous, Paractamol 1 g 8 hourly, and ringers lactate 6 hourly for 24 h. Post-operative management was done by a multidisciplinary team including a neurologist, cardiologist, intensive care physician, obstetrician, neonatologist and physiotherapist. On postoperative day 2 she was transferred from the intensive care unit to the maternity where she spends five additional days on nicardipine slow release 50 mg 12 hourly and paracetamol 1 g 8hourly and was later release after the ten days on nicardipine 50 mg daily and daily physiotherapy. Six weeks during routine postpartum visit the blood pressure was normal and patient was no longer aphasic and shet has regained the muscle strength partially. The baby was hospitalised in the neonatal unit for 10 days and discharged alongside the mother.

Discussion and conclusions
Recent studies have demonstrated that stroke is a rare event during pregnancy with incidence relatively lower in the antepartum period compared to non-pregnant women [5]. In one study risk factors of stroke during pregnancy were found to include: sociodemographic factors such as age ≥ 35 years($R = 2.2$, 95% CI = 1.2–2.2), African-American(OR = 1.5, 95% CI = 1.2–1.9); medical and obstetric determinants such as migraine headache (OR = 16.9, 95% CI =9.7–29.5), thrombophilia (OR = 16.0, 95% CI = 9.4–27.2), systemic lupus erythematosus

(OR = 15.2, 95% = CI 7.4–31.2), heart disease (OR 13.2, 95% = CI 10.2–17.0), sickle cell disease (OR = 9.1, 95% CI = 3.7–22.2), hypertension (OR = 6.1, 95% CI 4.5–8.1) and thrombocytopenia (OR = 6.0, 95% = CI 1.5–24.1), postpartum haemorrhage (OR 1.8 95% CI = 1.2–2.8) pre-eclampsia and gestational hypertension (OR = 4.4 95% CI 3.6–5.4) [8]. Hypertension remain one of the main easily reversible risk factor and focus of treatment of stroke in pregnancy [9, 10]. In the indexed case presented, the only risk factor identified was pre-eclampsia / hypertension. Her haemoglobin electrophoresis was AA and platelet count normal, however due to the limited capacity of the laboratory we could not assess for thrombophilia and systemic lupus erythematosus.

Compared with women without hypertension, women with a hypertensive disorder in pregnancy are six- to nine-fold more likely to develop stroke in pregnancy [8, 11].The role of pre-eclampsia in stroke has earlier been described in a review in 2013 which showed that pre-eclampsia / eclampsia is usually associated with about a third of stroke cases in pregnancy [12]. The most common type of stroke associated with pre-eclampsia / eclampsia is haemorrhagic stroke [13, 14].

The diagnosis is usually confirmed by a cerebral non-contrast computed tomography (CT) scan which will show a region of spontaneous hyper-density in the case of haemorrhagic stroke [15]. Contrary to public opinions, cerebral CT scan is not contraindicated in pregnancy because the radiation doses exposed to during a cerebral CT scan are well below the threshold of risk of foetal teratogenicity [16]. Cerebral (magnetic resonance imaging) MRI is the imaging modality of choice in case of suspicion of acute ischaemic stroke [16–18]. The regular unavailability and high cost of this imaging modality limited it use in favour for a cerebral CT scan which is readily available and affordable in our resource low-setting. In the indexed case cerebral CT scan showed spontaneous intracerebral haemorrhage in the parietal lobe. The management of stroke in pregnancy is multidisciplinary involving the obstetrician, neurologist, neurosurgeon, intensivist, anaesthetist, physiotherapist and paediatrician.

The main aim of management is to maintain cerebral perfusion pressure prevent secondary brain injuries [17] and deliver the baby and the placenta. Blood pressure should be reduced judiciously in the acute phase with a target of ≤160/110 [19]. Intravenous labetalol has been widely used as first line for the reduction of blood pressure in patients with stroke during pregnancy [12]. MgSO4 should be added in the acute management for eclampsia prophylaxis [17]. Our indexed case described herein received intravenous nicardipine for control of blood pressure due to the unavailability of intravenous labetalol in our resource-limited setting and MgSO4

using the Pritchard protocol for prevention of seizures [7]. The timing and mode of delivery is influenced by fetal condition, gestational age and severity of associated preeclampsia [17]. Historically, caesarean delivery has been advocated and is increasingly being used to circumvent the potential risks during labour and delivery [20, 21]. This was the mode of delivery in our patient which let to the extraction of a life female baby. The prognosis of haemorrhagic stroke occurring during pregnancy is more severe compared to ischaemic stroke [22].

Conclusion

Albeit the relative rarity of this condition in pregnancy, this case highlights the importance of a good neurological examination in a pregnant woman presenting with neurological symptoms and raised blood pressure. It also illustrate the importance of a well equip and multidisciplinary team in the management of emergencies. Finally it demonstrates the importance of early and aggressive management in life threatening conditions such as haemorrhagic stroke. The initiation of clinical registries are a potential avenue to increase awareness around these fatal conditions and thereby contribute to reduction of cardiovascular related morbidity and mortality. The author suggests a case control study should be carried out in order to well describe determinants of intracerebral haemorrhage in pregnancy.

Abbreviations
ANC: Antenatal Care; CT Scan: Computed tomography scan; MRI: Magnetic resonance imaging

Acknowledgements
We express our sincere gratitude to all doctors, nurses and medical students who took part in the management of the patient.

Funding
None.

Author's contributions
PNT conceived and wrote the draft manuscript, NSA & JZM corrected the original manuscript and provided important intellectual information; all authors corrected and approved the final manuscript.

Competing interests
"The authors declare that they have no competing interests" in this section.

References
1. Aho K, Harmsen P, Hatano S, Marquardsen J, Smirnov VE, Strasser T. Cerebrovascular disease in the community: results of a WHO collaborative study. Bull World Health Organ. 1980;58(1):113–30.
2. Sacco RL, Kasner SE, Broderick JP, Caplan LR, Connors JJ. (buddy), Culebras a, et al. an updated definition of stroke for the 21st century: a statement for healthcare professionals from the American Heart Association/American Stroke Association. Stroke. 2013 Jul 1;44(7):2064–89.

3.   Jaigobin C, Silver FL. Stroke and pregnancy. Stroke. 2000 Dec;31(12):2948–51.
4.   Ban L, Sprigg N, Sultan AA, Nelson-Piercy C, Bath PM, Ludvigsson JF, et al. Incidence of first stroke in pregnant and nonpregnant women of childbearing age: a population-based cohort study from England. J Am Heart Assoc. 2017 Apr 1;6(4):e004601.
5.   Mapoure YN, Kuate C, Tchaleu CB, Ngahane HBM, Mounjouopou GN, Ba H, et al. Stroke epidemiology in Douala: three years prospective study in a teaching Hospital in Cameroon. World J Neurosci. 2014 Oct 23;04(05):406.
6.   Gagnier JJ, Kienle G, Altman DG, Moher D, Sox H, Riley D, et al. The CARE guidelines: consensus-based clinical case reporting guideline development. BMJ Case Rep. 2013 Oct;23:2013.
7.   Joshi S. Algorithm and Standard Management Protocol for Eclampsia. [cited 2017 Aug 17]; Available from: https://www.academia.edu/4497772/Algorithm_and_Standard_Management_Protocol_for_Eclampsia
8.   James AH, Bushnell CD, Jamison MG, Myers ER. Incidence and risk factors for stroke in pregnancy and the puerperium. Obstet Gynecol. 2005 Sep; 106(3):509–16.
9.   Fairhall JM, Stoodley MA. Intracranial haemorrhage in pregnancy. Obstet Med. 2009 Dec 1;2(4):142–8.
10. Rezai S, Faye J, Hughes A, Cheung M-L, Cohen JR, Kaia JA, et al. Hemolysis, elevated liver enzymes, and low platelets, severe fetal growth restriction, postpartum subarachnoid hemorrhage, and craniotomy: a rare case report and systematic review. Case Rep Obstet Gynecol. 2017;2017:1–5.
11. Lanska DJ, Kryscio RJ. Risk factors for peripartum and postpartum stroke and intracranial venous thrombosis. Stroke. 2000 Jun;31(6):1274–82.
12. Crovetto F, Somigliana E, Peguero A, Figueras F. Stroke during pregnancy and pre-eclampsia. Curr Opin Obstet Gynecol. 2013 Dec;25(6):425–32.
13. Bateman BT, Schumacher HC, Bushnell CD, Pile-Spellman J, Simpson LL, Sacco RL, et al. Intracerebral hemorrhage in pregnancy frequency, risk factors, and outcome. Neurology. 2006 Aug 8;67(3):424–9.
14. Bushnell C, Chireau M. Preeclampsia and Stroke: Risks during and after Pregnancy. Stroke Res Treat [Internet]. 2011 Jan 20 [cited 2017 Aug 16]; 2011. Available from: http://www.ncbi.nlm.nih.gov/pmc/articles/PMC3034989/
15. Sibai BM, Coppage KH. Diagnosis and management of women with stroke during pregnancy/postpartum. Clin Perinatol. 2004 Dec;31(4):853–68 viii.
16. Turan TN, Stern BJ. Stroke in pregnancy. Neurol Clin. 2004 Nov;22(4):821–40.
17. Kane SC, Dennis A, da Silva Costa F, Kornman L, Brennecke S. Contemporary Clinical Management of the Cerebral Complications of Preeclampsia [Internet]. Obstetrics and Gynecology International. 2013 [cited 2017 Aug 17]. Available from: https://www.hindawi.com/journals/ogi/2013/985606/
18. Zeeman GG. Neurologic complications of pre-eclampsia. Semin Perinatol. 2009;33(3):166–72.
19. Hart LA, Sibai BM. Seizures in pregnancy: epilepsy, eclampsia, and stroke. Semin Perinatol. 2013 Aug 1;37(4):207–24.
20. Cohen-Gadol AA, Friedman JA, Friedman JD, Tubbs RS, Munis JR, Meyer FB. Neurosurgical management of intracranial lesions in the pregnant patient: a 36-year institutional experience and review of the literature. J Neurosurg. 2009 Dec;111(6):1150–7.
21. Grear KE, Bushnell CD. Stroke and pregnancy: clinical presentation, evaluation, Treatment and Epidemiology. Clin Obstet Gynecol. 2013 Jun;56(2):350–9.
22. Laadioui M, Bouzoubaa W, Jayi S, Fdili FZ, Bouguern H, Chaara H, et al. Spontaneous hemorrhagic strokes during pregnancy: case report and review of the literature. Pan Afr Med J [Internet]. 2014 Dec 11 [cited 2017 Aug 17];19. Available from: http://www.ncbi.nlm.nih.gov/pmc/articles/PMC4427470/

19

Delayed Lactogenesis II and potential utility of antenatal milk expression in women developing late-onset preeclampsia

Jill Demirci[1,2]* [iD], Mandy Schmella[1], Melissa Glasser[1], Lisa Bodnar[3,4] and Katherine P. Himes[5,4]

Abstract

Background: Preeclampsia is a multi-system, hypertensive disorder of pregnancy that increases a woman's risk of later-life cardiovascular disease. Breastfeeding may counteract the negative cardiovascular sequela associated with preeclampsia; however, women who develop preeclampsia may be at-risk for suboptimal breastfeeding rates. In this case series, we present three cases of late-onset preeclampsia and one case of severe gestational hypertension that illustrate a potential association between hypertensive disorders of pregnancy and suboptimal breastfeeding outcomes, including delayed onset of lactogenesis II and in-hospital formula supplementation.

Case presentation: All cases were drawn from an ongoing pilot randomized controlled trial investigating the impact of antenatal milk expression versus an education control on breastfeeding outcomes. All study participants were healthy nulliparous women recruited at 34–36$^{6/7}$ gestational weeks from a hospital-based midwife practice. The variability in clinical presentation among the four cases suggests that any effect of hypertensive disorders on breastfeeding outcomes is likely multifactorial in nature, and may include both primary (e.g., preeclampsia disease course itself) and secondary (e.g., magnesium sulfate therapy, delayed at-breast feeding due to maternal-infant separation) etiologies. We further describe the use of antenatal milk expression (AME), or milk expression and storage beginning around 37 weeks of gestation, as a potential intervention to mitigate suboptimal breastfeeding outcomes in women at risk for preeclampsia and other hypertensive disorders of pregnancy.

Conclusions: Additional research is needed to address incidence, etiology, and interventions, including AME, for breastfeeding issues among a larger sample of women who develop hypertensive disorders of pregnancy.

Keywords: Pre-eclampsia, Hypertension, Pregnancy-induced, Breast feeding, Lactation, Breast milk expression

Background

Preeclampsia is a heterogeneous and multi-system hypertensive disorder of pregnancy that affects ≈3–5% of pregnancies globally, causing significant maternal and neonatal/infant morbidity and mortality [1, 2]. The development of preeclampsia stems from the interactions between a dysfunctional placenta and maternal constitutional factors, which culminate in systemic endothelial dysfunction (e.g., maternal hypertension, proteinuria, activation of coagulation cascade) [3–5]. Preeclampsia is diagnosed when a woman presents with new onset hypertension after 20 weeks' gestation with proteinuria and/or signs of multi-system involvement (e.g., thrombocytopenia, renal insufficiency). Preeclampsia is characterized as early (< 34 weeks' gestation) or late (≥ 34 weeks' gestation) and with/without severe features indicative of multi-system organ involvement [6]. Certain pre-pregnancy and pregnancy related factors, including pre-pregnancy obesity, chronic hypertension, type 1 and 2 diabetes mellitus, advanced maternal age, and nulliparity are associated with an increased risk of preeclampsia [7].

* Correspondence: jvr5@pitt.edu
Jill Demirci and Mandy Schmella are co- first authors.
[1]Department of Health Promotion & Development, University of Pittsburgh School of Nursing, 440 Victoria Building, Pittsburgh, PA 15261, USA
[2]Department of Pediatrics, University of Pittsburgh School of Medicine, Pittsburgh, PA, USA

Although the acute signs/symptoms generally resolve in the days and weeks following delivery [8], preeclampsia is associated with an increased risk for cardiovascular disease remote from pregnancy. In women with a history of preeclampsia, the risk of ischemic heart disease and cerebrovascular events is doubled, the risk of hypertension is tripled, and the risk of incident heart failure is quadrupled [9–12]. Women with hypertensive disorders of pregnancy also have a significantly higher risk of mortality related to diabetes, ischemic heart disease, and diabetes [13, 14]. Children exposed to a preeclamptic pregnancy may be at increased risk for cardiovascular dysfunction in adolescence and adulthood [15–17].

Breastfeeding may be one way to counteract the negative cardiovascular sequelae associated with preeclampsia. Increased duration of lactation in women is associated with reduced later life risk of hypertension, type II diabetes, hyperlipidemia, metabolic syndrome, subclinical and clinical cardiovascular disease, and cardiovascular mortality [18–22]. Breastfed children have a reduced risk of childhood obesity and diabetes [23, 24]. Paradoxically, however, women who develop preeclampsia appear to be at-risk for premature breastfeeding discontinuation and early formula use [25, 26], for reasons which have not been previously described.

Here, we present three cases of late-onset preeclampsia and one case of severe gestational hypertension that illustrate a potential association between hypertensive disorders of pregnancy and suboptimal breastfeeding outcomes, including delayed onset of lactogenesis II and in-hospital formula supplementation. Lactogenesis II is defined as the onset of copious milk production, which typically occurs between 48 and 72 h postpartum; onset after 72 h is considered delayed and is associated with unintended breastfeeding reduction and cessation [27, 28]. Furthermore, we describe the use of antenatal milk expression (AME), or milk expression and storage beginning around 37 weeks of gestation, as a potential intervention to increase breastfeeding success in women at risk for preeclampsia and other hypertensive disorders of pregnancy.

All cases were drawn from an ongoing pilot randomized controlled trial investigating the impact of antenatal milk expression versus an education control on breastfeeding outcomes. All trial participants were healthy nulliparous women with singleton pregnancies recruited at 34–36$^{6/7}$ gestational weeks from a hospital-based midwife practice in the northeastern United States. Participants were recruited via study flyer and at their prenatal appointments after review of electronic medical records for eligibility criteria. At enrollment, women had no major risk factors for insufficient milk (e.g., breast hypoplasia, polycystic ovarian syndrome, diabetes) or preterm labor (e.g., vaginal bleeding after the first trimester, congenital anomalies, polyhydramnios). The AME protocol was modeled after an

existing randomized controlled trial of AME in women with diabetes [29] and involved demonstration of hand-expression of milk beginning at 37 weeks of gestation with a study lactation consultant, weekly visits with the same lactation consultant to reinforce technique, and at-home, independent milk expression and collection one to two times per day for up to 10 min, for up to 40 gestational weeks. Women were provided containers in which to collect and freeze milk. Among women who brought milk to the hospital, they were advised to transport it in an insulated bag or cooler with two icepacks, and milk was subsequently stored in the hospital refrigerator for a maximum of 24 h. Women in the education group received weekly hand-outs addressing common breastfeeding problems from gestational weeks 37 to 40. We followed-up with all study participants at 1–2 weeks and 3–4 months postpartum to assess breastfeeding status and conduct interviews about experiences with AME.

Cases were obtained from the first third of participants recruited in the study, as an early trend was observed soon after enrollment commenced regarding development of hypertensive disorders of pregnancy and suboptimal breastfeeding outcomes. Case data was compiled from study participants' electronic medical records (e.g., details on labor and delivery, feedings in hospital), study surveys (e.g., breastfeeding plans, timing of lactogenesis II, feedings after hospital discharge), antenatal breast milk expression logs (e.g., volume and timing of milk collection), and interviews (e.g., perceived impact of AME). Data were organized in tables to facilitate comparison across participants. In the presentation of all cases, we adhered to CARE case report guidelines guidelines, which specify inclusion of particular elements to increase transparency and accuracy of data (e.g., inclusion of dose/strength/duration of intervention, patient perspective).

Case presentation
A summary of the cases can be found in Table 1.

Case 1: M
M was a healthcare professional with some formal lactation training. During pregnancy, she experienced normal, physiologic changes to her breasts, including breast growth and soreness, darkening of the areola, and leaking milk. After delivery, M planned to exclusively breastfeed for six months and continue any breastfeeding to one year postpartum.

Assigned to the AME study intervention, M expressed milk at least daily at home from 37 weeks of gestation to delivery (14 days, 15 total expression sessions, 60 mL total milk volume). All expressed milk was stored in her home freezer, and approximately half of stored milk was brought to the hospital by her partner on Day 2 after

Table 1 Case subject characteristics

CASES				
	1: "M"	2: "C"	3: "K"	4: "S"
STUDY DATA				
Study group assignment	AME	Education	AME	AME
Number of intervention study visits prior to delivery (max of 4)	3	0	1	0
DEMOGRAPHICS				
Age	26	34	36	35
Race & ethnicity	Non-Hispanic, White	Non-Hispanic, White	Hispanic, Other	Non-Hispanic, White
Marital status	Married	Married	Married	Married
Highest level of education	Bachelors	Some college	Bachelors	PhD
OBSTETRIC & HEALTH HISTORY				
Pre-pregnancy BMI	22.6	20.2	24.7	30.0
Gestational weight gain (lbs)	33	57	33	32
Relevant health history	Supraventricular tachycardia	Anxiety, depression (no medications)	N/A	Anxiety, depression (75 mg sertraline daily)
Gravida status	1 (previous spontaneous abortion in first trimester)	0	0	0
PREECLAMPSIA/HYPERTENSIVE DISORDER				
Classification	Preeclampsia with severe features (thrombocytopenia)	Preeclampsia without severe features	Preeclampsia without severe features	Gestational hypertension (with severe range blood pressures)
Weeks at diagnosis	$39^{3/7}$	$36^{6/7}$	$39^{0/7}$	$37^{4/7}$
Magnesium sulfate administration	56.4 g over 49 h	n/a	n/a	83.8 g over 44 h
Placenta pathology report[a]	No diagnostic abnormalities; 557 g, 75th percentile	390 g, 10th percentile; Features of maternal vascular malperfusion	No diagnostic abnormalities; 383 g, 10th percentile	No diagnostic abnormalities; 353 g, 10th percentile
LABOR & DELIVERY				
Weeks gestation at delivery	$39^{4/7}$	$37^{0/7}$	$39^{1/7}$	$37^{5/7}$
Onset of labor	Natural	Induced	Induced	Induced
Augmentation of labor	Pitocin, misoprostol, foley bulb, artificial rupture of membranes	Misoprostol	Dinoprostone, Pitocin	Pitocin, misoprostol, foley bulb, artificial rupture of membranes
Labor anesthesia	Epidural	Spinal, general	Epidural, spinal	Epidural
Type of delivery (and indication)	Cesarean section (arrested dilation and worsening preeclampsia)	Cesarean section (fetal intolerance)	Cesarean section (fetal intolerance)	Vaginal
Duration of labor in hospital (hours)	36	15	25	24
Duration of second stage of labor (hours)	N/A	N/A	N/A	0.5
Total intravenous fluids during labor and postpartum (mL)	8148 over 85 h	6620 over 81 h	3408 over 7 h	6816 over 41 h
POSTPARTUM				
Maternal disposition after birth	ICU	Mother-baby unit	Mother-baby unit	Mother-baby unit

Table 1 Case subject characteristics *(Continued)*

CASES

	1: "M"	2: "C"	3: "K"	4: "S"
Infant disposition after birth	NICU	Well-baby nursery	Well-baby nursery	Well-baby nursery
Infant birthweight (g)	3766	2927	2947	2580
Infant weight change from birthweight at hospital discharge	−7.6%	− 6.6%	− 6.1%	− 6.2%
Infant Apgar scores 1 & 5 mins	2, 7	8, 9	7, 9	6, 8
Maternal hospital LOS (days)	4	5	4	2
Infant hospital LOS (days)	3	4	3	2
BREASTFEEDING				
Lactation consult(s) in hospital	No	Yes (×4)	Yes (×1)	Yes (×2)
Total volume of formula in hospital (mL)	0	455	0	199
First at-breast feed in hospital after delivery (hours)	1.5	3.5	1.3	1.5
First use of formula in hospital after delivery (hours)	N/A	1.5	N/A	15.5
Milk expression in hospital (e.g., hand expression or pump)	Yes	Yes	Yes	Yes
Maternal perception of onset of lactogenesis II	Day 5	Day 5	Day 2	Day 4
Breastfeeding status at 1–2 weeks[b]	Exclusive breastfeeding	Exclusive breastfeeding	Exclusive breastfeeding	Medium partial breastfeeding
Breastfeeding status at 3–4 months[b]	Exclusive breastfeeding	High partial breastfeeding	Exclusive breastfeeding	Exclusive breastfeeding

[a]Percentiles are placental weights-for-gestation

LOS = length of stay

[b]Breastfeeding status classifications based upon definitions provided by Labbok and Krasovec, where exclusive breastfeeding equates with 100% of all feeds as breast milk, high partial breastfeeding is 80% or more of all feeds as breast milk, and medium partial breastfeeding is 20–80% of all feeds as breast milk Labbok M, Krasovec K. Toward consistency in breastfeeding definitions. *Studies in Family Planning.* 1990;21(4):226–230

delivery. M experienced no problems with AME, such as physical discomfort or issues related to privacy, convenience, or milk transport to/use in the hospital.

At $39^{3/7}$ weeks' gestation, M presented to labor and delivery triage with painful contractions every five minutes. Her blood pressure was also elevated (reaching 140 s/ 110 s mmHg) and labs revealed thrombocytopenia (platelet count = 94,000/μl). Protein/creatinine (p/c) ratio was equivocal at 0.17. M was diagnosed with preeclampsia with severe features and intravenous magnesium sulfate treatment was initiated according to protocol. An epidural was placed approximately 17 h into labor.

Despite augmentation of labor, including up-titration of oxytocin (Pitocin, Par Pharmaceutical Inc., Spring Valley, New York) and artificial rupture of membranes, 24 h into

labor there was minimal cervical change and worsening preeclampsia-related laboratory values (e.g., liver and renal function labs trending upward, decreased urine output). This prompted a decision to proceed with a cesarean section, which was completed without maternal complication. At delivery, M's infant (female) was apneic and bradycardic, requiring bag and mask resuscitation. Resuscitation efforts were successful, and the infant was transferred to the neonatal intensive care unit (NICU) with continuous positive airway pressure (CPAP) for further monitoring. In the NICU, the infant was weaned to room air, and after one hour, was transferred to the well-baby nursery. Postoperatively, M was transferred to the intensive care unit (ICU) for further monitoring and magnesium sulfate continuation for approximately 24 h. On postpartum day two, M was transferred to the mother-baby unit with improving preeclampsia-related laboratory values.

The first feed, which was at-breast, occurred about 1.5 h after delivery in the ICU. M reported the infant latched on "decently" (no LATCH score available; note that LATCH scores are used in the clinical context to document success of individual breastfeeding sessions according to five criteria; scores range from 0 to 10, with a higher score indicative of a more successful breastfeeding session [30]). During M's ICU stay, she alternated between at-breast feeds and bottle-feeding fresh colostrum that she hand-expressed or pumped. M breastfed exclusively the rest of hospitalization with LATCH scores of 9–10 and supplemented once overnight with a bottle of breast milk she expressed antenatally (25 mL), due to fatigue. She did not have a lactation consult in the hospital.

Upon discharge at three days, M did not perceive an increase in milk supply, and that night she supplemented with an additional 25 mL of the antenatally expressed milk due to her concern about lack of wet diapers. At M's follow-up interview at seven days postpartum, she noted that her milk did not fully "come in" until Day 5.

During the interview, M was enthusiastic about her experience with AME; she attributed a progressively increasing volume of milk expressed and leaking during pregnancy to AME, which increased her breastfeeding confidence. She also noted that AME created a "back-up" milk supply and seemed to increase the availability of colostrum in the postpartum period before her milk came in. M credited AME with avoiding formula supplementation after birth, within contexts that typically result in unintended formula supplementation (e.g., exhaustion with prolonged labor, mother-infant separation, impaired mental clarity with magnesium sulfate administration). In her interview she stated, "I pumped that night in the ICU and was able to get 8cc's out and give that to [my baby] so I could rest. And I thoroughly believe that would never have happened had I not been doing the study and AME, because just of what I've seen in the hospital, the first time you pump, you get like drops." At the 3–4 month follow-up interview, M reported continued exclusive breastfeeding.

Case 2: C

C was randomized to the education only study group. She planned to exclusively breastfeed for 6 months and continue any breastfeeding up to 1 year. During pregnancy, she experienced breast growth and soreness.

C presented to labor and delivery triage at $36^{6/7}$ weeks gestation after a routine obstetrical visit exam revealed elevated blood pressure of 138/94 mmHg and 1+ protein on a urine dipstick. Upon exam in triage, C's blood pressure rose to 140 s/90s, and she had an elevated urine p/c ratio of 0.98. She was diagnosed with preeclampsia without

severe features, and induction of labor commenced. Approximately 8 hours into the induction, repetitive late decelerations in fetal heart rate were noted, and the decision was made to proceed with a cesarean section. After delivery of a healthy male infant, C developed uterine atony and carboprost and misoprostol were administered, along with a Pitocin drip and a uterine B-Lynch suture. Due to waning effect of spinal anesthesia, C was placed under general anesthesia during operative closure. After recovery, C and her infant were transferred to the mother-baby unit.

C's postoperative course was complicated by general malaise, persistent nausea and vomiting, and tachycardia. The latter two issues were attributed to postoperative ileus and under-resuscitation after significant blood loss at delivery. While C was in the operating room 1.5 h after delivery, her partner fed the infant a bottle of formula (undocumented volume). Approximately 3.5 h after delivery, C fed her infant at-breast for the first time, with an 8/10 LATCH score. For the next 40 h, C fed her infant at-breast with LATCH scores of 7–9, with the exception of 30 mL of formula overnight on the second night in the hospital due to infant hypoglycemia (undocumented if symptomatic). Early the following morning and for the next 24 h, the infant was fed only bottles of formula; per maternal self-report at the study hospital visit, this was due to her malaise. During this period, C was provided with a breast pump, and on days 3 to 4 after delivery, the infant then received a combination of at-breast feeds and formula or breast milk via bottle. C received daily lactation consults during her hospitalization, beginning 34 h after delivery. During consults, basic breastfeeding education was provided, including anticipatory guidance about potential issues feeding an early term infant, as well as assistance at breast.

C's symptoms gradually improved, and she was discharged on post-operative Day 4. She remained normotensive during the postpartum period. At study follow-up at 12 days postpartum, C reported that she felt her milk "came in" on postpartum Day 5, and she was exclusively breastfeeding at-breast. At the 3–4 month follow-up, C was breastfeeding at-breast for most feeds. She estimated that formula made up about 10% of her infant's total feeds in a 24 h period.

Case 3: K

K planned to breastfeed exclusively for 6 months and continue any breastfeeding for 12 months postpartum. During pregnancy, she experienced breast growth, soreness, and darkening of areola. K was randomized to receive AME but completed only the first study visit with AME instruction and 5 days of AME at home (seven milk expression sessions) prior to delivery. During milk expression sessions, several drops of milk were expressed, but not saved. K reported no problems with AME, with the exception of minor physical discomfort during expression related to breast soreness in pregnancy and some concern that perceived lack of milk flow in pregnancy might be predictive of impaired milk supply postpartum.

K presented to labor and delivery triage after a growth ultrasound at $39^{0/7}$ weeks gestation, which revealed fetal tachycardia, a non-reactive non-stress test and elevated maternal blood pressure. Upon arrival in triage, K was found to have new-onset hypertension in the 140 s–150 s/ 90s–100 s and a p/c ratio of 1.03. She was diagnosed with preeclampsia without severe features. K was admitted for an induction of labor, and cervical ripening proceeded with dinoprostone placement. As labor progressed, platelets began to trend down slightly with a low of 114,000/μL approximately 1 hour prior to delivery. Approximately 17 h into the induction, a Pitocin drip was begun and K received an epidural. At 20 h after the induction commenced, fetal heart monitoring revealed reduced variability, tachycardia, and recurrent late decelerations. Intrauterine resuscitation efforts (e.g., maternal repositioning, oxygen) did not improve the tracing, and when a vaginal exam was attempted, spontaneous rupture of membranes occurred with thick meconium-stained fluid. Given concern for fetal status and limited labor progress, the obstetric team proceeded with a cesarean section and delivered a healthy male infant. During the closure, K experienced mild uterine atony requiring uterotonic agents (carboprost, Pitocin, misoprostil). Both K and infant were transferred to the well mother-baby unit after recovery, with normotensive maternal blood pressure readings.

K breastfed her infant for the first time approximately 1.3 h after delivery, with a LATCH score of 6/10. She continued to exclusively breastfeed throughout the 3-day postpartum hospitalization, with LATCH scores ranging from 6 to 9/10. A lactation consult occurred at 48 h postdelivery. The lactation consultant note indicated that K was breastfeeding well and hand-expressing milk easily. "Pointers" were provided on latch and positioning.

At study follow-up at 12 days postpartum, K reported that her milk "came in" at 2 days postpartum and that she had no breastfeeding concerns. She was exclusively breastfeeding, and felt that AME had increased her confidence in her ability to produce milk after birth and allowed her to "practice" handling breasts and the mechanics of breastfeeding prior to birth. She also attributed AME to her milk "coming in sooner" after birth. At 3–4 months postpartum, K was exclusively breastfeeding at-breast.

Case 4: S

S experienced normal, physiologic changes to her breasts during pregnancy, including growth, areola darkening, increased breast vascularization, and leaking milk. S planned to breastfeed without formula in the postpartum period for as long as possible. Although randomized to AME, S's exam at her obstetric visit at $37^{4/7}$ weeks gestation revealed new-onset hypertension in the range of 130 s/90s mmHg, and she did not receive the intervention.

Upon admission to triage for further evaluation, her blood pressure increased to 160 s/110 s, with no other signs or symptoms of preeclampsia. She received a single dose of labetalol 20 mg IV. Induction of labor then commenced, and S received a 2 g/h magnesium sulfate drip for seizure prophylaxis. A Pitocin drip was begun approximately 6 h into labor, and membranes were artificially ruptured 10 h later. S received an epidural approximately 20 h into labor. Shortly thereafter, S delivered a female infant who required no resuscitation. S and her infant remained together throughout the recovery period and were later transferred to the well mother-baby unit. S continued to receive magnesium sulfate for approximately 24 h post-delivery, and her blood pressures returned to the 120 s/70s mmHg.

S first attempted at-breast feeding 1.5 h after delivery, with a LATCH score of 6/10. In the ensuing hours, nursing notes indicated no LATCH scores above 6 and several unobserved breastfeeding sessions where no sustained latch was achieved. S first supplemented with formula during the night following her morning delivery (22 mL), after an unsuccessful breastfeeding attempt. Formula was continued in lieu of breastfeeding the remainder of the night, with attempts to breastfeed the following morning followed by formula supplementation. A similar pattern was followed during the remainder of the hospitalization. S saw a hospital lactation consultant approximately 24 h after delivery who provided basic breastfeeding education, including feeding cues and instructions for pumping after unsuccessful breastfeeding attempts. She returned 5 hours later to observe a feed and demonstrate hand-expression of colostrum and the use of a nipple shield. The lactation consultant returned the following morning, and noted that S reported the infant "'frustrated and screaming [during breastfeeding].' [Mother] then gives a bottle [of formula] and pumps."

At study follow-up at 11 days of life, S reported feeling her milk "come in" at approximately 4 days postpartum. After hospital discharge, she had continued to feed a combination of breast milk (at-breast and via bottle) and formula, with approximately a third of feeds in the past 24 h being breast milk. She continued to use the nipple shield and had received breastfeeding help from family and friends. She continued to pump after formula feeding, roughly six times in a 24 h period, with about 4 oz. of breast milk expressed and fed to the infant. She attributed milk supply issues to a five-day course of furosemide (Lasix, Sanofi Aventis, Bridgewater, New Jersey) she was prescribed 5 days after delivery for peripheral edema and continued elevated blood pressures ("It has to be the Lasix.

It's drying you up everywhere."). At 3–4 months postpartum, S reported exclusive breast milk feedings, with the majority of feedings as expressed milk via bottle. She continued to use the nipple shield for at-breast feedings.

Discussion and conclusions

Three of the cases presented here illustrate a potential relationship between late-onset preeclampsia and other hypertensive disorders of pregnancy and early breastfeeding problems, including delayed onset of lactogenesis II and in-hospital formula use. Case 3 represents an exception to this association, with normal timing of lactogenesis II and exclusive breastfeeding in-hospital. The variability in clinical presentation among the four cases supports that any potential effect of preeclampsia or other hypertensive disorders of pregnancy on breastfeeding outcomes is likely multifactorial in nature, with possible primary etiology (e.g., preeclampsia disease course itself) and secondary causal factors (e.g., underlying maternal issue contributing to both preeclampsia and lactation problems, preeclampsia treatments).

We found two studies addressing the relationship between hypertensive disorders of pregnancy and breastfeeding outcomes, but none examining timing of lactogenesis II. Cordero et al. [25] found in their retrospective medical record analysis of 281 women diagnosed with severe preeclampsia and delivering ≥ 34 weeks of gestation, 51% of the overall sample and 78% of those intending to breastfeed initiated breastfeeding; however, only 33% of the sample was exclusively breastfeeding and 22% receiving any breast milk at the time of hospital discharge, which was lower than U.S. averages at the time but perhaps comparable to the region in which the study occurred [31, 32]. In a retrospective cohort study involving mothers with hypertensive disorders of pregnancy and matched controls, breastfeeding intention and continuation at 1 month postpartum was significantly lower among women with preeclampsia than control women [26]. These studies lend credence to a potential negative effect of preeclampsia or related factors on breastfeeding, though mechanism of action is unclear.

Three of four cases presented with lactogenesis II occurring after 3 days postpartum. Onset of lactogenesis II is triggered by a complex hormonal cascade, initiated by delivery of the placenta and a concomitant precipitous drop in progesterone. The methods by which various factors facilitate or impede this process are not well understood. Delays in lactogenesis occur at a rate of 23–44% in the U.S. [28, 33]. This is clinically significant, as delayed lactogenesis, and its corollary—formula supplementation, are both are strong prognosticators of early, unintended breastfeeding cessation [28, 34]. Delayed lactogenesis is more likely to occur among primiparous, obese, and diabetic women, as well as those who have a prolonged

second stage of labor (greater than 2–3 h for nulliparous women) [35], stressful labor or delivery, cesarean section, higher birthweight infant, postpartum edema, or a perception of ineffective breastfeeding during the first 24 h postpartum [33, 36–39]. Women in the presented cases possessed a number of these risk factors, many of which are also associated with preeclampsia and/or its treatment, including primipara status, delivery by cesarean section, stressful/prolonged labor and delivery, and early breastfeeding problems, including formula use.

While postpartum edema was not tracked as a potential cause of delayed lactogenesis II, it is a common occurrence in preeclampsia as vasculature becomes "leaky," resulting in third-spacing of fluids [40]. It is thus possible that lower intravascular volume contributed to poor diffusion of water into mammary alveoli and delayed the onset of copious milk production until fluid balance was restored. Alternately, postpartum breast edema can contribute to difficulty in early breast milk removal, a risk factor for delayed lactogenesis II [41].

Other factors related to hypertensive disorders of pregnancy may contribute to an unfavorable endocrine profile for establishment of lactation, including stress [38, 42] and obesity [43, 44], the latter potentially relevant for Case 4 with a BMI of 30. Placental dysfunction, which typifies preeclampsia, has been generically noted as a potential contributor to delayed onset of lactation [45]; it is theoretically possible that placental hormones impacting proliferation of glandular breast tissue in preparation for breastfeeding (e.g., progesterone) are compromised in preeclampsia.

Postpartum hemorrhage, as occurred for Case 2, has the potential to contribute to delayed or insufficient milk and negative breastfeeding outcomes through several mechanisms. These include anemia and necrotic damage or shock to the pituitary gland from hypovolemia. Pituitary dysfunction affects secretion of key lactation hormones, including prolactin necessary for milk production [46]. Labor complications associated with preeclampsia, including inductions, cesarean sections, and prolonged labors are also risk factors for postpartum hemorrhage.

It is possible that medications used to treat and manage preeclampsia impacted milk supply in these cases. For example, diuretics such as Case 4 received, may contribute to a fluid deficit in relation to the volume needed for adequate milk production [47]. Case 4 was also taking a selective serotonin reuptake inhibitor (SSRI) daily; SSRIs are associated with delayed lactogenesis, potentially through perturbation of the mammary gland epithelial cells [48]. Magnesium sulfate therapy is routinely utilized for seizure prophylaxis in women with preeclampsia during the intrapartum and postpartum periods. A case report from 1993 describes a woman who received ≈ 4 days of magnesium sulfate therapy (102 g total) for management of preeclampsia and experienced delayed lactogenesis to postpartum day 10 [49]. Traditional reasons for delayed lactogenesis (e.g., delayed at-breast feeding, decreased breast stimulation) were ruled out, and it was hypothesized that the disease process or the magnesium therapy itself impacted lactogenesis. Other studies have found a dose-dependent association of magnesium sulfate therapy with delayed initiation of breastfeeding [50] and factors that impact delayed breastfeeding, including decreased infant suckling behavior, lower Apgar scores, hypotonia, and NICU admissions [51, 52]. Two of the four cases presented in this case series received magnesium sulfate therapy (Case 1: 56.4 g total; Case 4: 83.8 g total) and experienced delayed lactogenesis II. Unfortunately, research investigating the impact of magnesium sulfate therapy on lactogenesis is still lacking.

Reduced opportunity for early and effective breast stimulation and emptying, as may occur with maternal infant separation and medical complications in preeclampsia management, are known risk factors for reduced breast milk production [33, 53]. Research suggests that the earlier postnatal milk removal and suckling occurs, the more rapid the conversion to lactogenesis II (copious mature milk) post-birth and the larger the postpartum milk supply [54, 55]. One explanation is the prolactin receptor theory, which posits that early breast stimulation increases the number of prolactin receptors in breast tissue; these receptors set the theoretical maximum volume of milk production and may only be amenable within a short period around birth [56]. This may be particularly relevant for Cases 2 and 4 who delivered prior to 39 weeks gestation, as preterm and early term infants generate reduced negative pressure during suckling and removal of less milk [57].

As illustrated in Cases 1 and 3, antenatal milk expression (AME) may address a number of breastfeeding complications experienced by women with late onset preeclampsia. For example, milk stored in pregnancy can be used as supplemental feeding when at-breast feeds are not possible or successful following a complicated birth. AME may also increase prenatal confidence and commitment to breastfeeding, allowing mothers to persevere despite early postpartum setbacks (however, AME may also have unintended consequences of decreasing confidence if mothers are not able to express any milk or only small volumes). Finally, existing research [58, 59] and anecdotal feedback in our study suggest that AME may contribute to increased volume of milk both prior to and following lactogenesis II and improved short-term breastfeeding outcomes. Forster et al. [58] found that AME beginning at 36 weeks of gestation among diabetic women at low-risk for birth complications did not increase risk of NICU admission or rate of preterm birth. Because nipple stimulation in pregnancy

can theoretically lead to uterine contractions and perhaps placental perfusion problems, the authors advised against unsupervised AME implementation in other high-risk groups. In our study, AME was not continued after women were diagnosed with any pregnancy complications. More research is warranted to understand the risks and benefits of AME among women who develop preeclampsia and other issues associated with postnatal breastfeeding problems. In the interim, women with prenatal *risk factors* for these problems, including nulliparity, with an otherwise low-risk pregnancy, may benefit from AME prior to onset of disease.

In this sample of women with hypertensive disorders of pregnancy, despite early setbacks and formula use, all were breastfeeding with little to no formula use by three to 4 months postpartum. It is unclear whether this would have been the case in a more diverse sample of women with less breastfeeding education and support. Thus, limitations of this analysis include the generalizability of findings based on the case study format and the demographically homogenous sample of women. Strengths include utilization of multiple data sources enabling methodological triangulation (e.g., electronic medical record data and maternal self-report of in-hospital feedings) and the prospective nature of data collection from pregnancy through the postpartum period, minimizing the potential for recall bias. Future research should address incidence, etiology, and interventions for breastfeeding issues among larger samples of women who develop late onset preeclampsia, while controlling for confounding variables.

Abbreviations

AME: Antenatal milk expression; CPAP: Continuous positive airway pressure; ICU: Intensive care unit; LATCH: breastfeeding scoring system based on five criteria represented by the LATCH acronym: L: latching of infant onto breast; A: audible swallows; T: type of nipple; C: comfort of the mother during breastfeeding; H-hold/position used during breastfeeding and assistance required; NICU: Neonatal intensive care unit; p/c ratio: Protein/creatinine ratio; SSRI: Selective serotonin reuptake inhibitor

Acknowledgements

We thank Debra Bogen for her contributions to the study design and Erin Caplan for her assistance with data collection.

Funding

This study was funded through the American Nurses Foundation (ANA Presidential Scholar Award; PI: Demirci). Data collection was also supported through NIH grant UL1TR001857. Funding sources had no role in the design of the study; data collection, analysis, or interpretation; or in writing the manuscript.

Author's contributions

JD conceived the study design, reviewed medical records and mother interviews for each case, and composed the first draft of the manuscript. MS assisted in interpretation of case data, reviewed of relevant background research, and assisted JD in drafting the first version of the manuscript. MG assisted JD in reviewing medical records and mother interviews for each case. KH assisted in interpretation of medical record data for each case. LB assisted in interpretation of data in the context of current literature in the population of interest. All authors were involved in critical revision of manuscript content, approved the final version of the manuscript, and are accountable for all aspects of the work.

Competing interests

The authors declare that they have no competing interests.

Author details

[1]Department of Health Promotion & Development, University of Pittsburgh School of Nursing, 440 Victoria Building, Pittsburgh, PA 15261, USA. [2]Department of Pediatrics, University of Pittsburgh School of Medicine, Pittsburgh, PA, USA. [3]Department of Epidemiology, University of Pittsburgh Graduate School of Public Health, Pittsburgh, PA, USA. [4]Department of Obstetrics, Gynecology and Reproductive Sciences, University of Pittsburgh School of Medicine, Pittsburgh, PA, USA. [5]Magee-Womens Research Institute, Pittsburgh, USA.

References

1. Abalos E, Cuesta C, Grosso AL, Chou D, Say L. Global and regional estimates of preeclampsia and eclampsia: a systematic review. Eur J Obstet Gynecol Reprod Biol. 2013;170(1):1–7.
2. Ananth CV, Keyes KM, Wapner RJ. Pre-eclampsia rates in the United States, 1980-2010: age-period-cohort analysis. BMJ. 2013;347:f6564.
3. Redman C. The six stages of pre-eclampsia. Pregnancy Hypertens. 2014;4(3):246.
4. Roberts JM, Hubel CA. The two stage model of preeclampsia: variations on the theme. Placenta. 2009;30(Suppl A):S32–7.
5. Roberts JM, Taylor RN, Musci TJ, Rodgers GM, Hubel CA, Preeclampsia MLMK. An endothelial cell disorder. Am J Obstet Gynecol. 1989;161(5):1200–4.
6. Hypertension in pregnancy. Report of the American College of Obstetricians and Gynecologists' task force on hypertension in pregnancy. Obstet Gynecol. 2013;122(5):1122–31.
7. Bartsch E, Medcalf KE, Park AL, Ray JG. Clinical risk factors for pre-eclampsia determined in early pregnancy: systematic review and meta-analysis of large cohort studies. BMJ. 2016;353:i1753.
8. August P, Sibai BM. Preeclampsia: Clinical features and diagnosis. Waltham, MA: UpToDate Inc. Available from: https://www.uptodate.com/contents/preeclampsia-clinical-features-and-diagnosis. [cited 11 Aug, 2017]
9. Wu P, Haththotuwa R, Kwok CS, Babu A, Kotronias RA, Rushton C, et al. Preeclampsia and future cardiovascular health: a systematic review and meta-analysis. Circ Cardiovasc Qual Outcomes. 2017;10(2):e003497.
10. Bellamy L, Casas JP, Hingorani AD, Williams DJ. Pre-eclampsia and risk of cardiovascular disease and cancer in later life: systematic review and meta-analysis. BMJ. 2007;335(7627):974.
11. Brown MC, Best KE, Pearce MS, Waugh J, Robson SC, Bell R. Cardiovascular disease risk in women with pre-eclampsia: systematic review and meta-analysis. Eur J Epidemiol. 2013;28(1):1–19.
12. McDonald SD, Malinowski A, Zhou Q, Yusuf S, Devereaux PJ. Cardiovascular sequelae of preeclampsia/eclampsia: a systematic review and meta-analyses. Am Heart J. 2008;156(5):918–30.
13. Theilen LH, Fraser A, Hollingshaus MS, Schliep KC, Varner MW, Smith KR, et al. All-cause and cause-specific mortality after hypertensive disease of pregnancy. Obstet Gynecol. 2016;128(2):238–44.
14. Theilen L, Meeks H, Fraser A, Esplin MS, Smith KR, Varner M. Long-term mortality risk and life expectancy following recurrent hypertensive disease of pregnancy. Am J Obstet Gynecol. 2017;216(1):S32–S3.
15. Fraser A, Nelson SM, Macdonald-Wallis C, Sattar N, Lawlor DA. Hypertensive disorders of pregnancy and cardiometabolic health in adolescent offspring. Hypertension. 2013;62(3):614–20.
16. Kajantie E, Eriksson JG, Osmond C, Thornburg K, Barker DJ. Pre-eclampsia is associated with increased risk of stroke in the adult offspring: the Helsinki birth cohort study. Stroke. 2009;40(4):1176–80.
17. Timpka S, Macdonald-Wallis C, Hughes AD, Chaturvedi N, Franks PW, Lawlor DA, et al. Hypertensive disorders of pregnancy and offspring cardiac structure and function in adolescence. J Am Heart Assoc. 2016;5(11):e003906.
18. Gunderson EP, Quesenberry CP Jr, Ning X, Jacobs DR Jr, Gross M, Goff DC Jr, et al. Lactation duration and midlife atherosclerosis. Obstet Gynecol. 2015; 126(2):381–90.
19. McClure CK, Catov JM, Ness RB, Schwarz EB. Lactation and maternal subclinical cardiovascular disease among premenopausal women. Am J Obstet Gynecol. 2012;207(1):46.e1–8.
20. Natland Fagerhaug T, Forsmo S, Jacobsen GW, Midthjell K, Andersen LF, Ivar Lund Nilsen T. A prospective population-based cohort study of lactation and cardiovascular disease mortality: the HUNT study. BMC Public Health. 2013;13:1070.
21. Perrine CG, Nelson JM, Corbelli J, Lactation SKS. Maternal cardio-metabolic health. Annu Rev Nutr. 2016;36:627–45.
22. Schwarz EB, Ray RM, Stuebe AM, Allison MA, Ness RB, Freiberg MS, et al. Duration of lactation and risk factors for maternal cardiovascular disease. Obstet Gynecol. 2009;113(5):974–82.
23. Ip S, Chung M, Raman G, Trikalinos TA, Lau J. A summary of the Agency for Healthcare Research and Quality's evidence report on breastfeeding in developed countries. Breastfeed Med. 2009;4(Suppl 1):S17–30.
24. Victora CG, Bahl R, Barros AJ, Franca GV, Horton S, Krasevec J, et al. Breastfeeding in the 21st century: epidemiology, mechanisms, and lifelong effect. Lancet. 2016;387(10017):475–90.
25. Cordero L, Valentine CJ, Samuels P, Giannone PJ, Nankervis CA. Breastfeeding in women with severe preeclampsia. Breastfeed Med. 2012;7(6):457–63.
26. Leeners B, Rath W, Kuse S, Neumaier-Wagner P. Breast-feeding in women with hypertensive disorders in pregnancy. J Perinat Med. 2005;33(6):553–60.
27. Lawrence RA. Lawrence RM. physiology of lactation. Breastfeeding a guide for the medical profession. 8th ed. Philadelphia: Elsevier; 2016. p. 56–63.
28. Brownell E, Howard CR, Lawrence RA, Dozier AM. Delayed onset lactogenesis II predicts the cessation of any or exclusive breastfeeding. J Pediatr. 2012;161(4):608–14.
29. Forster DA, Jacobs S, Amir LH, Davis P, Walker SP, McEgan K, et al. Safety and efficacy of antenatal milk expressing for women with diabetes in pregnancy: protocol for a randomised controlled trial. BMJ Open. 2014;4(10):e006571.
30. Jensen D, Wallace S, Kelsay PLATCH. A breastfeeding charting system and documentation tool. J Obstet Gynecol Neonatal Nurs. 1994;23(1):27–32.
31. Centers for Disease Control and Prevention. Breastfeeding among U.S. children born 2002–2014, CDC National Immunization Surveys 2017 [Available from: http://www.cdc.gov/breastfeeding/data/NIS_data/.
32. Centers for Disease Control and Prevention. Breastfeeding report card-United States, 2007 2007 [Available from: https://www.cdc.gov/breastfeeding/pdf/2007breastfeedingreportcard.pdf.
33. Nommsen-Rivers LA, Chantry CJ, Peerson JM, Cohen RJ, Dewey KG. Delayed onset of lactogenesis among first-time mothers is related to maternal obesity and factors associated with ineffective breastfeeding. Am J Clin Nutr. 2010;92(3):574–84.
34. Chantry CJ, Dewey KG, Peerson JM, Wagner EA, Nommsen-Rivers LA. In-hospital formula use increases early breastfeeding cessation among first-time mothers intending to exclusively breastfeed. J Pediatr. 2014;164(6):1339–45.
35. Laughon SK, Berghella V, Reddy UM, Sundaram R, Lu Z, Hoffman MK. Neonatal and maternal outcomes with prolonged second stage of labor. Obstet Gynecol. 2014;124(1):57–67.
36. Dewey KG, Nommsen-Rivers LA, Heinig MJ, Cohen RJ. Risk factors for suboptimal infant breastfeeding behavior, delayed onset of lactation, and excess neonatal weight loss. Pediatrics. 2003;112(3 Pt 1):607–19.
37. Chen DC, Nommsen-Rivers L, Dewey KG, Lonnerdal B. Stress during labor and delivery and early lactation performance. Am J Clin Nutr. 1998;68(2):335–44.
38. Dewey KG. Maternal and fetal stress are associated with impaired lactogenesis in humans. J Nutr. 2001;131(11):3012S–5S.
39. Matias SL, Dewey KG, Quesenberry CP Jr, Gunderson EP. Maternal prepregnancy obesity and insulin treatment during pregnancy are independently associated with delayed lactogenesis in women with recent gestational diabetes mellitus. Am J Clin Nutr. 2014;99(1):115–21.
40. Taylor RN, Roberts JM, Cunningham FG, Lindheimer MD, editors. Chesley's hypertensive disorders in pregnancy. Fourth ed. New York: Academic Press; 2015.

41. Hoover K. Perinatal and intrapartum care. In: Wambach K, Riordan J, editors. Breastfeeding and human lactation. Fifth ed. Burlington, MA: Jones & Bartlett Learning; 2016. p. 227–70.

42. Lau C. Effects of stress on lactation. Pediatr Clin N Am. 2001;48(1):221–34.

43. Bever Babendure J, Reifsnider E, Mendias E, Moramarco MW, Davila YR. Reduced breastfeeding rates among obese mothers: a review of contributing factors, clinical considerations and future directions. Int Breastfeed J. 2015;10:21.

44. Rasmussen KM, Kjolhede CL. Prepregnant overweight and obesity diminish the prolactin response to suckling in the first week postpartum. Pediatrics. 2004;113(5):e465–71.

45. Kellymom. When will my milk come in? 2016 [Available from: http://kellymom.com/ages/newborn/when-will-my-milk-come-in/.

46. Lawrence RA, Lawrence RM. Medical complications of mothers. In: Lawrence RA, Lawrence RM, editors. Breastfeeding a guide for the medical profession. Eighth ed. Philadelphia: Elsevier; 2016.

47. Cominos DC, van der Walt A, van Rooyen AJ. Suppression of postpartum lactation with furosemide. S Afr Med J. 1976;50(8):251–2.

48. Marshall AM, Nommsen-Rivers LA, Hernandez LL, Dewey KG, Chantry CJ, Gregerson KA, et al. Serotonin transport and metabolism in the mammary gland modulates secretory activation and involution. J Clin Endocrinol Metab. 2010;95(2):837–46.

49. Haldeman W. Can magnesium sulfate therapy impact lactogenesis? J Hum Lact. 1993;9(4):249–52.

50. Vigil-De Gracia P, Ramirez R, Duran Y, Quintero A. Magnesium sulfate for 6 vs 24 hours post delivery in patients who received magnesium sulfate for less than 8 hours before birth: a randomized clinical trial. BMC Pregnancy Childbirth. 2017;17(1):241.

51. Abbassi-Ghanavati M, Alexander JM, McIntire DD, Savani RC, Leveno KJ. Neonatal effects of magnesium sulfate given to the mother. Am J Perinatol. 2012;29(10):795–9.

52. Das M, Chaudhuri PR, Mondal BC, Mitra S, Bandyopadhyay D, Pramanik S. Assessment of serum magnesium levels and its outcome in neonates of eclamptic mothers treated with low-dose magnesium sulfate regimen. Indian J Pharmacol. 2015;47(5):502–8.

53. Parker LA, Sullivan S, Krueger C, Mueller M. Association of timing of initiation of breastmilk expression on milk volume and timing of lactogenesis stage II among mothers of very low-birth-weight infants. Breastfeed Med. 2015;10(2):84–91.

54. Neville MC, Morton J. Physiology and endocrine changes underlying human lactogenesis II. J Nutr. 2001;131(11):3005S–8S.

55. Parker LA, Sullivan S, Krueger C, Kelechi T, Mueller M. Effect of early breast milk expression on milk volume and timing of lactogenesis stage II among mothers of very low birth weight infants: a pilot study. J Perinatol. 2012; 32(3):205–9.

56. Wambach K, Watson GC. Anatomy and physiology of lactation. In: Wambach K, Riordan J, editors. Breastfeeding and human lactation. 5th ed. Burlington: Jones and Bartlett Learning; 2016. p. 79–120.

57. Medoff-Cooper B, McGrath JM, Bilker W. Nutritive sucking and neurobehavioral development in preterm infants from 34 weeks PCA to term. MCN Am J Matern Child Nurs. 2000;25(2):64–70.

58. Forster DA, Moorhead AM, Jacobs SE, Davis PG, Walker SP, McEgan KM, et al. Advising women with diabetes in pregnancy to express breastmilk in late pregnancy (diabetes and antenatal milk expressing [DAME]): a multicentre, unblinded, randomised controlled trial. Lancet. 2017;389(10085):2204–13.

59. Singh G, Chouhan R, Sidhu K. Effect of antenatal expression of breast milk at term in reducing breast feeding failures. Med J Armed Forces India. 2011; 65(2):131–3.

20

Increased postpartum haemorrhage, the possible relation with serotonergic and other psychopharmacological drugs

Hanna M. Heller[1*], Anita C. J. Ravelli[2], Andrea H. L. Bruning[3], Christianne J. M. de Groot[4], Fedde Scheele[5,6], Maria G. van Pampus[7] and Adriaan Honig[8,9]

Abstract

Background: Postpartum haemorrhage is a major obstetric risk worldwide. Therefore risk factors need to be investigated to control for this serious complication. A recent systematic review and meta-analysis revealed that the use of both serotonergic and non-serotonergic antidepressants in pregnancy are associated with a higher risk of postpartum haemorrhage. However, use of antidepressants in pregnancy is often necessary because untreated depression in pregnancy is associated with adverse maternal and neonatal outcome, such as postpartum depression, preterm birth and dysmaturity. Therefore it is of utmost importance to unravel the possible association between postpartum haemorrhage and the use of serotonergic and other psychopharmacological medication during pregnancy.

Methods: We performed a matched cohort observational study consecutively including all pregnant women using serotonergic medication (n = 578) or other psychopharmacological medication (n = 50) visiting two teaching hospitals in Amsterdam between 2010 and 2014. The incidence of postpartum haemorrhage in women using serotonergic medication or other psychopharmacological medication was compared with the incidence of postpartum haemorrhage in 641,364 pregnant women not using psychiatric medication selected from the database of the Netherlands Perinatal Registry foundation (Perined). Matching took place 1:5 for nine factors, i.e., parity, maternal age, ethnicity, socioeconomic status, macrosomia, gestational duration, history of postpartum haemorrhage, labour induction and hypertensive disorder.

Results: Postpartum haemorrhage occurred in 9.7% of the women using serotonergic medication. In the matched controls this was 6.6% (p = 0.01). The adjusted odds ratio (aOR) before matching was 1.6 (95% CI 1.2–2.1) and after matching 1.5 (95% CI 1.1–2.1). Among the women using other psychopharmacological medication, the incidence of postpartum haemorrhage before matching was 12.0% versus 6.1% (p = 0.08) with OR 2.1 (95% CI 0.9–4.9), and after matching 12.1% versus 4.4% (p = 0.03) with aOR of 3.3 (95% CI 1.1–9.8).

Conclusions: Pregnant women using serotonergic medication have an increased risk of postpartum haemorrhage, but this high risk is also seen in pregnant women using other psychopharmacological medication. We suggest that this higher risk of postpartum haemorrhage could not only be explained by serotonin, but also by other mechanisms. An additional explanation could be the underlying psychiatric disorder.

Keywords: Postpartum haemorrhage, Antidepressants, Serotonin, Postpartum blood loss, Pregnancy, Selective serotonin reuptake inhibitors, Psychopharmacological medication

* Correspondence: hm.heller@vumc.nl
[1]Department of Hospital Psychiatry, VU University Medical Centre, De Boelelaan 1117, 1081 HV Amsterdam, The Netherlands
Full list of author information is available at the end of the article

Background

Postpartum haemorrhage (PPH) is a major obstetric risk worldwide, with an increasing incidence in developed countries [1, 2]. In the Netherlands the overall incidence of PPH defined as blood loss of more than 1000 ml was around 6% in 2014 [3]. Despite the growing knowledge about risk factors, we are still unable to fully explain the increasing incidence of this obstetric complication. Recent studies suggest that the use of serotonergic antidepressants in pregnancy might be associated with a higher risk of PPH [4–8].

Several studies have investigated the association of serotonergic antidepressant exposure during pregnancy and PPH, with varying outcomes [4]. Some studies concluded that pregnant women using serotonergic antidepressants have an almost two times higher risk of PPH [5–9] whilst others reported no increased risk [10–13]. A recent systematic review and meta-analysis revealed that not only SSRI's, but also non serotonergic antidepressants are associated with a higher risk on PPH [14].

Treatment with antidepressants is often discontinued or not started or resumed during pregnancy because of possible foetal and obstetric complications [15]. On the other hand, untreated depression in pregnancy is associated with adverse neonatal outcome, such as an increased risk of prematurity, dysmaturity, decreased breastfeeding initiation [16, 17], increased risk of operative delivery [18–20], increased risk of caesarean delivery or rupture of the anal sphincter [21], increased risk of postpartum depression [22, 23] and affective and behavioural consequences for the offspring [24, 25]. Some of these complications are associated with postpartum haemorrhage. Therefore, the use of antidepressants in pregnancy mostly outweighs its potential risks; its use is increasing in more highly developed countries [26–28]. This underscores the need to investigate the effectiveness and safety of treatment options for depression in pregnancy and postpartum.

The most frequently prescribed antidepressants, the serotonin reuptake inhibitors (SSRIs), are estimated to be used by 2 to 3% of the pregnant women in Europe and by 10% in North America [15]. A frequently proposed hypothesis for the aetiology of PPH in these women is that the use of serotonergic medication, more specifically the serotonergic action of these drugs on platelets, causes diminished blood clotting [29].

However, the varying incidence of PPH in these women may also relate to confounding due to the large number of other factors that contribute to this complication. It is therefore important to properly adjust for these confounding factors [4]. The first aim of our study was to investigate the role of serotonergic medication on the development of PPH reducing as much as possible the effect of potential confounders by performing a matched paired cohort analysis.

Our secondary aim was to determine the effect of other psychopharmacological medication, such as lithium and antipsychotics on the development of PPH. However, we didn't expect antipsychotics to increase PPH, because most studies show that the use of especially second generation antipsychotics leads to an increased risk of platelet aggregation. [30]. Some other psychopharmacological drugs are supposed to have also a kind of serotonergic action including contributing to the serotonin syndrome [31] but are not the affecting the blood clotting in the same way.

Based on previous studies, we hypothesized that the risk of PPH is higher for serotonergic drugs than for no drugs or for other psychopharmacological medication. This question about the contribution of serotonergic drugs to the development of PPH is of the utmost importance since use in pregnancy has increased and better knowledge of outcomes can help pregnant women and clinicians make more informed decisions concerning care.

Methods
Setting, population and study participants

We consecutively included all women in two hospitals, Sint Lucas Andreas Hospital and Onze Lieve Vrouwe Gasthuis, in Amsterdam, the Netherlands, between 2007 and 2014 who used psychopharmacological medication during pregnancy. In the Netherlands most pregnant women receive prenatal care from a midwife residing in or outside the hospital. Only women with (expected) complications during pregnancy or delivery are seen by a gynaecologist. Since taking psychotropic medication may cause for example withdrawal symptoms in the baby or postpartum haemorrhage in the mother this can be a (sole) reason for referral to a gynaecologist.

The data from their visits to the hospitals and their deliveries were extracted from the patient charts. The study was approved by the research and ethics board of both hospitals (registration number 14–096).

The cohort was defined as consisting of single pregnancies of women who used psychopharmacological medication in the third trimester. The first cohort group used serotonergic antidepressants (SSRIs, TCAs or SNRIs) with or without other psychopharmacological medication (cohort 1) and the second cohort group only used other psychopharmacological medication (antipsychotics, lithium) but no antidepressants, except for bupropion(cohort 2), all in the third trimester. Bupropion was classified in the non-serotonergic group since its action is related to the inhibition of dopamine and noradrenaline reuptake. All cohort members delivered from 32.0 weeks onwards.

Study design

We conducted a matched cohort study consisting of either pregnancies of women taking serotonergic medication or pregnancies of women taking other psychopharmacological medication. We matched these women to pregnancies of women without documented psychiatric problems and measured the outcome PPH, since data on the use of psychiatric medication in the control population were not available.

Controls

To identify matched controls, we used the linked national perinatal database of the Netherlands Perinatal Registry foundation (PRN or named PERINED since 2016; PERINED approvalnr. 15.34) The PERINED registry covers 96% of all deliveries in the Netherlands and contains anonymous information on pregnancies, deliveries ≥ 22 weeks of gestation and readmission of the child until 28 days after birth [32]. Because the definition of the PERINED database variables changed from 2010 onwards, we used the data set of the recent years 2010–2014.

Exclusion criteria for controls were documented psychiatric problems, delivery in either of the two hospitals or the primary care facility where the cohort members delivered, and women with a length of gestation of less than 32 weeks.

We matched for parity (nulliparity vs multiparity), maternal age (<35, ≥35 years), ethnicity (Caucasian, non-Caucasian), socioeconomic status (low, middle/high), macrosomia (birth weight above 90th percentile adjusted for gestational age and parity), gestational duration (≤37 or >37 weeks), history of PPH (yes/no), induction of labour and hypertensive disorder (yes/no) to make the characteristics of the "type of woman" who used serotonergic or other medication comparable to the controls. We selected 5 controls for each cohort member and matched on equality or nearest neighbour.

In the Netherlands the socioeconomic status (SES) is determined by the Netherlands Institute for Social Research based on the 4-digit zip code, and the score is divided into low SES versus mid/high. The zip code is used nationwide to classify neighbourhoods for example as disadvantaged based om population density, educational level and percentage of low income [33]. The 90th percentile is based on the Dutch reference curve for birthweight by gestational age, parity, ethnicity and gender [34].

The matching factors were based on the 2009 guidelines of the Royal College of Obstetricians and Gynaecologists (revised in 2011), identified factors in literature, clinical reasoning and availability in both databases.

Primary outcome measurements

Outcome was defined as PPH with postpartum blood loss exceeding 1000 ml.

Statistical analysis

At first, in the 'unmatched' cohort, we used traditional analysing techniques (i.e., crude and adjusted logistic regression) to control for confounders in the women who used serotonergic medication and compared them with the controls. Univariate analyses of the baseline characteristics were performed with a chi-square test for categorical variables. Next we matched on the nine factors and repeated the analysis. Maternal and pregnancy baseline characteristics of the women who used serotonergic antidepressants and all the controls were described.

Secondarily, we repeated the analysis, the matching and the analysis after matching for the patients who only used other (non-serotonergic) psychopharmacological medication and compared these with the controls. To estimate the influence of the serotonergic and other psychopharmacological medication on PPH, univariate and multivariate logistic regression analyses were performed both before and after matching. In the adjusted logistic regression analysis, the same nine matching variables were used, supplemented with year of birth of the child.

We could not match for intermediate variables in the causal path of postpartum haemorrhage. The intermediate factors were mode of delivery (operative vaginal delivery or delivery by emergency caesarean section), episiotomy, perineal laceration (defined as third- and fourth-degree tears "total rupture") and retained placenta. Therefore, in addition to the matching, we performed a stratified analysis only for the cohort using serotonergic medication due to the small numbers in the cohort of women using other psychopharmacological medication.

All statistical tests were two-sided, and a p value of 0.05 was chosen as the threshold for statistical significance. Data were analysed using SAS software version 9.3 (SAS institute Inc., Cary, NC, USA). The matching was analysed with R statistical software version 3.2.0 (T Foundation for Statistical computing, Vienna, Austria) using the Matchit package.

Results

In total, 628 singleton pregnancies in women using psychopharmacological medication during the third trimester of pregnancy were included. There were 578 pregnancies in cohort 1 (women who used serotonergic medication) and 50 pregnancies in cohort 2 (women who used other psychopharmacological drugs). Of cohort 2 group, 27 women used antipsychotics (haloperidol, quetiapine, olanzapine, clozapine or flupentixol), eight used a mood stabiliser (lithium or sodium valproate), five used antipsychotics and also a mood stabiliser, two used antipsychotics and also a benzodiazepine, three used only benzodiazepines, one used an antipsychotic and bupropion, and five used only bupropion. 86% of these used monotherapy only. There were 641,364 controls.

Women with serotonergic medication (cohort 1 group)

Women in cohort 1 were more likely to be older than 35 years and to have a low socioeconomic status (SES). They were less likely to have Caucasian ethnicity. This group also had a higher percentage of women with a previous pregnancy complicated by premature birth and/or PPH (Table 1). No differences were found between the two groups for parity, induction of labour, maternal hypertension and macrosomia in the index pregnancy.

Before matching, PPH was more frequent in cohort 1 than among the 641,364 controls (9.7% versus 6.1%, p <0.0003). The adjusted odds ratio (aOR) was 1.6 (95% CI 1.2–2.1) (Table 2).

After matching, cohort 1 was compared with 2890 controls and the differences in the baseline characteristics disappeared (all p-values were non-significant). In cohort 1, the percentage of PPH was significantly higher than controls, 9.7% versus 6.6% (p = 0.0086) (Table 1). The aOR was also significantly increased to 1.5 (95% CI 1.1–2.1) (Table 2).

Women using other psychopharmacological medication (cohort 2 group)

First, we compared cohort 2 with the 641,364 controls (Table 3).

Before matching, cohort 2 comprised more nulliparous women and more women with non-Caucasian ethnicity, low SES and increased maternal age than the control group. The percentage of PPH in cohort 2 did not differ significantly from the percentage in the controls (12.0% versus 6.1%, (p = 0.082). The adjusted odds ratio did not significantly increase: aOR 2.1 (95% CI 0.9–4.9) (Table 4).

After matching, cohort 2 was comparable to 250 controls, and the incidence of PPH among the target population with other psychopharmacological drugs was significantly higher than among these comparable controls (12.1% versus 4.4% (p = 0.034). The adjusted odds ratio was significantly higher: 3.3 (95% CI 1.1–9.8) (Tables 3 and 4).

Stratified analyses

We performed a stratified analysis for intermediate factors in cohort 1 with a PPH of 9.7% and the 2890 controls with a PPH of 6.6%. In cohort 1, PPH was more common among women with operative vaginal deliveries (15.7% versus 7.5%; p = 0.0083) than in controls with operative vaginal deliveries. PPH was also more common among women in cohort 1 who delivered via emergency caesarean delivery (19.6% versus 5.7%;p = 0.0009).

However, in cohort 1, women with a perineal laceration had a lower incidence of PPH than controls with a perineal laceration (3.8% versus 12.9%, p = 0.0266). Among women with retained placentas, the risk of PPH was very high, but this risk was lower in women of cohort 1 compared to the controls (36.7% versus 62.6%; p = 0.0034).

Discussion
Main findings

In our study we tried to unravel the influence the role of serotonergic medication on the development of PPH

Table 1 Baseline characteristics and the outcomes of the 578 women using serotonergic medication and the controls before and after matching

	Before matching					After matching with 5 controls				
	Women with SRmed		Controls (Perined)			Women with SRmed		Controls (Perined)		
	(n = 578)	%	(n = 641,364)	%	p-value	(n = 578)	%	(n = 2890)	%	p-value
Characteristics										
Nulliparity	258	44.6%	289,190	45.1%	NS	258	44.6%	1290	44.6%	NS
Caucasian ethnicity	351	60.7%	522,141	81.4%	<0.0001	351	60.7%	1750	60.6%	NS
Low socioeconomic status	286	49.5%	155,183	24.2%	<0.0001	286	49.5%	1429	49.4%	NS
Maternal age > = 35 years	195	33.7%	131,584	20.5%	<0.0001	195	33.7%	971	33.6%	NS
Previous PPH	16	2.8%	6782	1.1%	<0.0001	16	2.8%	80	2.8%	NS
Induction of labour	135	23.4%	135,251	21.1%	NS	135	23.4%	674	23.3%	NS
Hypertension	47	8.1%	52,763	8.2%	NS	47	8.1%	230	8.0%	NS
Macrosomia P90	59	10.2%	65,522	10.2%	NS	59	10.2%	290	10.0%	NS
Gestational duration <37 weeks	43	7.4%	34,322	5.4%	0.0258	43	7.4%	216	7.5%	NS
Outcome										
PPH (>1000 ml)	56	9.7%	39,171	6.1%	0.0003	56	9.7%	191	6.6%	0.009

SRmed: serotonergic medication

Table 2 Postpartum haemorrhage after use of serotonergic medication (N = 578) versus controls before and after matching

	Crude Odds		Adjusted Odds[a]	
		95% C.I.		95% C.I.
Outcome before matching				
postpartum haemorrhage	1.7	1.3–2.2	1.6	1.2–2.1
Outcome after matching				
postpartum haemorrhage	1.5	1.1–2.1	1.5	1.1–2.1

[a]Adjusted for parity, maternal age, ethnicity, socio-economic status, previous postpartum haemorrhage, hypertension, macrosomia, induction of labour, year of birth and prematurity

reducing as much as possible the effect of potential confounders by performing a matched paired cohort analysis. Secondary we tried to investigate the influence of other psychopharmacological medication on the development of PPH.

Our findings of a higher prevalence of PPH among women using serotonergic medication in the third trimester of pregnancy is in line with the hypothesis we based on previous studies.

On the other hand this prevalence was also increased in women using other psychopharmacological medication. In our population of women using medication with a serotonergic action, we found a 1.5-fold higher percentage of PPH than in a matched control population of women who did not take any psychopharmacological medication. In the group of women using other psychopharmacological medication, this percentage was almost 3 times larger than in the matched control population. In both groups of women using any psychopharmacological medication, the adjusted odds ratios of PPH were significantly higher than in the control group (1.5 resp. 3.3, Tables 2 and 4).

Strengths and limitations

Several strengths and limitations of our study design need to be addressed. The first strength is that we compared the incidence of PPH both in women using serotonergic antidepressants and in women using other psychopharmacological medication to the incidence in women not using any psychopharmacological medication. Secondly, by using a match cohort study we have matched our study population for nine possible confounding variables. In this way we could, despite our small study population, minimize the influence of well-established maternal and pregnancy confounders. Having 5 controls instead of 3 or 1 per participant increased the sample size [35]. A match cohort study can minimize observed measured differences in characteristics among the participants and the controls.

However they cannot rule out unmeasured and unknown factors. Therefore, a limitation is that we had to leave out two well established matching variables, BMI and smoking, since these variables unfortunately were not available in the national PERINED databases. However, the incidence of obesity and smoking in our population was low, 5% of the pregnant women smoked more than 1 cigarette a day and 1,5% smoked more than 10 cigarettes a day. Obesity, defined as BMI above 30 kg/m^2 occurred in 3.3% of our study population. These data suggest that these confounders probably did not have a considerable influence on our results.

A second limitation is that in the serotonergic cohort some of the matched factors could be also considered as intermediate factors, like hypertensive disorders in pregnancy, foetal growth retardation and preterm birth. Therefore we repeated the matching with only five

Table 3 Baseline characteristics and the outcomes of the 50 women using other psychopharmacological medication and the controls before and after matching

	Before matching					After matching with 5 controls				
	other ps.drugs		Controls (Perined)			other ps.drugs		Controls (Perined)		
	(n = 50)	%	(n = 641,364)	%	p-value	n = 50	%	n = 250	%	p-value
Characteristics										
Nulliparity	29	58.0%	289,190	45.1%	0.0666	29	58.0%	145	58.0%	NS
Caucasian ethnicity	26	52.0%	522,141	81.4%	<0.0001	26	52.0%	130	52.0%	NS
Low socioeconomic status	23	46.0%	155,183	24.2%	0.0003	23	46.0%	115	46.0%	NS
Maternal age > = 35 years	16	32.0%	131,584	20.5%	0.044	16	32.0%	80	32.0%	NS
Previous PPH	0	0.0%	6782	1.1%	NS	0	0.0%	0	0.0%	NS
Induction of labour	15	30.0%	135,251	21.1%	NS	15	30.0%	75	30.0%	NS
Hypertension	4	8.0%	52,763	8.2%	NS	4	8.0%	20	8.0%	NS
Macrosomia P90	6	12.0%	65,522	10.2%	NS	6	12.0%	30	12.0%	NS
Gestational duration <37 weeks	5	10.0%	34,322	5.4%	NS	5	10.0%	25	10.0%	NS
Outcome										
PPH (>1000 ml)	6	12.0%	39,171	6.1%	0.0819	6	12.0%	11	4.4%	0.0339

ps.drugs: other psycofarmacological drugs

Table 4 Postpartum haemorrhage after use of other psychopharmacological drugs (n = 50) before and after matching

	Crude Odds	95% C.I.	Adjusted Odds[a]	95% C.I.
Outcome before matching				
Postpartum haemorrhage	2.1	0.9–4.9	2.1	0.9–4.9
Outcome after matching				
Postpartum haemorrhage	3.0	1.0–8.4	3.3	1.1–9.8

[a]Adjusted for parity, maternal age, ethnicity, socio-economic status, previous postpartum haemorrhage, hypertension, macrosomia, induction of labour, year of birth and prematurity

factors and performed a conditional analysis for this group. The adjusted odds ratio of the women using serotoninergic drugs was 1.7 (CI 1.2–1.3) which is even higher than in the first matching and analysis. We performed the matching with five factors and conditional analysis in the other psychopharmacological cohort (n = 50), and the risk was also increased (12% versus 6%) but no longer significant i.e., 1.9 (CI 0.7–5.4). This can be explained through the fact that the numbers of PPH cases are small in this cohort. Another explanation could be that the previous mentioned intermediate factors in the serotonergic cohort are not in the same way applicable to the cohort of women using other psychopharmacological medication [36–38].

A third limitation is that the PERINED database does not have information on the actual medication of women during pregnancy nor on depression during pregnancy. Nevertheless, we excluded all women with records of psychological problems or diseases in the PERINED database, but we cannot completely rule out that some women among the controls may also have used serotonergic or other psychopharmacological medication. On the other hand, this limitation only means that we may have underestimated the effects found in this study. A third limitation is that cohort 2 was relatively small, which made it difficult to perform a stratified analysis in this group.

Interpretation

Our finding that the use of serotoninergic drugs increases the risk of PPH is in agreement with at least five previous studies [5–9]. Some of these studies compared the risk of PPH between women using the medication in different stages of pregnancy [9], and other studies examined women with a psychiatric illness without medication [5]. These approaches do not take into account the potential role of the severity of the underlying psychiatric disorder, since taking women with psychiatric complaints but not using medication as controls probably implies leaving out the more severely ill. Also in those investigations, the severity of psychiatric disorders rather than medication use could be the risk factor related to PPH, since women with

stress due to psychiatric problems may be more prone to prolonged labour [21, 39]. Prolonged labour in itself constitutes a risk factor for PPH [40], but also for delivery by emergency caesarean section and for operative vaginal delivery [18, 19], and both types of delivery also contribute to the development of PPH.

A second explanation for other psychopharmacological medication generating a higher incidence of PPH could be that even though this medication does not directly influence serotoninergic action, it might affect other neurotransmitters and thus create a shift in the neurotransmitter balance, which may indirectly affect the platelet function.

Conclusion

Our study sheds a new light on the possible influence of psychopharmacological medication on postpartum haemorrhage. The hypothesis that the serotonergic action of antidepressant medication plays a main role in the development of PPH probably does not constitute the complete explanation. The results of our study suggest that serotonergic medication but also other psychopharmacological medication during pregnancy can result in a higher risk of PPH. However, it could be plausible that the acting mechanism is not only the medication, but also the underlying disease.

Future research should focus on blood loss postpartum in women using all types of psychopharmacological medication compared to women with equally serious psychiatric illness who do not use any of this medication during pregnancy.

Abbreviations

PPH: Postpartum haemorrhage; SES: Social economic status; BMI: Body mass index; PERINED: Netherlands perinatal registry foundation; SSRIs: Selective serotonin reuptake inhibitors; TCAs: Tricyclic antidepressants; SNRIs: Serotonin and noradrenalin reuptake inhibitors; aOR: Adjusted odds ratio

Acknowledgements

We thank Ms Nancy van der Mark and Ms Ine van der Spek for their contribution to the data collection.

Funding

This research study received no specific funding.

Authors' contributions

The authors were involved as follows: HH, AR, AB, FS and AH, made substantial contributions to conception and design; HH, AH, CdG, MP, AR and FS participated in data acquisition; HH, AR, FS and AH performed the analysis and interpretation of data; HH, AB, AR, CdG, MP, FS and AH have been involved in drafting the manuscript and revising it critically for important intellectual content; HH, AB, AR, CdG, MP, FS and AH have given final approval of the version to be published. Each author has agreed to be accountable for all aspects of the work in ensuring that questions related to the accuracy or integrity of any part of the work are appropriately investigated and resolved.

Competing interests

All authors have completed the Unified Competing Interest form available on request from the corresponding author and declare the following: no author received financial support for the submitted work; no financial relationships with any organizations that might have an interest in the submitted work in the previous 3 years; no other relationships or activities that hat could appear to have influenced the submitted work.

Ethics approval and consent to participate

The advisory board of the scientific board of the OLVG approved the study (registration number 14–096). In 2015, when the research was carried out, the Onze Lieve Vrouwe Gasthuis and the Sint Lucas Andreas Hospital were already legally and administratively merged in one hospital named OLVG. The board of directors decided that from then on approval of the ethic committee of one hospital ensured approval at the other side.

Informed consent of participants was not obtained since, in the Netherlands administrative permission in order to access patient information from patient charts is not needed if the information used is not personally identifiable, the study is retrospective, concerns large numbers of participants and it is not feasible to trace and contact individual participants.

Perined (the Netherlands Perinatal Registry foundation) approved to use the data of the control population (registration number 15.34).

Author details

[1]Department of Hospital Psychiatry, VU University Medical Centre, De Boelelaan 1117, 1081 HV Amsterdam, The Netherlands. [2]Department of Medical Informatics, Academic Medical Centre, University of Amsterdam, Meibergdreef 9, 1105 AZ Amsterdam, The Netherlands. [3]Department of Pediatric Infectious Diseases, Emma Children's Hospital, Academic Medical Centre, University of Amsterdam, Meibergdreef 9, 1105 AZ Amsterdam, The Netherlands. [4]Department of Obstetrics and Gynaecology, VU University Medical Centre, De Boelelaan 1117, 1081 HV Amsterdam, The Netherlands. [5]Department of Obstetrics and Gynaecology, OLVG Hospital (West), Jan Tooropstraat 164, 1061 AE Amsterdam, The Netherlands. [6]Department of Obstetrics and Gynaecology, VU University Medical Centre, De Boelelaan 1117, 1081 HV Amsterdam, The Netherlands. [7]Department of Obstetrics and Gynaecology, OLVG Hospital (East), Oosterpark 9, 1091 AC Amsterdam, The Netherlands. [8]Department of Hospital Psychiatry, OLVG Hospital (West), Jan Tooropstraat 164, 1061 AE Amsterdam, The Netherlands. [9]Department of Hospital Psychiatry, VU University Medical Centre, De Boelelaan 1117, 1081 HV Amsterdam, The Netherlands.

References

1. Briley A, Seed PT, Tydeman G, Ballard H, Waterstone M, Sandall J, Poston L, Tribe RM, Bewleya S. Reporting errors, incidence and risk factors for postpartum haemorrhage and progression to severe PPH: a prospective observational study. BJOG. 2014;121:876–88.
2. Knight M, Callaghan WM, Berg C, Alexander S, Bouvier-Colle M-H, Ford JB, Joseph K, Lewis G, Liston RM, Roberts CL, et al. Trends in postpartum hemorrhage in high resource countries: a review and recommendations from the International Postpartum Hemorrhage Collaborative Group. BMC Pregnancy Childbirth. 2009;9:55–65.
3. Smit M, Chan K, Middeldorp J, van Roosmalen J. Postpartum haemorrhage in midwifery care in the Netherlands: validation of quality indicators for midwifery guidelines. BMC Pregnancy Childbirth. 2014;14:397–402.
4. Bruning AHL, Heller HM, Kieviet N, Bakker PCAM, de Groot CJM, Dolman KM, Honig A. Antidepressants during pregnancy and postpartum hemorrhage: a systematic review. Eur J Obstet Gynecol Reprod Biol. 2015;189:38–47.
5. Grzeskowiak LE, McBain R, Dekker GA, Clifton VL. Antidepressant use in late gestation and risk of postpartum haemorrhage: a retrospective cohort study. BJOG. 2016;123:1929–36.
6. Hanley GE, Smolina K, Mintzes B, Oberlander TF, Morgan SG. Postpartum hemorrhage and use of serotonin reuptake inhibitor antidepressants in pregnancy. Obstet Gynecol. 2016;127(3):553–61.
7. Joseph KS, Sheehy O, Mehrabadi A, Urquia ML, Hutcheon JA, Kramer M, Bérard A. Can drug effects explain the recent temporal increase in atonic postpartum haemorrhage? Paediatr Perinat Epidemiol. 2015;29:220–31.
8. Lindquist PG, Nasiell J, Gustafsson LL, Nordstrom L. Selective serotonin reuptake inhibitor use during pregnancy increases the risk of postpartum hemorrhage and anemia: a hospital-based cohort study. J Thromb Haemost. 2014;12(12):1986–92.
9. Palmsten K, Hernandez-Diaz S, Huybrechts KF, Williams PL, Michels KB, Achtyes ED, Mogun H, Setoguchi S. Use of antidepressants near delivery and risk of postpartum hemorrhage: cohort study of low income women in the United States. BMJ. 2013;347. doi:10.1136/bmj.f4877.
10. Kim DR, Pinheiro E, Luther JF, Eng HF, Dills JL, Wisniewski SR, Wisner KL. Is third trimester serotonin reuptake inhibitor use associated with postpartum hemorrhage? J Psychiatr Res. 2016;73:79–85.
11. Lupattelli A, Spigset O, Koren G, Nordeng H. Risk of vaginal bleeding and postpartum hemorrhage after use of antidepressants in pregnancy a study from the norwegian mother and child cohort study. J Clin Psychopharmacol. 2014;34(1):143–8.
12. Reis M, Källén B. Delivery outcome after maternal use of antidepressant drugs in pregnancy: an update using Swedish data. Psychol Med. 2010; 40(10):1723–33.
13. Salkeld E, Ferris LE, Juurlink DN. The risk of postpartum hemorrhage with selective serotonin reuptake inhibitors and other antidepressants. J Clin Psychopharmacol. 2008;28(2):230–4.
14. Jiang H, Xu L, Li Y, Deng M, Peng C, Ruan B. Antidepressant use during pregnancy and risk of postpartum hemorrhage: a systematic review and meta-analysis. J Psychiatr Res. 2016;83:160–7.
15. Zoega H, Kieler H, Nørgaard M, Furu K, Valdimarsdottir U, Brandt L, Haglund B. Use of SSRI and SNRI antidepressants during pregnancy: a population-based study from Denmark, Iceland, Norway and Sweden. PLoS One. 2015; 10(12). doi:10.1371/journal.pone.0144474.
16. Grigoriadis S, VonderPorten EH, Mamisashvili L, Tomlinson G, Dennis CL, Koren G, Steiner M, Mousmanis P, Cheung A, Radford K, et al. The impact of maternal depression during pregnancy on perinatal outcomes: a systematic review and meta-analysis. J Clin Psychiatry. 2013;74(4):321–41.
17. Grote NK, Bridge JA, Gavin AR, Melville JL, Iyengar S, Katon WJ. A meta-analysis of depression during pregnancy and the risk of preterm birth, low birth weight and intrauterine growth restriction. Arch Gen Psychiatry. 2010;67(10):1012–24.
18. Hu R, Li Y, Zhang Z, Yan W. Antenatal depressive symptoms and the risk of preeclampsia or operative deliveries: a meta-analysis. PLoS One. 2015;10(3). doi:10.1371/journal.pone.0119018.
19. Chung TKH, Lau TK, Yip ASK, Chiu HFK, Lee DTS. Antepartum depressive symptomatology is associated with adverse obstetric and neonatal outcomes. Psychosom Med. 2001;63:830–4.
20. Kinney DK, Yurgelun-Todd DA, Levy DL, Medoff D, Lajonchere CM, Radford-Paregol M. Obstetrical complications in patients with bipolar disorder and their siblings. Psychiatry Res. 1993;48(1):47–56.
21. Andersson L, Sundstrom-Poromaa I, Wulff M, Åstrom M, Bixo M. Implications of antenatal depression and anxiety for obstetric outcome. Obstet Gynecol. 2004;104(3):467–76.
22. Dennis CL, Dowswell T. Interventions (other than pharmacological, psychosocial or psychological) for treating antenatal depression (Review). Cochrane Database Syst Rev. 2013;31(7). doi:10.1002/14651858.CD006795.pub3.
23. Biaggi A, Conroy S, Pawlby S, Pariante CM. Identifying the women at risk of antenatal anxiety and depression: a systematicreview. J Affect Disord. 2016; 191:62–77.
24. Murray L, Sinclair D, Cooper P, Ducournau P, Turner P, Stein A. The socioemotional development of 5-year-old children of postnatally depressed mothers. J Child Psychol Psychiatry. 1999;40(8):1259–71.
25. Verbeek T, Bockting CLH, Pampus MG, Ormel J, Meijer JL, Hartman CA, Burger H. Postpartum depression predicts offspring mental health problems in adolescence independently of parental lifetime psychopathology. J Affect Disord. 2012;136(3):948–54.
26. Cooper WO, Willy ME, Pont SJ, Ray WA. Increasing use of antidepressants in pregnancy. Am J Obstet Gynecol. 2007;196(6):544.e541–545.
27. Jimenez-Solem E. Exposure to antidepressants during pregnancy-prevalences and outcomes. Dan Med J. 2014;61(9):B4916.

28. Andrade SE, Raebel MA, Brown J, Lane K, Livingston J, Boudreau D, Rolnick SJ, Roblin D, Smith DH, Willy ME, et al. Use of antidepressant medications during pregnancy: a multisite study. Am J Obstet Gynecol. 2008;198:194.e191–5.
29. Andrade C, Sandarsh S, Chethan KB, Nagesh KS. Serotonin reuptake inhibitor antidepressants and abnormal bleeding: a review for clinicians and a reconsideration of mechanisms. J Clin Psychiatry. 2010;71(12):1565–75.
30. Dietrich-Muszalska A, Wachowicz B. Platelet haemostatic function in psychiatric disorders: effects of antidepressants and antipsychotic drugs. World J Biol Psychiatry. 2016;11(2-2):293–299.
31. Boyer EW, Shannin M. The serotonin syndrome. N Engl J Med. 2005;352(11):1112–20.
32. Méray N, Reitsma JB, Ravelli AC, Bonsel GJ. Probabilistic record linkage is a valid and transparent tool to combine databases without a patient identification number. J Clin Epidemiol. 2007;60:883–91.
33. Devillé W, Wiegers TA. Recalibration deprived urban areas NIVEL 2012. 2015.
34. Visser GH, Eilers PH, Elferink-Stinkens PM, Merkus HM, Wit JM. New Dutch reference curves for birthweight by gestational age. Early Hum Dev. 2009;85(12):737–44.
35. Rosenbaum P. Impact of multiple matched controls on design sensitivity in observational studies. Biometrics. 2013;69:118–27.
36. Vigod SN, Gomes T, Wilton AS, Taylor VH, Ray JG. Antipsychotic drug use in pregnancy: high dimensional, propensity matched, population based cohort study. BMJ. 2015;350:10. doi:10.1136/bmj.h2298.
37. Boden R, Lundgren M, Brandt L, Reutfors J, Andersen M, Kieler H. Risks of adverse pregnancy and birth outcomes in women treated or not treated with mood stabilisers for bipolar disorder: population based cohort study. BMJ. 2012;345. doi:10.1136/bmj.e7085.
38. Reis M, Kallen B. Maternal use of antipsychotics in early pregnancy and delivery outcome. J Clin Psychopharmacol. 2008;28:10.
39. Gisladottir A, Luque-Fernandez MA, Harlow BL, Gudmundsdottir B, Jonsdottir E, Bjarnadottir RI, Hauksdottir A, Aspelund T, Cnattingius S, Valdimarsdottir UA. Obstetric outcomes of mothers previously exposed to sexual violence. PLOS ONE. 2015;11(3). doi:10.1371/journal.pone.0150726.
40. Royal College of Obstetricians and Gynaecologists: Postpartum Haemorrhage, Prevention and Management (Green-top Guideline No. 52). https://www.rcog.org.uk/en/guidelines-research-services/guidelines/gtg52/.

21

Determinants of pre-eclampsia/Eclampsia among women attending delivery Services in Selected Public Hospitals of Addis Ababa, Ethiopia

Teklit Grum[1*], Abiy Seifu[2], Mebrahtu Abay[1], Teklit Angesom[1] and Lidiya Tsegay[3]

Abstract

Background: Pre-eclampsia is a pregnancy-specific hypertensive disorder usually occurs after 20 weeks of gestation. It is one of the leading causes of maternal and perinatal morbidity and mortality worldwide. In Ethiopia, the major direct obstetric complications including pre-eclampsia/eclampsia account for 85% of the maternal deaths. Unlike deaths due to other direct causes, pre-eclampsia/ eclampsia related deaths appear to be increasing and linked to multiple factors, making prevention of the disease a continuous challenge. The aim of this study is to assess determinants of pre-eclampsia/eclampsiaamong women attending delivery services in selected public hospitals in Addis Ababa, Ethiopia.

Methods: Hospital based unmatched case control study design was employed. The study wasconducted in Addis Ababa among women attending delivery services in two public hospitals from December, 2015 G.C. to February, 2016 G.C. with sample size of 291 (97 cases and 194 controls). Women with pre-eclampsia/eclampsia were cases and women who had not diagnosed for pre-eclampsia/eclampsia were controls. Case-control incidence density sampling followed by interviewer administered was conducted using pretested questionnaire. The data was entered in Epi Info 7 software and exported to STATA 14 for cleaning and analysis. Descriptive statistics were used todisplay the data using tables compared between cases and controls. To compare categorical variables between cases and controls Chi-squared testwas used. Both bivariable and multivariable logistic regression analyses were computed to identify the determinants of pre-eclampsia/eclampsia.

Results: Factors that were found to have statistically significant association with pre-eclampsia or eclampsia were primigravida (AOR: 2.68, 95% CI: 1.38, 5.22), history of preeclampsia on prior pregnancy (AOR: 4.28, 95% CI: 1.61, 11.43), multiple pregnancy (AOR: 8.22, 95% CI: 2.97, 22.78), receiving nutritional counseling during pregnancy (AOR: 0.22, 95% CI: 0.1, 0.48) and drinking alcohol during pregnancy (AOR: 3.97, 95% CI: 1.8, 8.75).

Conclusions: The study identified protective and risk factors for pre-eclampsia/eclampsia. To promptly diagnose and treat pre-eclampsia, health workers should give special attention to women with primigravida and multiple pregnancy. Besides, health care providers should provide nutritional counseling during ANC, including avoiding drinking alcohol during their pregnancy.

Keywords: Determinants, Pre-eclampsia/Eclampsia, Women, Ethiopia

* Correspondence: teklitgwg@yahoo.com
[1]School of Public Health, College of Health Sciences, Aksum University, Aksum, Ethiopia
Full list of author information is available at the end of the article

Background

Pre-eclampsia is a pregnancy-specific hypertensive disorder usually occurs after 20 weeks of gestation. It is a rapidly progressive condition characterized by elevated blood pressure and protein in the urine [1]. If undetected early, it can lead to eclampsia which is severeand one of the top five direct causes of maternal and infant adverse outcome [1, 2].

The exact cause of pre-eclampsia/eclampsia remains unclear. However, abnormally implanted placenta is considered to be major predisposing. This abnormally implanted placenta is believed to result in poor uterine and placental perfusion, which results a state of hypoxia and increased oxidative stress and the release of anti-angiogenic proteins into the maternal plasma along with inflammatory mediators into the maternal plasma [3].

Pre-eclampsia/eclampsia is one of the leading causes of maternal and perinatal morbidity and mortality worldwide. It is an important cause of severe morbidity, long term disability and death among both mothers and their babies. In Africa and Asia, nearly one tenth of all maternal deaths are associated with hypertensive disorders of pregnancy, whereas one quarter of maternal deaths in Latin America have been associated with pre-eclampsia/eclampsia complications [3]. The majority of deaths due to pre-eclampsia/eclampsia are avoidable through the provision of timely and effective care to the women presenting with these complications. Optimizing health care to prevent and treat women with hypertensive disorders is a necessary step towards reducing maternal and infant mortality and morbidity [4].

In Ethiopia the major direct obstetric complications (hemorrhage, obstructed labor, pre-eclampsia/eclampsia, unsafe abortion, sepsis) account for 85% of the maternal deaths as well as many acute and chronic illnesses [5]. Among the five major causes of maternal death severe pre-eclampsia/ eclampsia(PE/E) accounts 11% [6]. The country has identified PE/E as one of the major causes of maternal mortality and is working on improvement of the main components of quality health services. These include capacity-building (ensuring pre-service and in-service training for health providers to detect and manage PE/E, including magnesium sulfate in the national obstetric service guidelines), logistics (making supplies available to health facilities for management of PE/E), and supportive supervision and mentorship with the Obstetrics & Gynecological Society and other partners. Nevertheless, the late antenatal care initiation and limited evidences on causes for pre-eclampsia made difficult on controlling it. As a result, it remains a serious and poorly understood complication of pregnancy, which can progress to maternal death [7].

Unlike maternal deaths due to other direct causes, pre-eclampsia/ eclampsiarelated deaths appear to be increasing and remains a major problem both in maternal and infants morbidity and mortality [8].Giving attention to such causes of maternal mortality could hasten the reduction of maternal mortality. But the determinants of pre-eclampsia/eclampsia have not been well documented in Ethiopia. Therefore, the aim of this study is to assess determinants of pre-eclampsia/eclampsia.

Methods

Study setting

Hospital based unmatched case control study design was conducted in Addis Ababa in two selected public hospitals from December, 2015 G.C. to February, 2016 G.C.The source population for the study was all women attending delivery service in Gandhi and Zewditu Memorial Hospitals. The study population was the selected pregnant women attending delivery services in both hospitals.

Inclusion criteria

The cases were women with blood pressure ≥ 140 mmHg systolic or ≥90 mmHg diastolic on two separate readings taken at least four hours apart with previously normal blood pressure and when proteinuria is greater than or equal to 300 mg per 24-h urine collection or dipstick reading of 1+ after 28 weeks' gestation [1]. The diagnosis involves history taking, physical examination and laboratory test. Cases were selected after the physicians made diagnosis as part of routine case for the women. The women's charts were reviewed, and women were included as cases if they fulfilled the aforesaid diagnostic criteria.

Controls were women who were attending delivery care from both hospitals and were not diagnosed as pre-eclampsia/eclampsia. All cases and controls were seen by obstetrician in the hospitals.

Exclusion criteria

Women with known hypertension and renal disease were excluded from the study. Even though the design was unmatched case control study, women who were not from Addis Ababa were excluded from both groupsto make it comparable. Women with serious medical conditions and who couldn't give consent were also excluded from the study.

Sample size determination

EPI INFO 7 was used to calculate the sample size using double population proportion formula by assuming primigravida as a risk factor with lowest odds ratio of 2.16 and 39% among controls from the literatures reviewed [9]. With assumptions 95% confidence interval, 5% marginal error and 80% power, the calculated sample size was 264. Considering 10% possible non-respondents final sample size of 291(97 cases and 194 controls) was estimated.

Sampling procedure

Zewditu and Gandhi Memorial Hospitals were purposely selected because these two Hospitals are the largest public Hospitals with maternal health service under the Addis Ababa city administration. All cases who came for delivery services consecutively to both hospitals were included until the required sample size was fulfilled. Thestudy used an incidence density sampling approach to selecttwo control women who came for delivery services in the same facilities for each case. Sample size was split between the two hospitals proportional to their delivery caseload. According to the 2014/15 G.C HMIS report, GMH has annual delivery of 5984 while ZMH has annual delivery of 4440.

- Total annual delivery in both Hospitals = 5984 + 4440 = 10,424
- So, the sample size allocated for each hospital was;
- For GMH = 5984*291/10424 = 167 (56 cases and 111 controls)
- For ZMH = 4440*291/10424 = 124(41 cases and 83 controls)

Accordingly 167 and 124 samples were assigned for GMH and ZMH, respectively.

Data collection procedure

Data was collected using pretested interviewer administered questionnaire (Additional file 1). Respondent's medical charts were also reviewed to extract clinical laboratory results. The questionnaire was written in English, translated into Amharic (national language), and then translated back into English to assure its consistency. Four Amharic speaking diploma level midwife nurses were hired as data collectors. Two supervisors with BSc inmidwife nurses supervised the data collection and the principal investigator coordinated them. The supervisors daily checked the consistency, clarity and completeness of the collected questionnaires.

Data analysis procedure

The collected questionnairewas checked manually and entered the data in to epi Info 7 software and exported to stata14 for cleaning and further analysis. Frequency run was made to check for accuracy, consistencies, missed values and variables. Descriptive statistics was used to describe the study populations using measures of frequency, central tendency and dispersion that was displayed using tables compared between cases and controls. To compare categorical variables between cases and controls Chi-squared testwas used.

Bivariable logistic regression analysis was used and variables with P-value < 0.05 in the Bivariable logistic regression analysis were considered for inclusion in to

the multivariable logistic regression analysis to control the effect of confounders.Forwards selection strategy was used to include the variables in the multivariable model. Multicollinearity was checked among the independent variables using variance inflation factor. The necessary assumption of logistic regression was checked using Hosmer and Lemeshow goodness of fit test statistics. Variables with P-value < 0.05 in the multivariable logistic regression analysis were considered as independently significant determinant of pre-eclampsia/eclampsia.

Data quality management

To ensure data quality, questionnaire was pretested, 2 days training was provided to the data collectors and the data collection was supervised. The consistency of data collection among the data collectors was check using Cronbach alpha before data collection. During the data collection supervisors checked each questionnaire for its completeness, consistency and accuracy. Data collectors were informed to correct for any missing values or reconcile inconsistency before discharging the respondents from that hospital. In addition, during data entry range values and pattern analysis that comply with certain regular expression format pattern found in the attributes was used to ensure the quality.Missing value was handled using cases pairwise statistical technique during data analysis.

Results
Socio-demographic characteristics of study participants

From a total of 291 (97 cases and 194 controls) selected from both hospitals, 6(2 cases and 4 controls) refused to participate in the study. A total of 285(95 cases and 190 controls) women who came for delivery care service in GMH and ZMH completed the interview with response rate of 97.9% for both groups.

The mean age of cases 25.42(SD: ±5.33) was lower than that of the controls 27.96(SD: ±4.67). Seventy-four 74(77.89%) of the cases and 158(83.16%) of the controls were with in age group of 20-34 years.Thirty-nine (41.1%) of the cases and 62 (32.6%) of the controls belong to Amhara ethnicity. The dominant religion of the study participants was orthodox with 57(60%) of the cases. Concerning to marital status of study participants, 71 (74.7%) of the cases and 161(84.7%) of the controls were married or living together with their partner. With regards to their occupation, majority of the participants were housewives 47(49.5%) of the cases and 69(36.3%) of the controls.

The median house hold monthly income of study participants was $143 with minimum of $19 and maximum of $476 with range of $457. Forty-six (48.42%) of the cases and 104(54.74%) of the controls of house hold monthly income were above the median of the study subjects (Table 1).

Variables which had significant association with preeclampsia/eclampsia on bivariable analysis and were taken to multivariable analysis for controlling possible confounders were; marital status, family history of hypertension, history of pre-eclampsia, gravidity, pregnancy multiplicity,

Table 1 Socio-demographic characteristics of study participants in selected public hospitals of Addis Ababa, Ethiopia, 2016

Variables	Cases	Controls	Pearson chi^2	p-value
	Number (%)	Number (%)		
Age				
< 20	11(11.58)	10(5.26)		
20-34	74(77.89)	158(83.16)	3.7066	0.157
≥ 35	10(10.53)	22(11.58)		
Mean(SD)	25.42(±5.33)	27.96(±4.67)		
Ethnicity				
Amhara	39(41.1)	62(32.6)	3.2019	0.525
Oromo	23(24.2)	56(29.5)		
Tigray	12(12.6)	29(15.3)		
Gurage	12(12.6)	30(15.8)		
Others	9(9.5)	13(6.8)		
Religion				
Orthodox	57(60)	106(55.8)		
Muslim	17(17.9)	47(24.7)	3.0962	0.377
Protestant	11(11.6)	25(13.2)		
Others	10(10.5)	12(6.3)		
Marital status				
Never married	13(13.7)	13(6.8)	4.6947	0.096
Married/Living together	71(74.7)	161(84.7)		
Others	11(11.6)	16(8.4)		
Occupation				
House wife	47(49.47)	69(36.32)		
Merchant	11(11.56)	41(21.58)	10.4362	0.015
Employee	26(27.37)	69(36.32)		
Student	11(11.56)	11(5.79)		
Educational status				
No formal education	10(10.5)	17(8.9)		
Primary	24(25.3)	41(21.6)	3.8222	0.431
Secondary	33(34.7)	70(36.8)		
Vocational/Technical	14(14.7)	43(22.6)		
Higher education	14(14.7)	19(10)		
Monthly house hold income				
< $143	49(51.58)	86(45.26)	3.0672	0.080
≥ $143	46(48.42)	104(54.74)		

pregnancy planning, nutritional counseling during ANC, contraceptive use, alcohol and fruit intake during pregnancy.Even though attending ANC was significantly associated with preeclampsia on bivariable analysis, it was not included in the multivariable analysis due to collinearity.

Regarding to medical history related risk factors, multivariable analysis revealed that women who had previous history of preeclampsia had higher risk of preeclampsia. The odds of developing pre-eclampsia were 4 times higher for the women with history of preeclampsia comparing to their counter parts (AOR: 4.28, 95% CI: 1.61, 11.43). Primigravida was found to be risk factor for preeclampsia on the multivariable analysis. The odds of developing pre-eclampsia were 2.68 times higher in women with primigravida comparing to the women with multigravida (AOR: 2.68 95% CI: 1.38, 5.22). Women who had multiple pregnancies (twin) had higher risk of pre-eclampsia comparing to women with singleton pregnancy in the multivariable analysis (AOR: 8.22 95% CI: 2.97, 22.78). The multivariate analysis also revealed that receiving nutritional counseling during ANC contact was found to protect the women from preeclampsia. The risk of developing pre-eclampsia was lower among women who had received nutritional counseling (AOR: 0.22, 95% CI: 0.10, 0.48). Women who reported to have drunken alcohol during the pregnancy had also an increased risk of pre-eclampsia as compared to those women who did not drink alcohol in multivariable analysis (AOR = 3.97, 95% CI = 1.8, 8.75)(Table 2).

Discussion

We conducted facility based unmatched case control study with the aim of assessing medical disease, obstetric history and behavioral determinants of preeclampsia/eclampsia. We found that primigravida, having positive history of preeclampsia in previous pregnancy, multiplicity of pregnancy and alcohol drinking during pregnancy as risk factor whereas nutritional counseling during antenatal care was a protective factorfor preeclampsia/eclampsia.

Concerning to medical disease, family history of hypertension was statistically significant with pre-eclampsia/eclampsia on bivariate analysis only (COR: 2.6 95% CI: 1.08, 6.27) but on the Dessie cross sectional study [10] revealed that women with positive family history of hypertension had 7 times odds of developing pre-eclampsia/eclampsia. The study subjects in Dessie were pregnant women who came for ANC follow up so, the difference could be due to the difference of study design and study subjects.

Multivariable analysis revealed that women who had previous history of pre-eclampsia had higher risk of preeclampsia/eclampsia (AOR: 4.28, 95% CI: 1.61, 11.43). This finding is consistent with the studies conducted in Iran [11, 12]. This implies women with history of

Table 2 Bivariable and multivariable analyses on determinants of pre-eclampsia/eclampsia among womenattended delivery services in selected public Hospitalsof Addis Ababa, Ethiopia, 2016

Variables	Cases Number (%)	Controls Number (%)	COR(95%: CI)	AOR(95%: CI)
Marital status				
Never married	13(13.67)	13(6.84)	2.27(1.01, 5.14)	0.76(0.19, 2.88)
Married/Living together	71(74.74)	161(84.74)	1	1
Others	11(11.58)	16(8.42)	1.56(0.69, 3.53)	1.34(0.43, 4.11)
Occupation				
Employed	26(27.34)	69(36.32)	1	1
House wife	47(49.47)	69(36.32)	1.81(1.01, 3.24)	1.72(0.83, 3.58)
Merchant	11(11.58)	41(21.58)	0.71(0.32, 1.59)	0.55(0.18, 1.64)
Student	11(11.58)	11(5.79)	2.65(1.03, 6.86)	2.23(0.67, 7.46)
Family history of hypertension				
No	83(87.4)	180(94.7)	1	1
Yes	12(12.6)	10(5.3)	2.6(1.08, 6.27)	2.24(0.67, 7.46)
History of preeclampsia				
No	27(71.05)	106(89.1)	1	1
Yes	11(28.95)	13(10.9)	3.32(1.34, 8.23)	4.28(1.61, 11.43) *
Gravidity				
Primigravida	57(60)	71(37.37)	2.5(1.52, 4.17)	2.68(1.38, 5.22) *
Multigravida	38(40)	119(62.63)	1	1
Pregnancy multiplicity				
Singleton	78(82.1)	181(95.3)	1	1
Twin	17(17.9)	9(4.7)	5.03(2.18, 11.62)	8.22(2.97, 22.78) **
Planned pregnancy				
No	21(22.11)	14(7.37)	3.57(1.72, 7.39)	2.1(0.68, 7.46)
Yes	74(77.89)	176(92.63)	1	1
Receiving nutritional counseling during ANC				
No	34(40)	23(12.6)	1	1
Yes	51(60)	160(87.4)	0.22(0.12, 0.4)	0.22(0.1, 0.48) **
Using contraceptives				
Non-users	32(33.68)	85(44.74)	1	1
Hormonal	56(58.95)	81(42.63)	1.84(1.08, 3.12)	1.07(0.52, 2.2)
Mechanical	5(5.26)	10(5.26)	1.32(0.42, 4.19)	0.87(0.15, 5.17)
Alcohol intake				
No	62(65.26)	169(88.95)	1	1
Yes	33(34.74)	21(11.05)	4.28(2.3, 7.9)	3.97(1.8, 8.75) *
Fruit intake				
No	15(15.79)	11(5.79)	3.05(1.34, 6.94)	1.57(0.47. 5.26)
Yes	80(84.21)	179(94.21)	1	1

COR crud odds ratio, AOR adjusted odds ratio, * p-value <0.05, **p-value <0.001

preeclampsia/eclampsia on their prior history need to have a focus and could be an acceptable means of screening for pre-eclampsia, especially in limited resourced locations.

Primigravida was independently associated with pre-eclampsia/eclampsia in the multivariable analysis. This study is in agreement with studies conducted in Egypt [9], Nigeria [13], Uganda [14] and England (Krishnachetty, B.

and F. Plaat: Managment of hypertensive disorders of pregnancy, unpublished) which declares primigravida was a risk factor for pre-eclampsia/eclampsia. Pre-eclampsia generally is considered a disease of the first pregnancy [15] which is due to the immunological incompetence seen in first pregnancy between fetoplacental and maternal tissues [16].

In this study, multivariable analysis revealed that multiplicity of pregnancy was independently associated with pre-eclampsia/eclampsia. Another studies conducted in Pakistan [17], India [18] and England also has a finding which is in light of this study. This is explained by women with multiple pregnancy obstetric conditions had a large placenta which results in decreased placental perfusion. The excess of placenta tissues could not be perfused adequately [19] comparing to the women with singleton pregnancy which lead both the mother and the fetus contribute to the risk of pre-eclampsia/eclampsia.

Multivariate analysis revealed that preeclampsia was lower on women who had received nutritional counseling comparing to the women who had not received nutritional counseling (AOR: 0.22 95% CI: 0.1, 0.48). This finding was in agreement with the study conducted in India [18] which showed received advice on pregnancy nutrition during ANC visit was a protective for pre-eclampsia/eclampsia. The protective factor of receiving nutritional counseling during ANC could be explained by the counseling on the healthy diet during pregnancy by the health workers which can be protective factor for pre-eclampsia. The content of nutritional counseling of the two hospitals include antioxidant and calcium rich dietary habits. Besides, there is a need for further studies to assess preventive nutritional factors for pre-eclampsia/eclampsia.

The multivariable analysis in this study indicates that alcohol intake during pregnancy was a significant risk factor for pre-eclampsia/eclampsia. This current finding is in contrast of the studies conducted in Uganda [14] and India [18] in which alcohol drinking during pregnancy had no significant association with pre-eclampsia/eclampsia. The cross-sectional study conducted in India, unlike the current study, was based on the women's report of clinical manifestation for pre-eclampsia and were not diagnosed by physicians. More over the study subjects conducted in Uganda study were pregnant women who came for ANC follow up and labor ward with complications unlike to the current study which could be the reason for the difference.

This study could be seen in light of the limitations that the diagnosis for pre-eclampsia depend on the competency of obstetricians since this study used the diagnosed women. There might be introduced selection bias since cases were selected consecutively as they appear for diagnosis. Preeclampsia can be developed later on the postpartum period and the study subjects were not followed after discharge from hospitals. There might be also introduces recall bias for some information acquired using the memory of participants. Besides, the institutional study cannot represent the population.

Conclusions

The results of this studysuggest that there are preventive and risk factors for preeclampsia. Some factors such as primigravida, twin pregnancy, having history of pre-eclampsia and drinking alcohol during pregnancy were the risk factors for the pre-eclampsia/eclampsia.Since identification of the riskfactors will enhance the ability to diagnose and monitor women likely to develop preeclampsia before the onset of disease for timely interventions and better maternal and fetal outcomes. Receiving nutritional counseling during pregnancy on ANC follow up were found that protective for the pre-eclampsia/eclampsia.It is recommended that health workers should use primigravida, preeclampsia in previous pregnancy and women with twin pregnancy factors as a screening tool for pre-eclampsia prediction and early diagnoses. Health care providers should give nutritional counseling including avoiding drinking alcohol for the pregnant women during their ANC visits. Further research is needed to understand more for the risk factors for pre-eclampsia/eclampsia particularly on dietary habits.

Abbreviations

ANC: Antenatal Care; AOR: Adjusted Odds Ratio; CI: Confidence Interval; COR: Crude Odds Ratio; GMH: Gandhi Memorial Hospital; HMIS: Health Management Information System; PE/E: Preeclampsia/Eclampsia; SD: Standard Deviation; ZMH: Zewditu Memorial Hospital

Acknowledgments

We would like to thank school of Public Health College of health science Addis Ababa University for financially supporting the research.
Our sincere thanks also go to Addis Ababa regional health bureau, Zewditu Memorial Hospital and Gandhi Memorial Hospital health management information systemofficers for giving us the necessary information.Last but not least, we would like to thank the study participants, data collector and supervisors for their volunteers and participating actively during the data collection.

Funding

The research reported in this manuscript has been funded through the school of Public Health College of health science Addis Ababa University.

Authors' contributions

TG and AS have contributed in the design, data collection, data analysis, write up and manuscript development. TA, MA and LT have contributed in data collection, edition and revision of the final manuscript. All authors read and approved the final manuscript.

Competing interests

The authors declare that they have no competing interests

Author details

[1]School of Public Health, College of Health Sciences, Aksum University, Aksum, Ethiopia. [2]School of Public Health, College of Health Sciences, Addis Ababa University, Addis Ababa, Ethiopia. [3]School of Nursing, College of Health Sciences, Aksum University, Aksum, Ethiopia.

References

1. American College of Obstetricians and Gynecologists. Hypertension in Pregnancy,Task force on hypertension in pregnancy. Obstet Gynecol. 2013; 122(5):1122–31.
2. Green P.Update in the Diagnosis and Management of Hypertensive Disorders in Pregnancy. Michigan: Wayne State University School of Medicine; 2014.
3. Al-Jameila N, et al. A brief overview of preeclampsia. J Clin Med Res. 2014;6(1):1–7.
4. World health organization. Recommendations for prevention and treatment of pre-eclampsia and eclampsia. Geneva: World health organization; 2011.
5. Federal Democratic Republic of Ethiopia Ministry of Health, Health sector development Programme IV 2010/11 – 2014/15, 2010.
6. Federal Democratic Republic of Ethiopia Ministry of Health. Maternal death surveillance and response (MDSR) technical guideline. Addis Ababa: Federal Democratic Republic of Ethiopia Ministry of Health; 2013.
7. Maternal and Child Health Integrated Program (MCHIP). Interventions for impact in essential obstetric and newborn care. Addis Ababa: Maternal and Child Health Integrated Program (MCHIP); 2011.
8. JSI Research & Training Institute, Addressing community maternal and neonatal health in Ethiopia. Report from National Scoping Exercise and National Workshop to increase demand, accesses and use of community maternal and neonatal health services, 2009.
9. El-Moselhy EA, Khalifa HO, Amer SM, Mohammad KI, Abd El-Aal HM. Risk factors and impacts of pre-Eclampsia: an epidemiological study among pregnant mothers in Cairo, Egypt. J Am Sci. 2011;7(5):311–23.
10. Tessema GA, Tekeste A, Ayele TA. Preeclampsia and associated factors among pregnant women attending antenatal care in Dessie referral hospital, Northeast Ethiopia: a hospital-based study. BMC Pregnancy and Childbirth. 2015;15:73.
11. Direkvand-Moghadam A, Khosravi A, Sayehmiri K. Predictive factors for preeclampsia in pregnant women: a unvariate and multivariate logistic regression analysis. Biochimica Polonica. 2012;59(4):673–7.
12. Kashanian M, et al. Risk factors for pre-Eclampsia: a study in Tehran, Iran. Arch Iran Med. 2011;4(6):412–5.
13. Guerrier G, et al. Factors associated with severe preeclampsia and eclampsia in Jahun, Nigeria. Int J Women's Health. 2013;5:509–13.
14. Kiondo P, et al. Risk factors for pre-eclampsia in Mulago hospital, Kampala, Uganda. Trop Med Int Health. 2012;17(4):480–7.
15. Harutyunyan A. Investigation of risk factors for preeclampsia development among reproductive age women living in Yerevan, Armenia: a case-control study. 2009.
16. Sibai BM. Diagnosis and managment of gestational hypertension and pre-eclampsia. Obstet Gynecol. 2003;102(1):181–92.
17. Shamsi U, Saleem S, Nishter N. Epidemiology and risk factors of preeclampsia; an overview of observational studies. US Natl Libr Med Enlisted J. 2013;6(4):292-300.
18. Agrawal S, Walia GK. Prevalence and Risk Factors for Symptoms Suggestive of PreEclampsia in Indian Women. J Women's Health, Issues & Care. 2014; 3(6). http://dx.doi.org/10.4172/2325-9795.1000169.
19. Robert JM and Gammil HS, Preeclampsia: recent insights. American Heart Association. USA: Magee-Womens Research Institute; 2005.

22

Haematological and fibrinolytic status of Nigerian women with post-partum haemorrhage

Ian Roberts[1]* , Haleema Shakur[1], Bukola Fawole[2], Modupe Kuti[3], Oladapo Olayemi[4], Adenike Bello[4],
Olayinka Ogunbode[4], Taiwo Kotila[5], Chris O. Aimakhu[4], Tolulase Olutogun[5], Beverley J. Hunt[6] and Sumaya Huque[1]

Abstract

Background: Early treatment with tranexamic acid reduces deaths due to bleeding after post-partum haemorrhage. We report the prevalence of haematological, coagulation and fibrinolytic abnormalities in Nigerian women with postpartum haemorrhage.

Methods: We performed a secondary analysis of the WOMAN trial to assess laboratory data and rotational thromboelastometry (ROTEM) parameters in 167 women with postpartum haemorrhage treated at University College Hospital, Ibadan, Nigeria. We defined hyper-fibrinolysis as EXTEM maximum lysis (ML) > 15% on ROTEM. We defined coagulopathy as EXTEM clot amplitude at 5 min (A5) < 40 mm or prothrombin ratio > 1.5.

Results: Among the study cohort, 53 (40%) women had severe anaemia (haemoglobin< 70 g/L) and 17 (13%) women had severe thrombocytopenia (platelet count < 50 × 10⁹/L). Thirty-five women (23%) had ROTEM evidence of hyper-fibrinolysis. Based on prothrombin ratio criteria, 16 (12%) had coagulopathy. Based on EXTEM A5 criteria, 49 (34%) had coagulopathy.

Conclusion: Our findings suggest that, based on a convenience sample of women from a large teaching hospital in Nigeria, hyper-fibrinolysis may commonly occur in postpartum haemorrhage. Further mechanistic studies are needed to examine hyper-fibrinolysis associated with postpartum haemorrhage. Findings from such studies may optimize treatment approaches for postpartum haemorrhage.

Keywords: Fibrinolysis, Coagulation, Postpartum haemorrhage

Background

Tranexamic acid (TXA) administration reduces death due to bleeding in trauma patients. Among patients treated within 3 h of injury, TXA reduces death due to bleeding by one third [1–3]. Early activation of fibrinolysis is common after serious injury and contributes to the coagulation abnormalities seen in bleeding trauma patients [4, 5]. Hypo-perfusion and tissue injury are thought to start the coagulopathy, although we do not understand the molecular pathways [6].

Results from the WOMAN trial, a large randomised trial conducted primarily in low and middle income countries, show that early tranexamic acid use reduces death due to bleeding after postpartum haemorrhage (PPH) [7]. This suggests that fibrinolysis is also an important pathophysiological mechanism in obstetric bleeding. However, whereas increased fibrinolysis is common in trauma, its association with PPH is less well known [8]. We report the prevalence of hyper-fibrinolysis in women with PPH in Nigeria.

Methods

The WOMAN trial was a randomised placebo controlled trial of the effect of tranexamic acid on death, hysterectomy and other surgical interventions in women

* Correspondence: Ian.roberts@lshtm.ac.uk
[1]Clinical Trials Unit, London School of Hygiene and Tropical Medicine, Keppel Street, London WC1E 7HT, UK
Full list of author information is available at the end of the article

with clinically diagnosed primary PPH [7]. Although the diagnosis was clinical, we specified that diagnosis of primary PPH could be based on an estimated blood loss of more than 500 mL after vaginal birth or 1000 mL after caesarean section, or any blood loss sufficient to compromise haemodynamic stability. The diagnosis of PPH could also be made using clinical judgement, independent of the volume of blood loss. We have described the methods in detail elsewhere [7]. We examined haematological (full blood count) and haemostatic parameters in a sample of 167 trial participants recruited at University College Hospital, Ibadan, Nigeria. A total of 309 women were recruited into the WOMAN trial at University College Hospital. Because of occasional equipment failures and lack of reagents the 167 (54%) women included in the ETAC study were not a consecutive series. Although most of the recruited women delivered at University College Hospital, some patients were transferred from outlying health facilities after they had developed PPH because they required urgent medical support. In these women, blood loss was estimated based on the history and observed blood loss.

After completing consent procedures but before giving the trial treatment (TXA or placebo), we drew approximately 15 mL of venous blood and divided the sample into three vacutainer tubes. We collected one 5 mL sample in a tube containing potassium EDTA for full blood count analysis and two 4.5 mL samples in tubes containing 0.5 mL sodium citrate (0.109 mol/L)

for coagulation and rotational thromboelastometry. We used a five-parameter particle counter Sysmex KN analyser (Sysmex Corporation, Kobe, Japan) for the blood count analysis. Anaemia was defined according to the World Health Organisation definition of anaemia in pregnancy as a haemoglobin below 110 g/L and below 70 g/L for severe anaemia [9].

After centrifuging the blood at 3000 g for 20 min, we measured prothrombin time (PT), normalised prothrombin ratio, activated partial thromboplastin time (aPTT), Clauss fibrinogen and D-dimers using a HumaClot Junior automated coagulation analyser. We measured ROTEM thromboelastometry parameters at 37 °C using two of the four channels (EXTEM, APTEM) of the ROTEM coagulation analyser [TEM®, Munich, Germany]). In EXTEM, coagulation is initiated using a small amount of tissue factor and the development of the clot is expressed in numbers and as a trace. In APTEM, coagulation is initiated in the same way, but the addition of aprotinin or tranexamic acid in the reagent inhibits fibrinolysis in vitro. By comparing the two traces, the extent of fibrinolysis can be assessed. If the sample is hyper-fibrinolytic, the same degree of clot lysis seen in EXTEM is not present in APTEM (Fig. 1). The following ROTEM variables were examined from the EXTEM and APTEM traces (Fig. 2): Clotting time (CT) which corresponds to the time required to trigger the process of coagulation, amplitude of the clot at 5 min and 10 min (CA5 and CA10, respectively), maximum clot firmness (MCF), clot lysis at

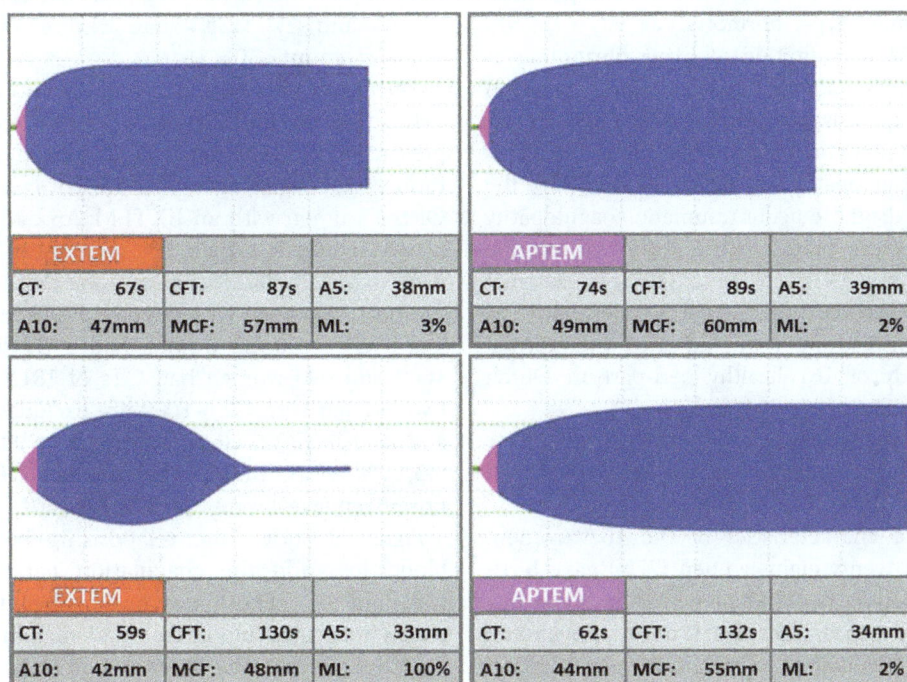

Fig. 1 ROTEM traces with (top) and without (bottom) hyper-fibrinolysis

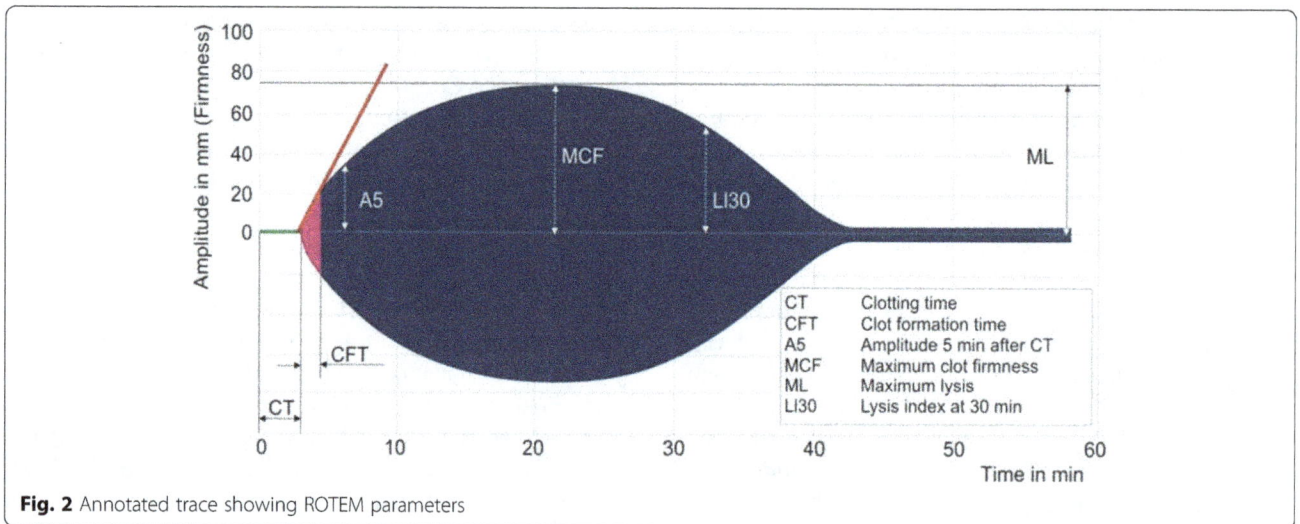

Fig. 2 Annotated trace showing ROTEM parameters

30 min and 60 min (LI30 and LI60, respectively), and maximum lysis (ML). We stored the ROTEM reagents at 2–8 °C with temperature monitoring and we used in date reagents.

We conducted quality control (QC) analyses as per the manufacturer's recommendations. Before starting the study, TEM staff trained the Nigerian study team to use the ROTEM machine. We stored the ROTEM data on the machine with a backup after each analysis. We collected, cleaned and analysed the study data at the Clinical Trials Unit of the London School of Hygiene & Tropical Medicine. Fibrinolysis was assessed as the amount of clot lysis on EXTEM (https://www.rotem.de/en/methodology/interpretation/). We defined hyper-fibrinolysis as ML > 15% on ROTEM EXTEM. This definition of hyper-fibrinolysis is provided by the manufacturer and is widely used in research studies [4]. Coagulopathy was defined as an EXTEM A5 < 40 mm or a prothrombin ratio > 1.5. This A5 definition of coagulopathy was based on studies of the use of ROTEM to diagnose acute traumatic coagulopathy in which a A5 < 40 mm predicted the receipt of massive blood transfusion in 73% of patients [10, 11]. Normal ROTEM values for peri-partum Nigerian women have not been studied, so instead we have indicated the normal values from a study of 161 healthy peri-partum Dutch women [12].

Results

Table 1 shows the characteristics of the 167 women. One hundred and twenty eight women (77%) gave birth in the hospital, whereas 39 (23%) gave birth in other settings and were admitted after PPH onset. Seventeen (10%) women received colloids during fluid resuscitation for PPH prior to sampling. The estimated mean blood loss at the time of randomisation and blood sampling

was 1531 mL. One hundred and eight (65%) women lost more than 1000 mL of blood.

Table 2 shows the full blood count and haemostatic parameters. One hundred and sixteen (88%) women were anaemic (haemoglobin < 110 g/L) and 53 (40%) were severely anaemic (haemoglobin < 70 g/L) at the time of sampling. Thirty eight women (33%) had a microcytic picture (defined as an mean corpuscular volume < 80 fl), although there was no further investigation to discover if this was due to iron deficiency or thalassemia traits or both. Twenty-six women (21%) were lymphopenic (lymphocyte count < 1×10^9/L). Forty-one (32%) women had thrombocytopenia (platelet count < 100×10^9/L) and 17 (13%) had severe thrombocytopenia (platelet count < 50×10^9/L).

Thirty five women (23%) had an EXTEM ML > 15%. If defined as an EXTEM A5 < 40 mm, coagulopathy was present in 49 (34%) mothers. If defined as a prothrombin ratio > 1.5, coagulopathy was present in 16 (12%) mothers. Of the women with an EXTEM A5 < 40 mm, 72% had a platelet count less than 100. The mean and median CT were markedly different suggesting that there are outliers. Of the 151 women with data for EXTEM CT, 127 women had a CT ≤ 100, 22 women had a CT between 101 and 1000 and two women had CTs of 1814 and 3468. If the two women with CT > 1000 are excluded, the mean (SD) and median (IQR) clotting times were 93.6 (138.7) and 54 (45, 70) respectively. The median (IQR) for plasma fibrinogen levels were 6.6 (3.2–12.3) g/L.

Figure 3 shows the relationship between estimated blood loss and the coagulation parameters (maximal lysis and A5). There was no significant correlation between estimated blood loss and maximal lysis ($r = 0.01$, $p = 0.86$). There was a weak but statistically significant negative correlation between estimated blood loss and A5 ($r = -0.35$, $p < 0.001$). After excluding women transferred

Table 1 Baseline characteristics of trial participants (N = 167)

	Count (%) / Mean(SD)
Age (years)	
Mean (SD)	31.9 (5.6)
Range	18–46
Time since delivery (hours)	
≤ 3	103 (61.7%)
> 3	64 (38.3%)
Mean (SD)	4.2 (5.4)
Type of delivery	
Vaginal	80 (47.9%)
Caesarean section	87 (52.1%)
Delivery in randomising hospital	
Yes	128 (76.7%)
No	39 (23.4%)
Cause of haemorrhage	
Uterine Atony	74 (44.3%)
Surgical trauma/tears	59 (35.3%)
Placenta praevia/accreta	21 (12.6%)
Other	12 (7.2%)
Unknown	1 (0.6%)
Systolic blood pressure (mm(Hg)	
< 90	31 (18.6%)
≥90	135 (80.8%)
Missing	1 (0.6%)
Mean (SD)	110 (27)
Estimated volume of blood loss (mL)	
≤ 1000	59 (35.3%)
> 1000	108 (64.7%)
Median (25th, 75th percentile)	1200 (1000, 2000)
Range	500–5530
Colloids given	
Yes	17 (10.2%)
No	150 (89.8%)

from outside health facilities, the results were essentially the same (Maximal Lysis $r = 0.06$, $p = 0.51$; A5 $r = -0.46$, $p < 0.001$).

Discussion

Although 99% deaths from PPH occur in low and middle income countries, most of the research on the haemostatic abnormalities in PPH is from high income countries [13–15].

Among this cohort of women who received care at a Nigerian hospital for PPH, nearly one quarter of women had findings suggestive of hyper-fibrinolysis (ML > 15%).

This contrasts with studies in high-income settings where hyper-fibrinolysis is considered less common in PPH [14] de Lange et al. reported that 9% of women after normal labour had ML of > 15% within 1 h of delivery of the placenta [12] with increased D-dimer levels. Older studies looking at peri-partum changes in fibrinolysis show increases in tissue plasminogen activator (t-PA) immediately after delivery, followed by increases in plasminogen activator inhibitor (PAI-1) [16, 17].

In patients with trauma, ROTEM appears to underestimate the prevalence of fibrinolytic activation compared with more sensitive measures such as plasmin-antiplasmin complexes [4]. Further studies are needed to examine which parameters are most sensitive in detecting fibrinolysis in obstetric bleeding. Although we did not find any correlation between estimated blood loss and fibrinolytic activity, inaccuracy in blood loss estimates could easily have obscured such an association. Indeed, evidence from the WOMAN trial that administration of tranexamic acid significantly reduces death due to bleeding and re-operation for bleeding, strongly suggests that fibrinolysis plays an important role in PPH. Furthermore, a randomised trial conducted in France has shown that there is an early increase in D-dimers and plasmin-antiplasmin complexes in women with active PPH and that this increase is attenuated among women who received tranexamic acid [18].

Fibrinogen levels would be expected to fall with increased fibrinolysis due to increased consumption and fibrinogenolysis. However, despite the high prevalence of hyper-fibrinolysis, the fibrinogen levels appeared to be elevated. Compared to non-pregnant women, fibrinogen levels are increased in pregnancy reaching their peak in the third trimester [19]. Nevertheless, the fibrinogen levels seen in our study are higher than in studies in high income settings. This might be related to the effects of inflammation due to acute and chronic infections including HIV and their treatments [20]. The prevalence of HIV in Nigeria is 3% and it is notable that 21% of our sample were lymphopenic. Further studies in low and middle income countries are need to confirm or refute our results.

Many women were anaemic and the degree of anaemia suggests that many were anaemic before developing PPH. Anaemia in Africa has multiple aetiologies including iron deficiency, functional iron deficiency (due infections such as malaria and HIV); genetic conditions such as sickle cell disease, thalassemia and glucose-6-phosphate dehydrogenase deficiency; parasitic infections leading to blood loss (e.g. hookworms); and drugs such as anti-retrovirals. Furthermore, due to the expansion of the plasma volume in pregnancy, haematocrit falls. Olatunbosun et al. found that 54% of women booking into an obstetric clinic in Uyo, Nigeria were anaemic, with most having evidence of

Table 2 Haematological parameters of trial participants at baseline ($N = 167$)

	n^a	Mean (SD) / Count (%)	Median (25th, 75th centile range)	Normal range[b]
Full Blood Count Variables				
Red blood cell count (×10^12/L)	130	2.9 (1.0)	3.0 (2.3, 3.7)	3.8–5.8
Haemoglobin (g/L)	132	78.1 (35.6)	79.5 (56, 97)	110–165
Haemoglobin < 110 g/L		116 (87.9%)		
Microcytic (MCV < 80)		38 (32.8%)		
Normocytic (MCV 80–100)		75 (64.7%)		
Macrocytic (MCV > 100)		3 (2.6%)		
Haemoglobin < 70 g/L		53 (40.2%)		
Hematocrit (%)	127	24.2 (7.7)	24.7 (19.2, 30)	35–50
Hematocrit < 33%		109 (85.8%)		
Hematocrit < 25%		64 (50.4%)		
White cell count (×10^9/L)	131	11.9 (8.1)	11.2 (5.3, 16.9)	3.5–10.0
White cell count > 25 (×10^9/L)		8 (6.1%)		
Lymphocyte count (×10^9/L)	122	2.6 (2.4)	1.9 (1, 3)	1.2–3.2
Lymphocyte count < 1 (×10^9/L)		26 (21.3%)		
Differential white cell count (monocytes) (×10^9/L)	100	1.8 (1.8)	1.3 (0.6, 2.2)	0.3–0.8
Differential white cell count (granulocytes) (×10^9/L)	100	8.7 (5.6)	7.7 (5.1, 11.5)	1.2–6.8
Platelet count (×10^9/L)	130	155.2 (101.7)	137 (86, 208)	150–390
Platelet count < 100 (×10^9/L)		41 (31.5%)		
Platelet count < 50 (×10^9/L)		17 (13.1%)		
Coagulation variables				
Prothrombin time (PT, seconds)	137	19.0 (12.6)	15.2 (13.5, 18.8)	9.6–12.9
Normalised prothrombin ratio	133	1.2 (0.7)	1.0 (0.9, 1.2)	
Normalised prothrombin ratio > 1.2		29 (21.8%)		
Normalised prothrombin ratio > 1.5		16 (12.0%)		
Activated partial thromboplastin time (APTT, seconds)	133	35.9 (22.9)	30.4 (27.1, 35.6)	
Thrombin time (TT, seconds)	124	13.1 (12.5)	10.4 (9.1, 12.6)	
Normalised thrombin ratio	124	0.9 (0.9)	0.7 (0.6, 0.9)	
Fibrinogen (g/L)	136	8.4 (6.6)	6.6 (3.2, 12.3)	
Fibrinogen (< 1 g/L)		4 (2.9%)		
Fibrinogen (< 2 g/L)		16 (11.8%)		
Fibrinogen (< 4 g/L)		45 (33.1%)		
D-Dimer (mg/L)	119	8.6 (8.2)	5.7 (2.3, 13.5)	
Thromboelastometry (ROTEM® EXTEM) variables				
Clotting time (CT, seconds)	151	127.4 (336.9)	54 (45, 72)	34–66
Amplitude at 5 mins (A5, mm)	146	42.1 (15.8)	47 (35, 53)	
A5 < 40 mm		49 (33.6%)		
Amplitude at 10 mins (A10, mm)	149	51.6 (17.5)	58 (47, 63)	44–73
Maximum clot firmness (MCF, mm)	146	59.3 (17.5)	65 (56, 70)	55–78
Clot lysis at 30 min (LI30, %)	145	98.0 (10.8)	100 (100, 100)	
Clot lysis at 60 min (LI60, %)	101	93.3 (10.1)	96 (92, 99)	

Table 2 Haematological parameters of trial participants at baseline (N = 167) (Continued)

	n^a	Mean (SD) / Count (%)	Median (25th, 75th centile range)	Normal range[b]
Maximum Lysis (ML, %)	150	14.7 (20.4)	9 (4, 15)	0–44
ML > 15%		35 (23.3%)		
Thromboelastometry (ROTEM® APTEM) variables				
Clotting time (CT, seconds)	152	245.2 (882.3)	58 (46, 81)	31–71
Amplitude at 5 mins (A5, mm)	143	44.0 (15.2)	48 (35, 54)	
A5 < 40 mm		49 (33.6%)		
Amplitude at 10 mins (A10, mm)	147	52.9 (16.8)	59 (46, 64)	43–72
Maximum clot firmness (MCF, mm)	144	61.4 (15.6)	67 (58, 71)	56–78
Maximum Lysis (ML, %)	147	5.9 (5.7)	5 (2, 8)	0–14

[a] Number of women with available data
[b] Reference ranges for full blood count variables were obtained from the Sysmex KN analyser output. Reference ranges for thromboelastometry variables were obtained from literature [11]

iron deficiency [21]. Women with antenatal anaemia may have an increased risk of PPH and an increased risk of severe anaemia after delivery [22, 23].

One third of women was thrombocytopenic and many were severely thrombocytopenic. This also contrasts with studies in high income countries in which thrombocytopenia is relatively uncommon [24]. The low platelet counts (in the context of the relatively well preserved coagulation factors) may explain why so many women had an EXTEM A5 < 40 mm since EXTEM A5 values are influenced by platelet and fibrinogen levels. Further studies are needed to assess the FIBTEM and EXTEM A5 levels in similar populations to differentiate the extent to which low platelet and/or fibrinogen levels impact on PPH progression. Several studies have shown that a low A5 using ROTEM FIBTEM measured during the early phase of bleeding is associated with an increased risk of severe PPH [25].

Our study has several weaknesses. Because we did not collect blood samples prior to PPH onset, we cannot determine whether the abnormal haematological values (anaemia and thrombocytopenia) observed in this study are a cause or consequence of the bleeding. Due to technical

problems with either blood samples or measurement instruments, the number of patients with available data was less than the number enrolled. We did not compare our results with a control group of women who did not experience PPH. Although the women in our study were a sample (54%) of all those recruited into the WOMAN trial at University College Hospital, we do not believe they were selected based on bleeding severity. The mean blood loss among the 167 women who were included was similar to that for the 142 women enrolled in the Woman trial but not included in this ROTEM study [1530 ml (SD) 897 for the included women versus 1548 (SD) 810] in women not included in the ROTEM study]. Their systolic blood pressures at baseline were also similar [110 mmHg (27) among included women versus 103 (33) in women who were not included]. It is possible that the reason for the high prevalence of coagulopathy found in our study is that our cohort had more severe PPH than studies in high income settings.

Conclusions

Based on findings from a convenience sample of women who delivered in a teaching hospital in Nigeria, hyper-

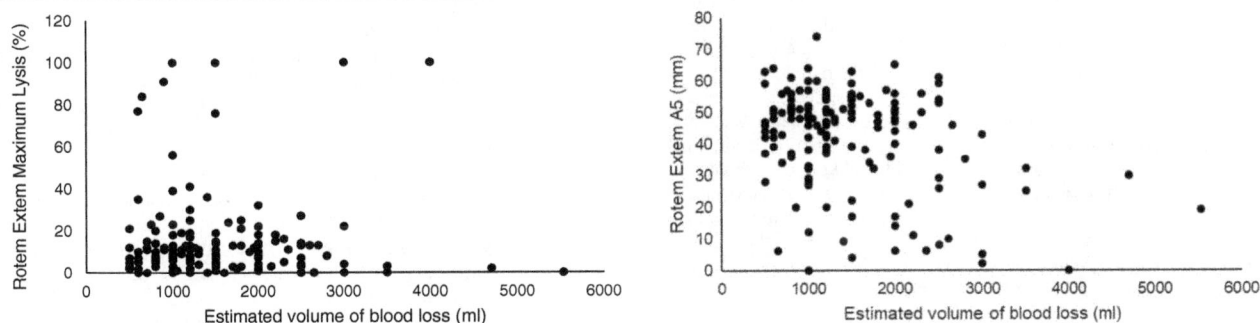

Fig. 3 Scatterplot of the relationship between estimated blood loss and ROTEM ML and A5

fibrinolysis occurs in nearly 25% of women with PPH. Further studies into the pathophysiological mechanisms for hyper-fibrinolysis should help us to identify better treatment strategies for women with PPH.

Abbreviations

A5: Clot amplitude (firmness) at five minutes; aPTT: Activated partial thromboplastin time; EDTA: Ethylene diamine triacetic acid; ETAC: Effect of tranexamic acid on coagulation sub-study of woman trial.; EXTEM: Extrinsic screening test on ROTEM; g/L: Grams per litre; HIV: Human immunodeficiency virus; INTEM: Intrinsic screening test on ROTEM; L: Litre; LSHTM: London school of hygiene and tropical medicine; MCV: Mean corpuscular volume; ML: Maximum Lysis; mL: Millilitre; mmHg: Millimetre of mercury; mol/L: Moles per litre; NAFDAC: National agency for food & drug administration and control; PAI-1: Plasminogen activator inhibitors; PPH: Postpartum haemorrhage; PT: Prothrombin time; QC: Quality control; ROTEM: Rotational thromboelastometry; t-PA: Tissue plasminogen activator; WOMAN Trial: World maternal anti-fibrinolytic trial

Funding

London School of Hygiene and Tropical Medicine, UK Department of Health, Wellcome Trust, Bill & Melinda Gates Foundation funded the WOMAN trial. An educational grant, equipment and consumables for ROTEM analysis was provided by tem innovations GmbH, M.-Kollar-Str. 13–15, 81829 Munich, Germany to LSHTM and utilised fully at the university college hospital, Ibadan. The funders had no role in the design of the study and collection, analysis, and interpretation of data or in writing the manuscript.

Authors' contributions

IR and HS conceived the study, contributed data cleaning, statistical analysis and writing of the manuscript. BK contributed to protocol development and had overall responsibility for the study at the trial site and review of the manuscript. OO contributed to protocol development and is the site principal investigator for WOMAN trial and review of the manuscript. MK contributed to the protocol development and was responsible for overseeing laboratory tests, laboratory standard operating procedures and staff training and review of the manuscript. AB contributed to protocol development and was responsible for data transfer and review of the manuscript. OO contributed to the protocol development, development of the standard operating procedures and was responsible for participant recruitment and review of the manuscript. CA contributed to the protocol development and was responsible for participant recruitment and review of the manuscript. TK contributed to the protocol development and was responsible for routine laboratory tests and review of the manuscript. BH contributed to data cleaning and writing of the manuscript. SH conducted the statistical analysis and contributed to the writing of the manuscript. TO was responsible for overseeing laboratory tests, laboratory standard operating procedures and staff training and review of the manuscript. All authors have read and approved the final version of the manuscript.

Ethics approval and consent to participate

Approvals to conduct this study were obtained from the Ethics Committees of London School of Hygiene and Tropical Medicine and the University of Ibadan & University College Hospital Ethics Committee. Regulatory approval was obtained from the Nigerian National Agency for Food and Drug Administration and Control (NAFDAC). The study was undertaken according to ICH-GCP guidelines. The consent procedures is detailed in the WOMAN Trial protocol [22]. Briefly, we obtained written consent from a patient if their physical and mental capacity allowed. If a patient could not give written consent, we obtained proxy consent from a relative or representative. If a proxy was unavailable, then if local regulation allows, we deferred or waived consent. In this situation, we informed the patient about the trial as soon as possible, and obtained written consent to use the data. The London School of Hygiene & Tropical Medicine is the sponsor.

Competing interests

The authors declare that they have no competing interests.

Author details

[1]Clinical Trials Unit, London School of Hygiene and Tropical Medicine, Keppel Street, London WC1E 7HT, UK. [2]Department of Obstetrics & Gynaecology, National Institute of Maternal and Child Health, College of Medicine, University of Ibadan, Orita-Mefa, Ibadan, Nigeria. [3]Department of Chemical Pathology, College of Medicine, University of Ibadan, Orita-Mefa, Ibadan, Nigeria. [4]Department of Obstetrics & Gynaecology, College of Medicine, University of Ibadan, Orita-Mefa, Ibadan, Nigeria. [5]Department of Haematology, College of Medicine, University of Ibadan, Orita-Mefa, Ibadan, Nigeria. [6]Thrombosis & Haemophilia Centre, Guy's & St Thomas' Trust, St Thomas' Hospital, Lambeth Palace Road, London, UK.

References

1. CRASH-2 trial collaborators, Shakur H, Roberts I, Bautista R, Caballero J, Coats T, et al. Effects of tranexamic acid on death, vascular occlusive events, and blood transfusion in trauma patients with significant haemorrhage (CRASH-2): a randomised, placebo-controlled trial. Lancet. 2010;376(9734):23–32.
2. CRASH-2 collaborators, Roberts I, Shakur H, Afolabi A, Brohi K, Coats T, et al. The importance of early treatment with tranexamic acid in bleeding trauma patients: an exploratory analysis of the CRASH-2 randomised controlled trial. Lancet. 2011;377(9771):1096–101.
3. Roberts I, Prieto-Merino D, Manno D. Mechanism of action of tranexamic acid in bleeding trauma patients: an exploratory analysis of data from the CRASH-2 trial. Crit Care. 2014;18:685.
4. Raza I, Davenport R, Rourke C, Platton S, Manson J, Spoors C, Khan S, De'ath H, Allard S, Hart D, John Pasi K, Hunt BJ, Stanworth S, Maccallum P, Brohi K. The incidence and magnitude of fibrinolytic activation in trauma patients. J Thromb Haemost. 2013;11(2):307–14.
5. Chapman MP, Moore EE, Moore HB, Gonzalez E, Gamboni F, Chandler JG, Mitra S, Ghasabyan A, Chin TL, Sauaia A, Banerjee A, Silliman CC. Overwhelming tPA release, not PAI-1 degradation, is responsible for hyperfibrinolysis in severely injured trauma patients. J Trauma Acute Care Surg. 2016;80:16–25.
6. Cap A, Hunt BJ. The pathogenesis of traumatic coagulopathy. Anaesthesia. 2015;70(Suppl 1):e96–101.
7. The WOMAN Trial Collaborators. Effect of early administration of tranexamic acid on mortality, hysterectomy, other morbidities in women with postpartum haemorrhage (the WOMAN trial): a randomised, placebo-controlled trial. Lancet. 2017;389(10084):2105–16.
8. Wikkelsø AJ, Edwards HM, Afshari A, Stensballe J, Langhoff-Roos J, Albrechtsen C, Ekelund K, Hanke G, Secher EL, Sharif HF, Pedersen LM, Troelstrup A, Lauenborg J, Mitchell AU, Fuhrmann L, Svare J, Madsen MG, Bødker B, Møller AM, FIB-PPH trial group. Pre-emptive treatment with fibrinogen concentrate for postpartum haemorrhage: randomized controlled trial. Br J Anaesth. 2015;114:623–33.
9. World Health Organization (WHO). The prevalence of Anaemia in women: a tabulation of available information. Geneva: WHO; 1992. WHO/MCH/MSM/92.2
10. Brohi K, Singh J, Heron M, Coats T. Acute traumatic coagulopathy. J Trauma. 2003;54:1127–30.
11. Hagemo JS, Christiaans SC, Stanworth SJ, et al. Detection of acute traumatic coagulopathy and massive transfusion requirements by means of rotational thromboelastometry: an international prospective validation study. Crit Care. 2015;19(1):97.
12. de Lange NM, van Rheeneen-Flach LE, Lance MD, Mooyman L, et al. Peri-partum reference ranges for ROTEM®thromboelastometry. Br J Anaesth. 2014;112(5):852–9.
13. Ronsmans C, Graham WJ. Lancet maternal survival series steering group: maternal mortality: who, when, where, and why. Lancet. 2006;368(9542):1189–200.
14. Solomon C, Collis R, Collins P. Haemostatic monitoring during postpartum haemorrhage and implications for management. Br J Anaesth. 2012; 109(6):851–63.
15. Erhabor O, Isaac I, Muhammad A, Abdulrahman Y, Ezimah A, Adias T. Some hemostatis parameters in women with obstetric haemorrhage in Sokoto, Nigeria. Int J Womens Health. 2013;5:285–91.
16. Mackinnon S, Walker ID, Davidson JF, Walker JJ. Plasma fibrinolysis during and after normal childbirth. Br J Haematol. 1987;65:339–42.
17. Bremer HA, Brommer EJP, Wallenburg HCS. Effects of labour and delivery on fibrinolysis. Eur J Ob Gynaecol Repro Biol. 1994;55:163–8.
18. Ducloy-Bouthors AS, Duhamel A, Kipnis E, Tournoys A, Prado-Dupont A, Elkalioubie A, Jeanpierre E, Debize G, Peynaud-Debayle E, DeProst D,

Huissoud C, Rauch A, Susen S. Postpartum haemorrhage related early increase in D-dimers is inhibited by tranexamic acid: haemostasis parameters of a randomized controlled open labelled trial. Br J Anaesth. 2016;116:641–8.

19. Okwesili A, Ibrahim K, Nnadi D, Barnabas B, Abdulrahaman Y, Buhari H, Udomah F, Imoru M, Egenti B, Erhabor O. Fibrinogen levels among pregnant women of African descent in Sokoto north western Nigeria. Front Biomed Sci. 2016;1(2):7–11.

20. Madden E, Lee G, Kotler DP, et al. Association of Antiretroviral Therapy with fibrinogen levels in HIV infection. AIDS. 2008;22(6):707–15.

21. Olatunbosun O, Abasiattai A, Bassey E, James R, Ibanga G, Morgan A. Prevalence of anaemia among pregnant women at booking in the University of Uyo Teaching Hospital. Uyo: Biomed Research International; 2014. Article ID: 849080

22. Nair M, Choudhry MK, Choudhry SS, Kakoty SD, Sarma UC, Webster P, et al. Association between maternal anaemia and pregnancy outcome: a cohort study in Assam, India. BMJ Global Health. 2016;1:e000026.

23. Butwick A, Walsh E, Kuzniewicz M, Li S, Escobar G. Patterns and predictors of severe postpartum anemia after cesarean section. Transfusion. 2017;57:36–44.

24. Jones RM, de Lloyd L, Kealaher EJ, Lilley GJ, Precious E, Burckett st Laurent D, Hamlyn V, Collis RE, Collins PW, collaborators. Platelet count and transfusion requirements during moderate or severe postpartum haemorrhage. Anaesthesia. 2016;71:648–56.

25. Collins PW, Lilley G, Bruynseels D, et al. Fibrin-based clot formation as an early and rapid biomarker for progression of postpartum hemorrhage: a prospective study. Blood. 2014;124:1727–36.

23

The third delay: understanding waiting time for obstetric referrals at a large regional hospital in Ghana

David M. Goodman[1], Emmanuel K. Srofenyoh[2], Adeyemi J. Olufolabi[3], Sung Min Kim[4] and Medge D. Owen[5*]

Abstract

Background: Delay in receiving care significantly contributes to maternal morbidity and mortality. Much has been studied about reducing delays prior to arrival to referral facilities, but the delays incurred upon arrival to the hospital have not been described in many low- and middle-income countries.

Methods: We report on the obstetric referral process at Ridge Regional Hospital, Accra, Ghana, the largest referral hospital in the Ghana Health System. This study uses data from a prospectively-collected cohort of 1082 women presenting with pregnancy complications over a 10-week period. To characterize which factors lead to delays in receiving care, we analyzed wait times based on reason for referral, time and day of arrival, and concurrent volume of patients in the triage area.

Results: The findings show that 108 facilities refer patients to Ridge Regional Hospital, and 52 facilities account for 90.5% of all transfers. The most common reason for referral was fetal-pelvic size disproportion (24.3%) followed by hypertensive disorders of pregnancy (9.8%) and prior uterine scar (9.1%). The median arrival-to-evaluation (wait) time was 40 min (IQR 15–100); 206 (22%) of women were evaluated within 10 min of arrival. Factors associated with longer wait times include presenting during the night shift, being in latent labour, and having a non-time-sensitive risk factor. The median time to be evaluated was 32 min (12–80) for women with hypertensive disorders of pregnancy and 37 min (10–66) for women with obstetric hemorrhage. In addition, the wait time for women in the second stage of labour was 30 min (12–79).

Conclusions: Reducing delay upon arrival is imperative to improve the care at high-volume comprehensive emergency obstetric centers. Although women with time-sensitive risk factors such as hypertension, bleeding, fever, and second stage of labour were seen more quickly than the baseline population, all groups failed to be evaluated within the international standard of 10 min. This study emphasizes the need to improve hospital systems so that space and personnel are available to access high-risk pregnancy transfers rapidly.

Keywords: Low-middle income countries, Obstetric triage, Obstetric referral, Ridge regional hospital, Ghana

Background

As the global health community works to achieve the Sustainable Development Goals (SDG), it is evident that reducing the worldwide maternal mortality ratio to <70/100,000 live births will require significantly improved systems of healthcare delivery [1]. In low-income countries, obstetric care is focused on providing skilled care for home births and encouraging institutional delivery at community and district hospitals [2, 3]. However, 15% of women will develop complications such as obstructed labour, hypertensive disorders of pregnancy (HDoP), or obstetric hemorrhage (OH) that require transfer to a tertiary level of care capable of performing the signal functions of comprehensive emergency obstetric care (CEmOC) [4]. The inevitable need for escalating care introduces delay into the system and, for many years now, delay has been recognized as one of the root causes of maternal deaths [5, 6].

* Correspondence: mowen@wakehealth.edu
[5]Department of Anesthesiology, Wake Forest School of Medicine, Medical Center Boulevard, Winston-Salem, NC 27157-1009, USA

Much has been written about reducing delays in deciding for referral and reaching referral sites, but less attention has been given to reducing delays once a woman has reached tertiary care [6]. The necessity of frequently receiving high-acuity patients led to the development of obstetric triage as a function of high-quality labour wards. Obstetric triage is defined as "the brief, thorough, and systematic maternal and fetal assessment performed when a pregnant woman presents for care, to determine priority for full evaluation" [7]. This function is most frequently performed by nurses and nurse-midwives. It is more thorough than the type of triage performed in trauma situations as it includes periods of monitoring for labour evaluation, fetal well-being, and laboratory assessment of obstetric complications.

Over the last 30 years, the practice of obstetric triage has been implemented throughout the United States and other high-income countries. In many obstetric units in these hospitals, there is a separate triage area with dedicated staff to receive and rapidly assess women in order to quickly treat complications [8]. The Association of Women's Health Obstetric and Neonatal Nurses (AWHONN) recommends that the triage assessment begin within 10 min of arrival to a facility [7]. The goal for triage is to conclude the evaluation with a disposition so that the woman can either be discharged home safely or continue with inpatient care. Understanding referral reasons and triage practices is critical for improving maternal health in the new SDG era.

From 2007 to 2011, obstetric admissions increased from 6049 to 9357 at Ridge Regional Hospital (RRH) in Accra, Ghana, a major obstetric referral center for the Ghana Health Service (GHS). An initial pilot survey (data not included) and an analysis of care processes identified bottleneck areas within the labour ward and a decision was taken to study referrals and timeliness of care upon patient arrival [9]. This study characterizes obstetric referrals received at RRH and analyzes the timeliness through which women enter CEmOC.

Methods

RRH in Accra, Ghana was selected as the site for this study as the highest volume obstetric unit of 10 regional referral hospitals in the GHS. Regional hospitals primarily manage complicated pregnancies and as such, approximately 70% of deliveries at RRH are high-risk antenatal or peripartum referrals. The maternity unit at RRH has a 90-bed capacity and provides comprehensive services from antenatal care through postpartum discharge. In 2012, there were 10 labour and delivery beds, one obstetric operating room, and four general operating rooms shared among surgical services and located remotely from the labour ward. The obstetric triage area was an open hallway with a bench and a small adjacent

examination room. Staffing consisted of only two obstetricians, an average of four medical officers/residents, and 22 midwives to manage the operating room and labour ward. Despite these challenges, the unit maintained an open-door policy of not turning away patients needing maternity care. Morning shifts were conducted from 0800 to 1400, afternoon shifts from 1400 to 2000 and night shifts from 2000 to 0800, during which there were typically 4 midwives scheduled during the day shifts and 3 midwives during the night shifts.

Prior to this study, we conducted a small pilot survey among patients that identified waiting time as a significant modifiable factor that negatively affected patient experience and outcome [9]. We developed a data collection and analysis plan to further understand this issue. The a priori goal of the study was to document the wait time and triage time for women when they arrive. We also wanted to identify factors that led to prolonged delays so that an educational and systems-based intervention could be developed. Four non-staff nurses were hired and trained to collect data on obstetric patients admitted to RRH during a 10-week period from September 9 to November 11, 2012. This sample time represented a time of the year with intermediate patient volume based on monthly census data and was selected to reduce the potential influence of peak or low volume periods. Data collectors were scheduled to work throughout the day and night to gather time-sequence information at patient arrival and from patient records and logbooks within 24 h. Data included patient and labour characteristics, referral information, and the timeliness of triage. Timeliness was based on direct observation of patient-provider interactions by the data collection nurses and recorded on a data sheet. We defined wait time as the difference in minutes from arrival at the facility to the first interaction with a midwife. Triage time was defined as the time from first interaction with a midwife to departure from the triage area en route to a treatment area (women's ward, labour ward, operating theatre, etc.).

Data analysis

For variables that were normally distributed, Student's t-test and one-way ANOVA was used for continuous variable, and Pearson chi-squared test was used for categorical variables. Results are shown with means and 95% confidence intervals (CI) where applicable. For variables, such as wait time, that are nonparametric, more appropriate tests were chosen. The Wilcox rank-sum (also known as Mann-Whitney U) test was used for continuous variables and Krukal-Wallis test for categorical variables. These results are reported using medians and interquartile ranges. Statistical analyses were done using STATA version 14.0 software (StataCorp, College Station, TX).

Results

Over a 10-week period from September 9 to November 11, 2012, data were captured for 1082 women who presented to RRH as transfers from other facilities or self-referrals. This represents 80% of the 1351 deliveries at RRH that occurred during this period. Twenty percent of women were not captured due to the following reasons: admitted directly from clinic, thus bypassing triage; admitted prior to study period, but delivering during the 10-week window; presenting during lapses in data collection nurse coverage. There were 108 sites that referred patients to RRH during the data collection period. There was a wide array of referring facilities ranging from private maternity homes to academic medical centers. The most distant referral sites were 50 km from RRH, a trip that would likely require several hours to complete depending on the time of day. Half of the referrals to RRH came from 9 facilities and the remaining half came from 99 other facilities.

Table 1 shows maternal and labour characteristics upon admission for this population. There were notable gaps in compliance in recording maternal vital signs and in labour assessment. Most notably, maternal temperature was poorly recorded, as well as the presence or absence of uterine contractions. Table 2 shows the reasons for referral as provided by the referring institution. The most common reason for referral was fetal-pelvic disproportion. In a subset of these, 90 patients were referred for prolonged first or second stage of labour, yet 41 arrived with intact membranes. Also, the local vernacular "big abdomen" or "big baby" was used in 90 of these referrals. Twenty-five of these were potentially inappropriate referrals because the fundal height was <40 cm, which would not support this diagnosis. Of the 139 patients referred for hypertension,

13 had normal blood pressure at the time of admission. Two-hundred (18%) of referred women came in advanced labour (>7 cm cervical dilation) and of those, 83 (8%) arrived completely dilated.

For women presenting to RRH, the median wait time from arrival until initial assessment by a labour ward midwife was 40 min (interquartile range 15–100 min) (Table 3). Two-hundred and six (22%) women were evaluated within 10 min of arrival, and 41% percent of women were evaluated within 30 min. Seven percent of women were not evaluated within at least 3 h and two women waited longer than a day. A doctor was consulted for 288 (27%) of patients (consultant 42, medical officer 151, house officer 93, 2 unknown). Only 62% of women had a plan of care documented in the chart.

Factors associated with wait times and triage times

We hypothesized that several factors might correlate with faster initial evaluation. We evaluated the time differences from arrival to initial assessment as the "wait" time, and the time from initial assessment to transition beyond the triage assessment as "triage" time. We compared performance around these metrics with respect to the following: time of day, day of the week, volume on a given day, presence of risk factors, and labour status (Table 3, Fig. 1). Arrival times were evenly distributed according to number of hours/shift during the morning (25%), evening (22%), and night (53%) shifts. The median wait time for evaluation was significantly longer at night [55 min (15–120)], than was the morning [35 min (10–83) and evening [28 min (12–51)] shifts ($P = 0.0004$) (Table 3). There was no difference based on day of the week either in volume or wait times ($P = 0.38$).

Table 1 Maternal and obstetric characteristics

Variable	Number (%) observed	Mean	S.D.	Min	Max
Maternal age (yr)	1066 (99)	28.1	5.7	15	46
Maternal heart rate	702 (65)				
Systolic blood pressure (mmHg)	950 (88)	123	25.3	0	220
Diastolic blood pressure (mmHg)	950 (88)	77	16.2	0	140
Temperature (°C)	791 (73)	36.6	0.94	30	40.5
Gravidy	1047 (97)	2.6	1.6	1	13
Parity	1040 (96)	1.4	1.5	0	8
Gestational age (wk)	1000 (93)	39 + 1	24.7	24 + 0	49 + 0
Fundal Height (cm)	954 (88)	37.1	3.72	22	57
Uterine contractions	118 (11)				
Cervical examination (cm)	941 (87)	4.1	2.6	0	10
Fetal heart rate (beats/min)	912 (84)				
Membrane status	926 (86)				
Presentation	1017 (94)				

Table 2 Indications for referral

Indication	Number	Percent (%)
Fetal-pelvic size disproportion[a]	346	24.3
Hypertensive disorders of pregnancy[b]	139	9.8
Prior uterine scar[c]	129	9.1
Maternal miscellaneous[d]	115	8.1
Anemia[e]	103	7.2
Self-referral/Ridge Hospital patient	92	6.5
Fetal compromise[f]	69	4.8
Fetal malpresentation[g]	62	4.4
Rupture of membranes[h]	54	3.8
Labour	45	3.2
Lack of resources at referral site[i]	43	3.0
Infectious causes[j]	39	2.7
Acute haemorrhage[k]	39	2.7
Prematurity[l]	29	2.0
Previous poor obstetric outcome[m]	27	1.9
Multiple gestation[n]	26	1.8
Record illegible	22	1.5
Maternal age extremes (≤15 or >35 yr)	18	1.3
Intra-uterine fetal demise	14	1.0
No/poor prenatal care	12	0.8
Fetal miscellaneous[o]	2	0.1
Total	1425	100%
One referral indication	739	68.3%
Two referral indications	315	29.1%
Three referral indications	28	2.6%

There were 1082 referral records captured for deliveries occurring at Ridge Regional Hospital from September 9, 2012 to November 11, 2012
[a]Cephalopelvic disproportion, fetal macrosomia, large maternal abdomen, post-term pregnancy, over 40 weeks estimated gestational age, borderline pelvis, contracted pelvis, failure to progress (delayed or prolonged labour, arrest of labour, slow progress, failed induction, unfavorable cervix, high head in labour, obstructed labour)
[b]Chronic hypertension, PIH, pre-eclampsia, severe pre-eclampsia, or eclampsia
[c]Previous cesarean delivery, prior myomectomy, or previous uterine rupture
[d]Maternal asthma, diabetes, gestational diabetes, prior abdominal surgery, uterine fibroids, vaginal/vulvar growth or discharge, proteinuria, urinary tract infection, fever, generalized edema, short/long pregnancy interval, short maternal stature, maternal distress, sterilization request, grand multiparty, seizure disorder, mental illness, obesity, patient refusal for care, patient lacks labouratory or scan information, crippled, rhesus negative
[e]Maternal anemia or sickle cell disease
[f]Abnormal cardiotocography, fetal tachycardia, fetal distress, oligohydramnios, meconium stained amniotic fluid, decreased fetal movement, intrauterine growth restricition, umbilical cord prolapse
[g]Face/mentoposterior, brow, breech/footling breech, oblique, transverse, unstable lie, arm prolapse, leading twin breech, compound presentation
[h]Rupture of membranes, prolonged rupture of membranes, loosing liquor, gestations >37 weeks
[i]No electricity, no bed, no gloves, no water, no doctor, no anesthetist
[j]Hepatitis B, malaria, syphilis, human immunodeficiency virus
[k]Placenta previa, placental abruption, placenta accreta, ante-, intra- and postpartum bleeding, unclassified haemorrhage
[l]Gestation <37 weeks, prematurity, preterm labour or preterm premature rupture of membranes
[m]Bad obstetric history, prior stillbirth, prior ectopic pregnancy, unexplained history of intrauterine fetal death, previous failure to progress, prior cervical cerclage, previous peripartum haemorrhage
[n]Twin pregnancy, triplet pregnancy
[o]Anencephaly, severe hydrocephalus, polyhydramnios, fetal deformity

The impact of volume on wait and triage times showed a non-linear relationship. With respect to wait time, no difference was noted ($P = 0.23$) between groups stratified in groups of 10 patients/day. Moving women out of the triage area took significantly longer on high-volume days (>30 patients) when the median triage time was 83 min ($P = 0.0285$), possibly the result of occupied labor beds. The three most common causes of maternal death at RRH have been shown to be OH, HDoP, and sepsis [10]; thus, we identified women presenting with vaginal bleeding ($n = 39$), hypertension ($n = 139$), fever ($n = 1$), or prolonged rupture of membranes ($n = 54$) as having a time-sensitive risk factor. Women with these risk factors were seen more quickly, 35 min (12–80 min) compared to 45 min (15–110 min) ($P = 0.009$) for women without these risk factors (Table 3, Fig. 1).

Being in labour, either 1st stage or 2nd stage, was associated with being evaluated and being moved out of triage into the labour ward more quickly. Women in labour were evaluated within 35 min (10–83 min) and 30 min (12–79 min) ($P = 0.0279$) for the 1st and 2nd stages respectively, and moved out of triage within 24 (10–65 min) and 10 min (5–32 min) ($P = 0.0001$) respectively (Table 3, Fig. 1).

Discussion

The results of this study show that regional hospitals face significant challenges receiving, evaluating, and treating many high-risk obstetric referrals. To the best of our knowledge, we report the first large-scale evaluation of delays incurred with obstetric triage in a low-to-middle income country. The analysis presented is intended to describe referral characteristics and delays that occur while receiving patients at a high volume obstetric referral hospital and to inform the development of context specific obstetric triage and staffing strategies to overcome challenges.

The leading indications for referral to RRH were failure to progress (24%) and HDoP (10%). These were similar to the analysis by Nkyekyer et al. who found that the primary reason for referral to Korle Bu Teaching Hospital (KBTH), the main academic medical centre in Accra, was failure to progress (22%) and hypertensive disorders (16%) [11]. Referral for prior uterine scar was only seen in 8 (2%) of patients in the Nkyekyer study; however, this was the third leading indication for patients who presented to RRH constituting 9% of referrals. The increase in these referrals is concerning because it may indicate a rising cesarean delivery rate in Accra over the last few years. Many of these patients were referred from institutions without operating theatres and should have been identified and referred earlier in pregnancy and prior to labor. A continued rise will ultimately lead to an increase in the cesarean delivery burden on regional and large referral hospitals [12].

Table 3 Wait time and triage time analysis

Factor	N (%)	Wait time (minutes)	IQR (minutes)	p-value	N (%)	Triage time (minutes)	IQR (minutes)	p-value
Shift								
Morning	325 (32%)	37	11–84	0.0001	253 (28%)	41	13–200	0.0945
Evening	306 (30%)	30	12–84		352 (40%)	40	13–200	
Night	390 (38%)	55	15–135		282 (32%)	70	15–293	
Daily Volume								
< 10 pts	80 (9%)	50	19–92	0.2304	85 (9%)	45	20–380	0.0285
10–19 pts	554 (60%)	40	15–102		555 (60%)	44	15–250	
20–29 pts	210 (23%)	32	10–85		201 (22%)	33	11–143	
> 30 pts	81 (9%)	37	5–125		86 (9%)	83	10–361	
Day of the Week								
Sunday	130 (14%)	47	18–107	0.3767	121 (14%)	70	20–365	0.2316
Monday	122 (13%)	40	15–110		114 (13%)	40	15–213	
Tuesday	118 (13%)	36	12–100		113 (13%)	55	15–310	
Wednesday	129 (14%)	35	12–91		124 (14%)	43	15–231	
Thursday	147 (16%)	40	15–70		142 (16%)	33	10–235	
Friday	146 (16%)	39	10–95		144 (16%)	38	10–174	
Saturday	134 (14%)	44	12–120		130 (15%)	60	16–208	
Weekday	662 (72%)	40	14–192	0.1253	637 (72%)	40	12–227	0.0071
Weekend	263 (28%)	45	15–111		251 (28%)	65	20–298	
Risk Factor								
Other	529 (57%)	45	15–110	0.0299	486 (55%)	60	15–310	0.0079
Sepsis	65 (7%)	35	10–70		68 (8%)	51	18–182	
OH	44 (5%)	37	10–66		42 (5%)	24	12–185	
HDoP	285 (31%)	32	12–80		283 (32%)	34	11–171	
Labour Status								
Latent	489 (56%)	44	15–108	0.0279	476 (56%)	85	20–336	0.0001
1st Stage	275 (31%)	35	10–83		271 (32%)	24	10–65	
2nd Stage	42 (5%)	30	12–79	Ob	45 (5%)	10	5–32	
Not labouring	69 (8%)	38	15–90		51 (6%)	60	15–365	

The Greater Accra Region (GAR) has 17 districts and municipalities for which RRH is responsible. Within GAR there are 4 polyclinics, 31 health centers, and 38 community health and planning services that provide care to pregnant women within the public sector [13]. There are a host of other private and district-level institutions. Two other hospitals, 37 Military Hospital and KBTH, are capable of providing CEmOC and are located within the catchment area. The longest distance traveled by our patient population was 50 km, which was incurred prior to wait time and triage time. Inappropriate and unnecessary referrals also overburden referral hospitals and may contribute to delay in attending to more critically ill patients. Although we didn't specifically examine accuracy of the referring diagnosis, from the patient folders we found that 41 of 90 patients referred for prolonged labor had intact membranes; 25 of 90 parturients with "big baby" diagnosis had fundal height < 40 cm, and 13 of 139 with diagnosed hypertension had normal blood pressure on arrival. Our analysis indicates that further study and planning is required to optimize the referral patterns and indications and presents an opportunity to add structure to the referral process within the city.

Eighteen years ago, Nkyekyer et al. found that 27% of women reached KBTH by ambulance, whereas 59% relied on taxis for referral [11]. Interestingly, this is consistent with our preliminary 2010 pilot survey in which most patients reported arriving by taxi [9]. This is concerning because the present study found that 200 patients arrived at RRH in advanced labour, 93 of whom were completely dilated. The prospect is frightening of

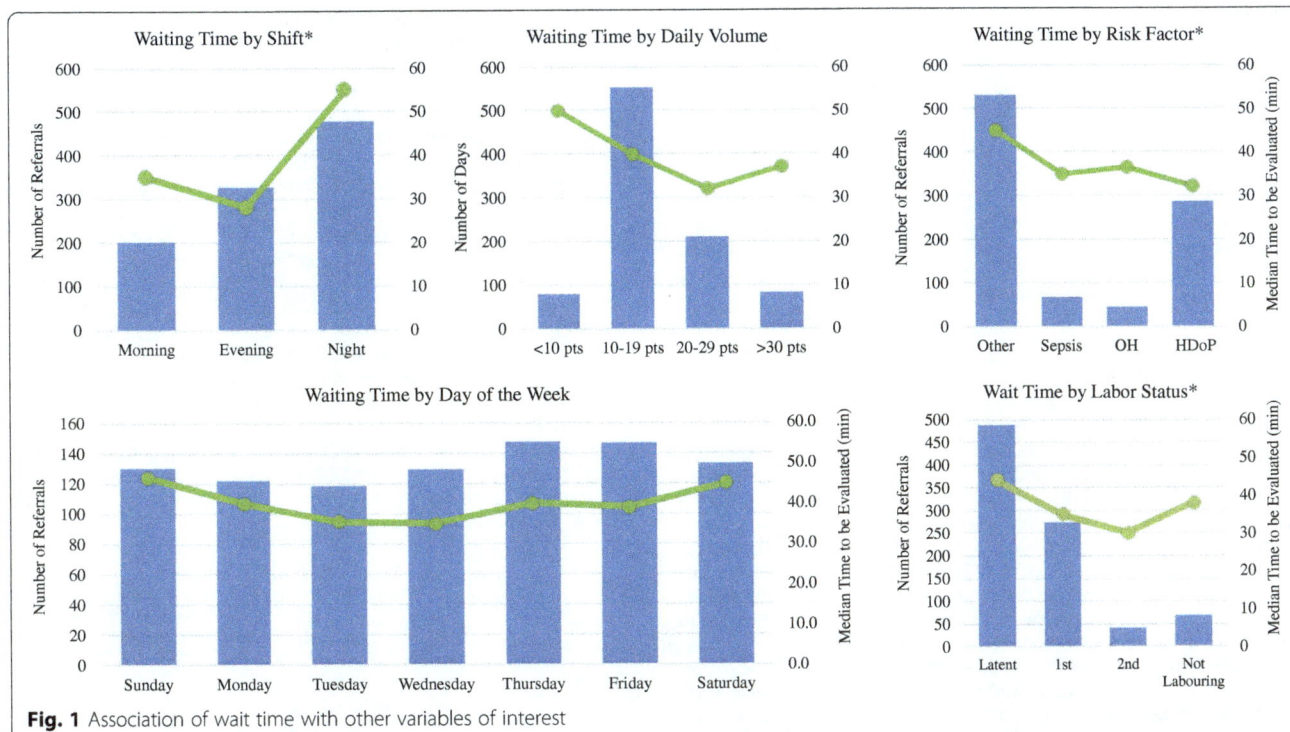

Fig. 1 Association of wait time with other variables of interest

high-risk, pregnant women in advanced labour being transported across the city in taxis and other non-medical vehicles to reach the referral hospital. This is another area where more information is needed in order to improve the referral processes in Accra.

In this study, the volume of patients ranged from 5 to 38 patients/day and there were no differences in volume based on day of the week. Wait times were similar each day of the week; however, it was more likely for patients to wait longer for assessment at night—during shifts with lower staffing. Our analysis shows that an equal number of patients present overnight as do during the daytime shifts. Nursing managers and administrators should make provisions for this observation in order to prevent delays from occurring during overnight. It is reassuring that having a time-sensitive reason for referral does increase the likelihood for quicker evaluation, but this does not reach the AWHONN goal of 10 min, or a more feasible 30-min goal between arrival and evaluation, which was the policy of the hospital.

Our study shows that there was at least a trend towards improved performance with respect to wait and triage times on days with moderately-high volume (20–29 patients) compared with low-volume or the high-volume days. It may be that days of moderately-high volume effectively activate the staff to move through the triage process more quickly. Based on these outcomes we hypothesized that the system should be modified to ensure a reduction of wait and triage times and this will be the focus of future reports.

Studying the outcomes immediately following obstetric referral in Accra can provide guidance to other major cities in Sub-Saharan Africa. Accra has a skilled antenatal care rate of 96% and skilled delivery coverage that ranges from 79 to 84% [13]. These are reassuring achievements and are building blocks for the country to reach their SDGs. As these goals are reached, hospitals will inevitably see an increase in referrals. The early work presented in this study can serve as baseline for planners and a comparison for future efforts.

Conclusions

Our study shows that RRH is capable of receiving and caring for large numbers of obstetric referrals on a daily basis. We demonstrated that they have a large number of referring facilities, some of which are remotely located, that present a significant burden to women and contributes to delay in their care. Although the median wait time prior to evaluation was 40 min, we believe training and systems improvement could enable the staff to reach a local goal of 30-min evaluation for all patients. Further research is needed in this area in order to establish triage as an integral part of the package of CEmOC in low-resource settings.

Abbreviations
AWHONN: Association of women's health obstetric and neonatal nurses; CEmOC: Comprehensive emergency obstetric care; GAR: Greater Accra Region; GHS: Ghana Health Service; HDoP: Hypertensive disorders of pregnancy; KBTH: Korle Bu Teaching Hospital; OH: Obstetric haemorrhage; RRH: Ridge regional hospital; SDG: Sustainable development goals

Acknowledgments
The study was supported by Kybele, Inc. (www.kybeleworldwide.org), a 501(c)(3) organization dedicated to improving childbirth safety worldwide. The authors wish to acknowledge Tobi Olufolabi and Louisa Oates for conducting the pilot survey and Sebnem Ucer and Erin Pfeiffer for compilation of data.

Funding
Funding for this project was received from the Lacy Foundation, the Society of Obstetric Anesthesia and Perinatology, and Obstetric Anaesthetists Association. The funders had no role in the study design, execution, or analysis. They have not modified or influenced the manuscript in any way.

Authors' contributions
DMG made significant contribution to data analysis and interpretation, was involved as primary drafter and editor of manuscript, gave final approval to this version, and agrees to be accountable for the accuracy and integrity of the work. EKS made significant contribution to study conception and design and acquisition of data, was involved with revising the manuscript for each draft, gave final approval to this version, and agrees to be accountable for the accuracy and integrity of the work. AJO made significant contribution to study conception and design, was involved with revising the manuscript for each draft, gave final approval to this version, and agrees to be accountable for the accuracy and integrity of the work. SMK made significant contribution to acquisition of data, was involved with revising the manuscript for the first draft, gave final approval to this version, and agrees to be accountable for the accuracy and integrity of the work. MDO made significant contribution to study conception and design and acquisition and interpretation of data, was heavily involved with revising the manuscript for each draft, gave final approval to this version, and agrees to be accountable for the accuracy and integrity of the work. All authors have read and approved the final version of this manuscript.

Competing interests
The authors declare that they have no competing interests.

Author details
[1]Department of Obstetrics & Gynecology, Duke University Medical Center, Box 3084, Durham, NC 27710, USA. [2]Ridge Regional Hospital, Accra, Ghana. [3]Department of Anesthesiology, Duke University Medical Center, Box 3094, Durham, NC 27710, USA. [4]Wake Forest School of Medicine, Medical Center Boulevard, Winston-Salem, NC 27157, USA. [5]Department of Anesthesiology, Wake Forest School of Medicine, Medical Center Boulevard, Winston-Salem, NC 27157-1009, USA.

References
1. Sustainable Development Goals: Goal 3, Ensure healthy lives and promote well-being for all at all ages. United Nations: Department of Economic and Social Affairs, Sustainable Development: Knowledge Platform. Available at: https://sustainabledevelopment.un.org/sdg3. Accessed 3 Aug 2016.
2. Althabe F, Bergel E, Cafferata ML, Gibbons L, Ciapponi A, Alemán A, Colantonio L, Palacios AR. Strategies for improving the quality of health care in maternal and child health in low- and middle-income countries: an overview of systematic reviews. Paediatr Perinat Epidemiol. 2008; 22(Suppl 1):42–60.
3. Campbell OM. Graham WJ; lancet maternal survival series steering group. Strategies for reducing maternal mortality: getting on with what works. Lancet. 2006;368:1284–99.
4. Otolorin E, Gomez P, Currie S, Thapa K, Dao B. Essential basic and emergency obstetric and newborn care: from education and training to service delivery and quality of care. Int J Gynaecol Obstet. 2015;130(Suppl 2):S46–53.
5. Thaddeus S, Maine D. Too far to walk: maternal mortality in context. Soc Sci Med. 1994;38:1091–110.
6. Gabrysch S, Campbell OM. Still too far to walk: literature review of the determinants of delivery service use. BMC Pregnancy Childbirth. 2009;9:34.
7. AWHONN. Women's Health Perinatal Nursing Care Quality Measures Specifications 2013. Available at: https://c.ymcdn.com/sites/www.awhonn.org/resource/resmgr/Downloadables/perinatalqualitymeasures.pdf. Accessed 3 Aug 2016.
8. Angelini D, Howard E. Obstetric triage: a systematic review of the past fifteen years: 1998-2013. MCN Am J Matern Child Nurs. 2014;39:284–97.
9. Olufolabi AJ, Atito-Narh E, Eshun M, Ross VH, Muir HA, Owen MD. Teaching neuroaxial anesthesia techniques for obstetric care in a Ghanaian referral hospital: achievements and obstacles. Anesth Analg. 2015;120:1317–22.
10. Srofenyoh EK, Kassebaum NJ, Goodman DM, Olufolabi AJ, Owen MD. Measuring the impact of a quality improvement collaboration to decrease maternal mortality in a Ghanaian regional hospital. Int J Gynaecol Obstet Off Organ Int Fed Gynaecol Obstet. 2016;134:181–5.
11. Nkyekyer K. Peripartum referrals to Korle Bu teaching hospital, Ghana—a descriptive study. Tropical Med Int Health. 2000;5:811–7.
12. Knight HE, Self A, Kennedy SH. Why are women dying when they reach hospital on time? A systematic review of the 'third delay'. PLoS One. 2013;8:e63846.
13. Amoakoh-Coleman M, Kayode GA, Brown-Davies C, Agyepong IA, Grobbee DE, Klipstein-Grobusch K, Ansah EK. Completeness and accuracy of data transfer of routine maternal health services data in the greater Accra region. BMC Res Notes. 2015;8:114.

Permissions

List of Contributors

Amy Brenner, Haleema Shakur-Still and Ian Roberts
Clinical Trials Unit, London School of Hygiene and Tropical Medicine, Keppel Street, London WC1E 7HT, UK

Rizwana Chaudhri
Holy Family Hospital, Gynaecology & Obstetrics Unit 1, F-762 Said Pur Road, Satellite Town, Rawalpindi, Pakistan

Bukola Fawole
Department of Obstetrics & Gynaecology, College of Medicine, University of Ibadan, Queen Elizabeth Road, Ibadan, Nigeria

Sabaratnam Arulkumaran
St George's University of London, Room 1.126, First Floor, Jenner Wing, Cranmer Terrace, London SW17 0RE, UK

Eniya Lufumpa and Antje Lindenmeyer
Institute of Applied Health Research, University of Birmingham, Edgbaston, Birmingham B15 2TT, UK

Lucy Doos
Institute for Research into Superdiversity, University of Birmingham, Edgbaston, Birmingham B15 2TT, UK

Leonardo Antonio Chavane
Jhpiego Mozambique, Rua A.W. Bayly, 61 Maputo, Mozambique

Patricia Bailey
RMNCH Unit, Global Health Programs, FHI, Durham, NC 360, USA

Osvaldo Loquiha
Department of Mathematics and Informatics, Eduardo Mondlane University, Maputo, Mozambique

Martinho Dgedge
Faculty of Medicine, Eduardo Mondlane University, Maputo, Mozambique

Marc Aerts
Interuniversity Institute for Biostatistics and Statistical Bioinformatics (I–BioStat), Hasselt University, Hasselt, Belgium

Marleen Temmerman
Centre of Excellence in Women and Child Health-East Africa, Aga Khan University, Karachi, Pakistan Ghent University Belgium, Ghent, Belgium

Angel Chimenea, Lutgardo García-Díaz, Ana María Calderón and María Moreno-De Las Heras
Department of Genetics, Reproduction, and Fetal Medicine, Institute of Biomedicine of Seville (IBIS), Hospital Universitario Virgen del Rocio/CSIC/University of Seville, Seville, Spain

Guillermo Antiñolo
Department of Genetics, Reproduction, and Fetal Medicine, Institute of Biomedicine of Seville (IBIS), Hospital Universitario Virgen del Rocio/CSIC/University of Seville, Seville, Spain
Centre for Biomedical Network Research on Rare Diseases (CIBERER), Seville, Spain

Flavia Ghouri, Amelia Hollywood and Kath Ryan
School of Pharmacy, University of Reading, Whiteknights, Reading RG6 6AP, UK

Qiu-Yue Zhong, Bizu Gelaye and Michelle A. Williams
Department of Epidemiology, Harvard T.H. Chan School of Public Health, Boston, 677 Huntington Avenue, Room Kresge 502A, Boston, MA 02115, USA

Gregory L. Fricchione
Division of Psychiatry and Medicine, Pierce Division of Global Psychiatry, Massachusetts General Hospital, Boston, Massachusetts, USA

Paul Avillach
Department of Epidemiology, Harvard T.H. Chan School of Public Health, Boston, 677 Huntington Avenue, Room Kresge 502A, Boston, MA 02115, USA
Department of Biomedical Informatics, Harvard Medical School, Boston, Massachusetts, USA
Children's Hospital Informatics Program, Boston Children's Hospital, Boston, Massachusetts, USA

Elizabeth W. Karlson
Division of Rheumatology, Allergy and Immunology, Brigham and Women's Hospital, Boston, Massachusetts, USA

Sarah Fogarty
School of Medicine, Western Sydney University, Locked Bag 1797, Penrith, NSW 2751, Australia

Rakime Elmir
Affiliate Ingham Institute for Applied Medical Research, Centre for Applied Nursing Research (CANR), Liverpool, NSW 2170, Australia
School of Nursing and Midwifery, Western Sydney University, Locked Bag 1797, Penrith, NSW 2751, Australia

Virginia Schmied
School of Nursing and Midwifery, Western Sydney University, Locked Bag 1797, Penrith, NSW 2751, Australia

Phillipa Hay
School of Medicine and Centre for Health Research, Western Sydney University, Locked Bag 1797, Penrith, NSW 2751, Australia

Eliane Saori Otaguiri, Ana Elisa Belotto Morguette, Alexandre Tadachi Morey, Eliandro Reis Tavares and Lucy Megumi Yamauchi
Departamento de Microbiologia, Centro de Ciências Biológicas, Universidade Estadual de Londrina, Londrina, Paraná, Brazil

Gilselena Kerbauy
Departamento de Enfermagem, Universidade Estadual de Londrina, Londrina, Paraná, Brazil

Rosângela S. L. de Almeida Torres
Laboratory of Bacteriology, Epidemiology Laboratory and Disease Control Division, Laboratório Central do Estado do Paraná – LACEN, Curitiba, PR, Brazil

Mauricio Chaves Júnior
Departamento de Medicina, Hospital Universitário de Maringá, Universidade Estadual de Maringá, Maringá, Brazil

Maria Cristina Bronharo Tognim
Departamento de Ciências Básicas da Saúde, Universidade Estadual de Maringá, Maringá, Brazil

Viviane Monteiro Góes and Marco Aurélio Krieger
Instituto Carlos Chagas, Fundação Instituto Oswaldo Cruz, Curitiba, Brazil

Marcia Regina Eches Perugini
Departamento de Patologia, Análises Clínicas e Toxicológicas, Centro de Ciências da Saúde, Universidade Estadual de Londrina, Londrina, Paraná, Brazil

Sueli Fumie Yamada-Ogatta
Departamento de Microbiologia, Centro de Ciências Biológicas, Universidade Estadual de Londrina, Londrina, Paraná, Brazil
Departamento de Microbiologia, Universidade Estadual de Londrina, Centro de Ciências Biológicas, Rodovia Celso Garcia Cid, PR 445, km 380. CEP, Londrina 86057-970, Brazil

T. Happillon, K. Azudin, J.-B. Tylcz, D. Istrate and C. Marque
Sorbonne Universités, Université de Technologie de Compiègne, CNRS, BMBI UMR 7338, 60200 Compiègne, France

C. Muszynski
Sorbonne Universités, Université de Technologie de Compiègne, CNRS, BMBI UMR 7338, 60200 Compiègne, France
Département de gynécologie et obstétrique, CHU Amiens-Picardie, avenue Laënnec, 80480 Salouël, France

Michael Girsberger and Michael Jan Dickenmann
Clinic for Transplantation Immunology and Nephrology, University Hospital Basel, Petersgraben 4, 4031 Basel, Switzerland

Catherine Muff and Irene Hösli
Department of Gynaecology and Obstetrics, University Hospital Basel, Spitalstrasse 21, 4031 Basel, Switzerland

Marianne Bertolet, Mansi Desai, Candace K. McClure, Akira Sekikawa, Ping Guo Tepper and Emma J. Barinas-Mitchell
Department of Epidemiology, Graduate School of Public Health, University of Pittsburgh, 130 De Soto Street, Pittsburgh, PA 15261, USA

Nancy Anderson Niemczyk
Department of Epidemiology, Graduate School of Public Health, University of Pittsburgh, 130 De Soto Street, Pittsburgh, PA 15261, USA
Department of Health Promotion and Development, School of Nursing, University of Pittsburgh, 3500 Victoria Street, 440 Victoria Building, Pittsburgh, PA 15261, USA

Janet M. Catov
Department of Epidemiology, Graduate School of Public Health, University of Pittsburgh, 130 De Soto Street, Pittsburgh, PA 15261, USA
Department of Obstetrics and Gynecology, School of Medicine, University of Pittsburgh, 3550 Terrace Street, Pittsburgh, PA 15213, USA
Department of Clinical and Translational Research, School of Medicine, University of Pittsburgh, 3550 Terrace Street, Pittsburgh, PA 15213, USA

James M. Roberts
Department of Epidemiology, Graduate School of Public Health, University of Pittsburgh, 130 De Soto Street, Pittsburgh, PA 15261, USA
Department of Obstetrics and Gynecology, School of Medicine, University of Pittsburgh, 3550 Terrace Street, Pittsburgh, PA 15213, USA
Department of Clinical and Translational Research, School of Medicine, University of Pittsburgh, 3550 Terrace Street, Pittsburgh, PA 15213, USA
Magee-Womens Research Institute, Magee-Womens Hospital of University of Pittsburgh Medical Center (UPMC), 204 Craft Avenue, Pittsburgh, PA 15213, USA

Shu-Han You, Po-Jen Cheng and Hsien-Ming Wu
Department of Obstetrics and Gynecology, Chang Gung Memorial Hospital, Linkou, Taiwan

Ting-Ting Chung
Big data research office, Chang Gung Memorial Hospital, Linkou, Taiwan

Chang-Fu Kuo
Division of Rheumatology, Allergy and Immunology, Chang Gung Memorial Hospital, Linkou, Taiwan

Pao-Hsien Chu
Department of Cardiology, Chang Gung Memorial Hospital, Linkou, Taiwan

Bothwell Takaingofa Guzha, Thulani Lesley Magwali, Bismark Mateveke and Stephen Peter Munjanja
Department of Obstetrics and Gynaecology, University of Zimbabwe, College of Health Sciences, Avondale, Harare, Zimbabwe

Maxwell Chirehwa
Department of Medicine, Division of Clinical Pharmacology, University of Cape Town, K45 Old Main Building, Groote Schuur Hospital, Observatory, Cape Town 7925, South Africa

George Nyandoro
Biomedical Research and Training Institute, 10 Seagrave Avenue, Avondale, Harare, Zimbabwe

Jimena Fritz, Héctor Lamadrid-Figueroa and Alejandra Montoya
Division of Reproductive Health, Research Center for Population Health, National Institute of Public Health (INSP), Av. Universidad 655, Col. Santa María Ahuacatitlán, 62100 Cuernavaca, Morelos, Mexico

Gustavo Angeles
Department of Maternal and Child Health, University of North Carolina at Chapel Hill (UNC), Chapel Hill, North Carolina, USA

Dilys Walker
Department of Obstetrics, Gynecology and Reproductive Sciences, Bixby Center for Global Reproductive Health, University of California in San Francisco, (UCSF), San Francisco, California, USA

José M. Belizán
Instituto de Efectividad Clínica y Sanitaria (IECS-CONICET), Emilio Ravignani, 2024 Buenos Aires, Argentina

Janetta Harbron
Division of Human Nutrition, Department of Human Biology, Faculty of Health Sciences, University of Cape Town, Cape Town, South Africa

Gabriela Cormick
Instituto de Efectividad Clínica y Sanitaria (IECS-CONICET), Emilio Ravignani, 2024 Buenos Aires, Argentina
Division of Human Nutrition, Department of Human Biology, Faculty of Health Sciences, University of Cape Town, Cape Town, South Africa

Ana Pilar Betrán
HRP – UNDP/UNFPA/UNICEF/WHO/World
Bank Special Programme of Research, Development
and Research Training in Human Reproduction,
Department of Reproductive Health and Research,
World Health Organization, Geneva, Switzerland

Tina Dannemann Purnat
WHO Regional Office for Europe, World Health
Organization, Copenhagen, Denmark

Catherine Parker and G. Justus Hofmeyr
Effective Care Research Unit, University of the
Witwatersrand, Johannesburg, South Africa
Effective Care Research Unit, Eastern Cape
Department of Health Walter Sisulu University,
Mthatha, South Africa
Effective Care Research Unit, University of Fort
Hare, East London, South Africa

David Hall
Department of Obstetrics and Gynaecology,
Stellenbosch University and Tygerberg Hospital,
Cape Town, South Africa

Armando H. Seuc
Epidemiología y Microbiología La Habana, Instituto
Nacional de Higiene, Havana, Cuba

James M. Roberts
Magee-Womens Research Institute, Department
of Obstetrics and Gynecology, University of
Pittsburgh, Pittsburgh, USA

Kirsten M. Dane
Mercy Perinatal, Mercy Hospital for Women,
Melbourne, VIC, Australia

Richard J. Hiscock
Department of Obstetrics and Gynaecology,
University of Melbourne, Melbourne, VIC, Australia

Anna L. Middleton
Mercy Perinatal, Mercy Hospital for Women,
Melbourne, VIC, Australia
Department of Obstetrics and Gynaecology,
University of Melbourne, Melbourne, VIC, Australia

Tu'uhevaha J. Kaitu'u-Lino and Ping Cannon
Department of Obstetrics and Gynaecology,
University of Melbourne, Melbourne, VIC, Australia
Translational Obstetrics Group, University of
Melbourne, Melbourne, VIC, Australia

**Teresa M. MacDonald, Susan P. Walker, Lisa Hui
and Stephen Tong**
Mercy Perinatal, Mercy Hospital for Women,
Melbourne, VIC, Australia
Department of Obstetrics and Gynaecology,
University of Melbourne, Melbourne, VIC, Australia
Translational Obstetrics Group, University of
Melbourne, Melbourne, VIC, Australia

Chuong Tran
Department of Laboratory Services, Royal Children's
Hospital, Melbourne, VIC, Australia

Shaun P. Brennecke
Department of Obstetrics and Gynaecology,
University of Melbourne, Melbourne, VIC, Australia
Department of Maternal-Fetal Medicine, Royal
Women's Hospital, Melbourne, VIC, Australia

Johanna Dahlberg
Department of Clinical and Experimental Medicine,
Linköping University, Linköping, Sweden

Marie Nelson
Department of Obstetrics and Gynecology,
Linköping University, Linköping, Sweden

Marie Blomberg
Department of Clinical and Experimental Medicine,
Linköping University, Linköping, Sweden
Department of Obstetrics and Gynecology,
Linköping University, Linköping, Sweden

Madeleine Abrandt Dahlgren
Department of Medicine and Health Sciences,
Linköping University, Linköping, Sweden

**Nkemnji Standley Awungafac and Jacqueline Ze
Minkande**
Faculty of Medicine and Biomedical Sciences,
University of Yaoundé 1, Yaoundé, Cameroon

Paul Nkemtendong Tolefac
Faculty of Medicine and Biomedical Sciences,
University of Yaoundé 1, Yaoundé, Cameroon
Mbalmayo District Hospita, Mbalmayo, Cameroon

Mandy Schmella and Melissa Glasser
Department of Health Promotion & Development,
University of Pittsburgh School of Nursing, 440
Victoria Building, Pittsburgh, PA 15261, USA

Jill Demirci
Department of Health Promotion & Development, University of Pittsburgh School of Nursing, 440 Victoria Building, Pittsburgh, PA 15261, USA
Department of Pediatrics, University of Pittsburgh School of Medicine, Pittsburgh, PA, USA

Lisa Bodnar
Department of Epidemiology, University of Pittsburgh Graduate School of Public Health, Pittsburgh, PA, USA
Department of Obstetrics, Gynecology and Reproductive Sciences, University of Pittsburgh School of Medicine, Pittsburgh, PA, USA

Katherine P. Himes
Department of Obstetrics, Gynecology and Reproductive Sciences, University of Pittsburgh School of Medicine, Pittsburgh, PA, USA
Magee-Womens Research Institute, Pittsburgh, USA

Hanna M. Heller
Department of Hospital Psychiatry, VU University Medical Centre, De Boelelaan 1117, 1081 HV Amsterdam, The Netherlands

Anita C. J. Ravelli
Department of Medical Informatics, Academic Medical Centre, University of Amsterdam, Meibergdreef 9, 1105 AZ Amsterdam, The Netherlands

Andrea H. L. Bruning
Department of Pediatric Infectious Diseases, Emma Children's Hospital, Academic Medical Centre, University of Amsterdam, Meibergdreef 9, 1105 AZ Amsterdam, The Netherlands

Christianne J. M. de Groot
Department of Obstetrics and Gynaecology, VU University Medical Centre, De Boelelaan 1117, 1081 HV Amsterdam, The Netherlands

Fedde Scheele
Department of Obstetrics and Gynaecology, OLVG Hospital (West), Jan Tooropstraat 164, 1061 AE Amsterdam, The Netherlands
Department of Obstetrics and Gynaecology, VU University Medical Centre, De Boelelaan 1117, 1081 HV Amsterdam, The Netherlands

Maria G. van Pampus
Department of Obstetrics and Gynaecology, OLVG Hospital (East), Oosterpark 9, 1091 AC Amsterdam, The Netherlands

Adriaan Honig
Department of Hospital Psychiatry, OLVG Hospital (West), Jan Tooropstraat 164, 1061 AE Amsterdam, The Netherlands
Department of Hospital Psychiatry, VU University Medical Centre, De Boelelaan 1117, 1081 HV Amsterdam, The Netherlands

Teklit Grum, Mebrahtu Abay and Teklit Angesom
School of Public Health, College of Health Sciences, Aksum University, Aksum, Ethiopia

Abiy Seifu
School of Public Health, College of Health Sciences, Addis Ababa University, Addis Ababa, Ethiopia

Lidiya Tsegay
School of Nursing, College of Health Sciences, Aksum University, Aksum, Ethiopia

Ian Roberts, Haleema Shakur and Sumaya Huque
Clinical Trials Unit, London School of Hygiene and Tropical Medicine, Keppel Street, London WC1E 7HT, UK

Bukola Fawole
Department of Obstetrics & Gynaecology, National Institute of Maternal and Child Health, College of Medicine, University of Ibadan, Orita-Mefa, Ibadan, Nigeria

Modupe Kuti
Department of Chemical Pathology, College of Medicine, University of Ibadan, Orita-Mefa, Ibadan, Nigeria

Oladapo Olayemi, Adenike Bello, Olayinka Ogunbode and Chris O. Aimakhu
Department of Obstetrics & Gynaecology, College of Medicine, University of Ibadan, Orita-Mefa, Ibadan, Nigeria

Taiwo Kotila and Tolulase Olutogun
Department of Haematology, College of Medicine, University of Ibadan, Orita-Mefa, Ibadan, Nigeria

Beverley J. Hunt
Thrombosis & Haemophilia Centre, Guy's & St Thomas' Trust, St Thomas' Hospital, Lambeth Palace Road, London, UK

David M. Goodman
Department of Obstetrics & Gynecology, Duke University Medical Center, Durham, NC 27710, USA

Emmanuel K. Srofenyoh
Ridge Regional Hospital, Accra, Ghana

Adeyemi J. Olufolabi
Department of Anesthesiology, Duke University Medical Center, Durham, NC 27710, USA

Sung Min Kim
Wake Forest School of Medicine, Medical Center Boulevard, Winston-Salem, NC 27157, USA

Medge D. Owen
Department of Anesthesiology, Wake Forest School of Medicine, Medical Center Boulevard, Winston-Salem, NC 27157-1009, USA

Index

www.ingramcontent.com/pod-product-compliance
Lightning Source LLC
Chambersburg PA
CBHW082038190326
41458CB00010B/3403